The Foundations of Shoulder and Elbow Surgery

The Foundations of Shoulder and Elbow Surgery

Editors

Surena Namdari, MD, MSc
Rothman Orthopaedic Institute
Thomas Jefferson University
Philadelphia, Pennsylvania

Benjamin Zmistowski, MD
Department of Orthopaedic Surgery
Washington University
St. Louis, Missouri

Reza Omid, MD
Department of Orthopaedic Surgery
Keck School of Medicine
University of Southern California
Los Angeles, California

CRC Press
Taylor & Francis Group
Boca Raton London New York

CRC Press is an imprint of the
Taylor & Francis Group, an **informa** business

First published 2020 by SLACK Incorporated

Published 2024 by CRC Press
2385 NW Executive Center Drive, Suite 320, Boca Raton FL 33431

and by CRC Press
4 Park Square, Milton Park, Abingdon, Oxon, OX14 4RN

CRC Press is an imprint of Taylor & Francis Group, LLC

Cover Artist: Justin Dalton

Library of Congress Cataloging-in-Publication Data

Names: Namdari, Surena, editor. | Zmistowski, Benjamin, editor. | Omid, Reza, editor.
Title: The foundations of shoulder and elbow surgery / [edited by] Surena Namdari, Benjamin Zmistowski, Reza Omid.
Description: Thorofare, NJ : SLACK Incorporated, [2020] | Includes bibliographical references and index.
Identifiers: LCCN 2020011512 | ISBN 9781630915322 (paperback) |
Subjects: MESH: Elbow Joint--anatomy & histology | Elbow Joint--injuries | Elbow Joint--surgery | Shoulder Joint--anatomy & histology | Shoulder Injuries--surgery | Athletic Injuries--surgery
Classification: LCC RD558 | NLM WE 820 | DDC 617.5/74044--dc23
LC record available at https://lccn.loc.gov/2020011512

ISBN: 9781630915322 (pbk)
ISBN: 9781003524243 (ebk)

DOI: 10.1201/9781003524243

Dedication

The editors dedicate this text to their families:

Vesta, Yara, and Noora Namdari

Heather, Luke, Matthew, Zachary, and Jacob Zmistowski

Raiden, Jaron, Karla, Hengi, Hart, and Ali Omid

Without their unwavering support, this effort certainly would have been futile.

Contents

Acknowledgments

We wish to acknowledge our mentors in shoulder and elbow surgery. Only through their teaching and guidance have we been able to meaningfully contribute to patient care and produce this text to disseminate what they have taught us.

About the Editors

Surena Namdari, MD, MSc completed his medical school at Brown Medical School in 2007. He went on to complete his orthopedic residency at the University of Pennsylvania and his shoulder and elbow fellowship at Washington University in St. Louis. He practices at the Rothman Orthopaedic Institute where he serves as co-director of Shoulder and Elbow Research. He is also an Associate Professor of Orthopaedic Surgery and the Shoulder and Elbow Surgery Fellowship Director at Thomas Jefferson University Hospital in Philadelphia, Pennsylvania.

Benjamin Zmistowski, MD graduated medical school from Thomas Jefferson University in 2014. He completed his orthopedic residency at Thomas Jefferson University in 2019 and his shoulder and elbow fellowship at Washington University in St. Louis in 2020. He now practices shoulder and elbow surgery at Washington University.

Reza Omid, MD graduated medical school from Chicago Medical School in 2005, his orthopedic residency at University of Southern California in 2010, and shoulder and elbow fellowship at Washington University in 2011. He is an Associate Professor and Associate Program Director at the Keck School of Medicine of the University of Southern California in Los Angeles, California.

Contributing Authors

Joseph A. Abboud, MD (Chapter 2)
Professor of Shoulder and Elbow Surgery
Rothman Orthopaedic Institute
Sidney Kimmel Medical College
Thomas Jefferson University
Philadelphia, Pennsylvania

Alexander W. Aleem, MD (Chapter 3)
Assistant Professor of Orthopaedic Surgery
Washington University in St. Louis
St. Louis, Missouri

Luke Austin, MD (Chapter 13)
Associate Professor of Orthopaedic Surgery
Sidney Kimmel Medical College
Thomas Jefferson University
Philadelphia, Pennsylvania

Wayne W. Chan, MD, PhD (Chapter 14)
Rothman Orthopaedic Institute
Thomas Jefferson University
Philadelphia, Pennsylvania

Talia Chapman, MD (Chapter 4)
Rothman Orthopaedic Institute
Thomas Jefferson University
Philadelphia, Pennsylvania

Michael C. Ciccotti, MD (Chapter 17)
Orthopaedic Sports Medicine Fellow
The Steadman Clinic
Steadman Philippon Research Institute
Vail, Colorado

Michael G. Ciccotti, MD (Chapter 17)
Everett J. and Marian Gordon Professor of Orthopaedic Surgery
Chief, Division of Sports Medicine
Rothman Orthopaedic Institute
Thomas Jefferson University
Philadelphia, Pennsylvania

Jason L. Codding, MD (Chapter 3)
The Everett Clinic
Everett, Washington

Daniel E. Davis, MD (Chapter 1)
Rothman Orthopaedic Institute
Thomas Jefferson University
Philadelphia, Pennsylvania

Vahid Entezari, MD, MMSc (Chapter 10)
Staff Shoulder and Elbow Surgeon
Orthopaedic and Rheumatologic Institute
Cleveland Clinic
Cleveland, Ohio

Seth Gamradt, MD (Chapter 12)
Director of Orthopaedic Athletic Medicine
Associate Professor of Clinical Orthopaedic Surgery
Keck School of Medicine
University of Southern California
Los Angeles, California

Charles L. Getz, MD (Chapter 15)
Associate Professor of Orthopaedic Surgery
Thomas Jefferson University
Philadelphia, Pennsylvania

Benjamin Hendy, MD (Chapter 8)
Rothman Orthopaedic Institute
Thomas Jefferson University
Philadelphia, Pennsylvania

J. Gabriel Horneff III, MD (Chapter 8)
Assistant Professor of Orthopaedic Surgery
Shoulder and Elbow Surgery
Rothman Orthopaedic Institute
Thomas Jefferson University
Philadelphia, Pennsylvania

Jason E. Hsu, MD (Chapter 16)
Shoulder and Elbow Surgery
University of Washington
Seattle, Washington

Asif Ilyas, MD, FACS (Chapter 4)
Rothman Orthopaedic Institute
Thomas Jefferson University
Philadelphia, Pennsylvania

Jason S. Klein, MD (Chapter 2)
Orthopaedic Surgeon
The Carrell Clinic
Dallas, Texas

Mark D. Lazarus, MD (Chapter 10)
Professor of Orthopaedic Surgery
Rothman Orthopaedic Institute
Sidney Kimmel Medical College
Thomas Jefferson University
Philadelphia, Pennsylvania

Christopher McDowell, DO (Chapter 13)
Department of Orthopedic Surgery
School of Osteopathic Medicine
Rowan University
Stratford, New Jersey

Eric M. Padegimas, MD (Chapter 15)
Connecticut Orthopaedic Specialists
Hamden, Connecticut
Connecticut Orthopaedic Institute
Midstate Medical Center
Meriden, Connecticut

Nilay A. Patel, MD (Chapter 5)
Department of Orthopaedic Surgery
Irvine Medical Center
University of California
Orange, California

E. Scott Paxton, MD (Chapter 7)
Department of Orthopaedic Surgery
Warren Alpert Medical School
Brown University
Providence, Rhode Island

Matthew L. Ramsey, MD (Chapter 6)
Professor of Orthopaedic Surgery
Chief, Shoulder and Elbow Service
Rothman Orthopaedic Institute
Sidney Kimmel Medical College
Thomas Jefferson University
Philadelphia, Pennsylvania

John Scolaro, MD, MA (Chapter 5)
Department of Orthopaedic Surgery
Irvine Medical Center
University of California
Orange, California

Kalpit N. Shah, MD (Chapter 7)
Department of Orthopaedic Surgery
Warren Alpert Medical School
Brown University
Providence, Rhode Island

Michael A. Stone, MD (Chapter 9)
Department of Orthopaedic Surgery
Cedars-Sinai Medical Center
Los Angeles, California

Jared R. Thomas, MD (Chapter 6)
IHA Orthopaedic Surgery Associates
Michigan Orthopaedic Center
Lansing, Michigan
St. Joseph Mercy Ann Arbor Orthopaedics
University of Michigan
Ypsilanti, Michigan

Nicholas A. Trasolini, MD (Chapter 12)
Department of Orthopaedic Surgery
Keck School of Medicine
University of Southern California
Los Angeles, California

Alexis Williams, MD (Chapter 1)
Orthopaedic Surgery Resident Physician
Rothman Orthopaedic Institute
Thomas Jefferson University
Philadelphia, Pennsylvania

Gerald R. Williams Jr, MD (Chapter 14)
John M. Fenlin Jr. Professor of Shoulder and Elbow Surgery
Department of Orthopaedic Surgery
Rothman Orthopaedic Institute
Sidney Kimmel Medical College
Thomas Jefferson University
Philadelphia, Pennsylvania

Preface

Surgery of the shoulder and elbow has increased in prevalence over the past 3 decades as an understanding of anatomy, physiology, and pathology has increased. In addition, innovations in surgical techniques (eg, arthroscopic surgery) and implant design (eg, reverse shoulder arthroplasty) have given surgeons the tools to address a greater number of shoulder pathologies. To adequately care for this increased volume of patients, it is necessary that the basics of shoulder and elbow care be disseminated to those in training.

As its title implies, this book provides an introduction to the orthopedic surgical subspecialty of shoulder and elbow surgery by establishing the foundation for a thorough understanding. Giants of shoulder and elbow have left their mark on the field with irreplaceable works such as Rockwood and Matsen's *The Shoulder* and Williams and Ramsey's *Operative Techniques in Shoulder and Elbow Surgery.* This book is not meant to supplant those detailed texts. Rather, this text provides the surgeon-in-training—medical student, resident surgeon, fellow, or even young attending—an organized introduction to essential topics in the care of the shoulder and elbow.

With many experts in the field of shoulder and elbow contributing, readers are encouraged to review each chapter with detail. Throughout the text, important citations will be highlighted. These citations will include classic references and more recent research that will change the course of shoulder and elbow care. In conjunction with clinical experience, this text will serve as an invaluable tool to the surgeon developing the skills needed to care for patients with shoulder and elbow pathology at a high level.

SECTION I

Elbow

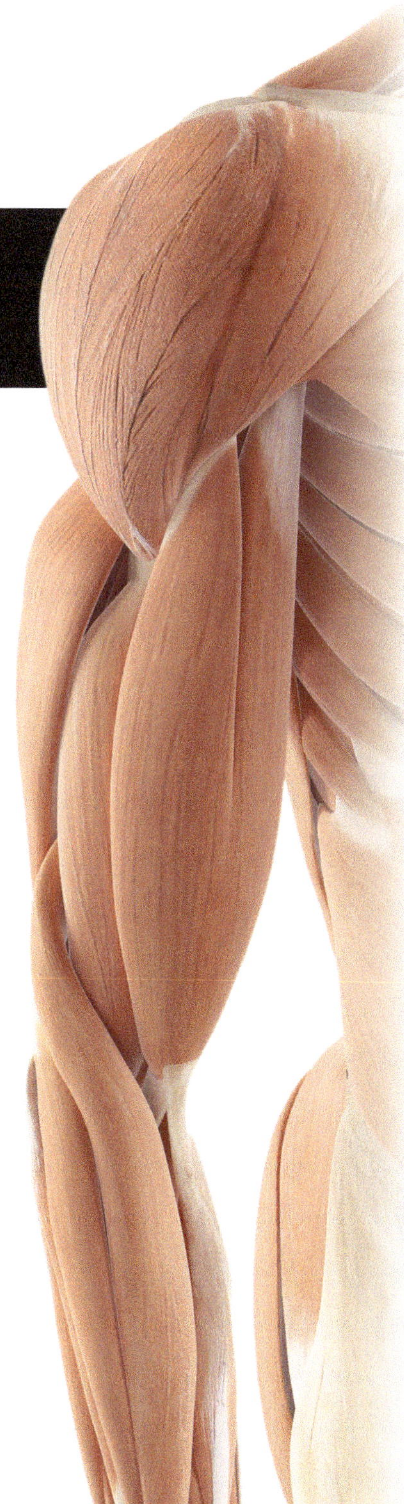

1

Elbow Anatomy and Physical Examination

Alexis Williams, MD and Daniel E. Davis, MD

Gross Anatomy

- Osteology: The 3 bones that comprise the elbow joint (distal humerus, proximal ulna, and proximal radius) allow it to function as a trochoginglymus joint, providing both flexion/extension as well as pronation-supination.
  - Distal humerus: transitions from the shaft to the medial and lateral columns, which support the articular surface (Figure 1-1)
    - Lateral column
      - Lateral supracondylar ridge: attachment of brachioradialis (BR) and extensor carpi radialis longus anteriorly and triceps posteriorly (Figure 1-2)
        - Avascular zone between BR and triceps marks the lateral column for surgical exposure
      - Lateral epicondyle: attachment of common extensor-supinator tendon and lateral ulnar collateral ligament (LUCL) posteriorly
        - Tendinitis of extensor carpi brachialis brevis (deep in common extensor mass) is cause of lateral epicondylitis[1] (Figure 1-3)
        - Lateral epicondyle debridement: must stay anterior to LUCL to avoid creating posterior rotatory instability
    - Medial column
      - The medial supracondylar ridge is more narrow than lateral, thus more prone to fracture
      - The medial epicondyle is more prominent than the lateral, serves as attachment of medial ulnar collateral ligament and flexor-pronator mass

Namdari S, Zmistowski B, Omid R, eds.
The Foundations of Shoulder and Elbow Surgery (pp 3-16).

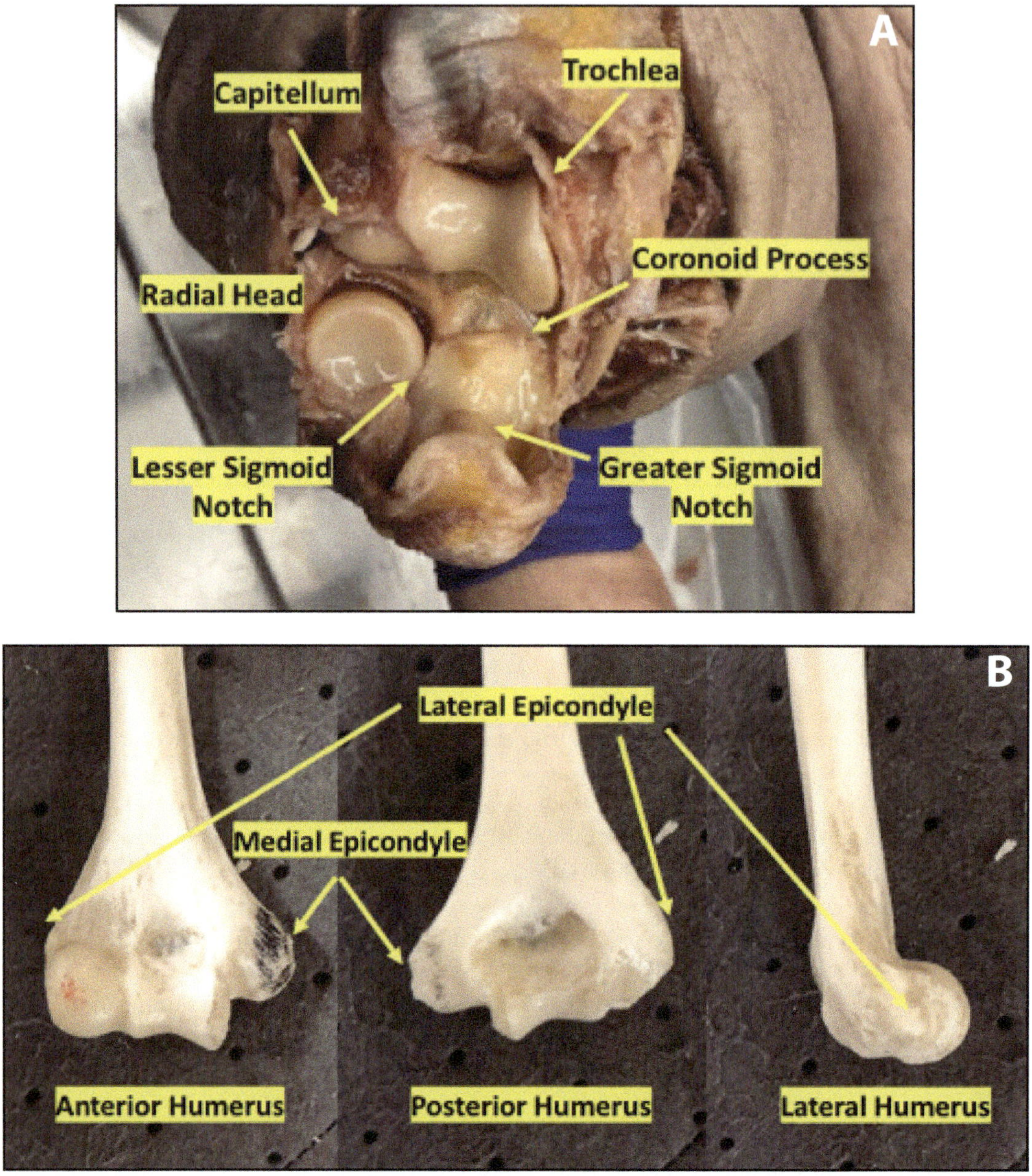

Figure 1-1. (A) The articular surfaces of the elbow joint. Note the anterior capsular attachment to the coronoid. This also demonstrates the more anterior/distal projection of the medial trochlea, which creates the valgus carrying angle in elbow extension. (B) Osteology of the distal humerus. Note the coronoid fossa and olecranon fossa anteriorly and posteriorly, respectively. The lateral view demonstrates the anterior angulation of the distal humerus to aid in full flexion.

    - Supracondylar process is seen in 1% to 3% of patients, attachment for ligament of Struthers may cause median nerve impingement (pronator syndrome)[2]
- Articular surfaces: angulated 30 degrees anteriorly, matches 30 degrees posterior angulation of greater sigmoid notch of the ulna
    - Trochlea: articulates with greater sigmoid notch of ulna, 300 degrees covered with articular cartilage, medial portion is more distal than lateral, bordered anterosuperiorly by coronoid fossa and posterosuperiorly by olecranon fossa

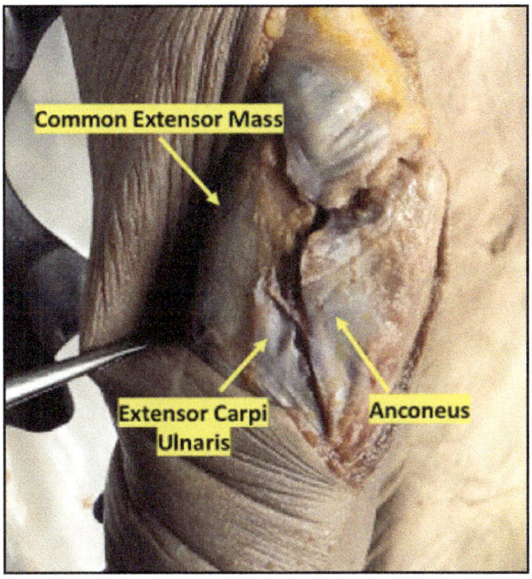

Figure 1-2. Superficial view of the lateral humerus demonstrates the fascial layer of the common extensor mass, the anconeus, and the triceps at the top of the figure.

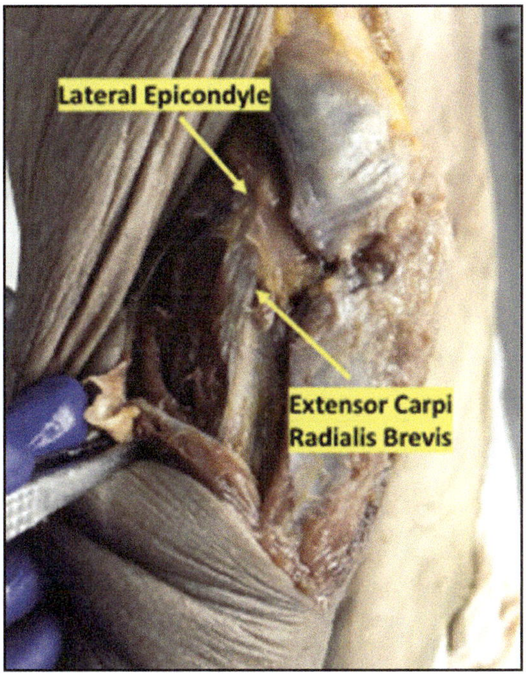

Figure 1-3. The superficial layer of the common extensor mass is reflected to demonstrate the deeper layer containing the tendinous insertion of the extensor carpi radialis brevis. This is the tendon affected by lateral epicondylitis at the tendon's insertion to the lateral epicondyle.

        - Capitellum: articulates with radial head, spheroidal in shape, thick cartilage layer (approximately 2 mm) anteriorly
- Proximal ulna: subcutaneous along posteromedial aspect of forearm (Figure 1-4)
    - Olecranon process: posterior and proximal portion of the ulna, serves as an attachment site for the triceps tendon
    - Coronoid process: anterior portion of ulnohumeral articulation, serves as a buttress to maintain anterior stability of the joint, attachment site of the brachialis tendon and anterior joint capsule
    - Greater sigmoid notch: cartilage-covered grooved surface that articulates with the trochlea of the distal humerus and allows flexion and extension of the joint, 30 degrees of posterior angulation to match that of the trochlea
    - Lesser sigmoid notch: distal-lateral to the greater sigmoid notch, small cartilage-covered groove that articulates the ulna with the radial head
        - Can serve as an alignment landmark for reconstruction or replacement of radial head fractures[3]
    - Supinator crest: raised area distal and posterior to lesser sigmoid notch, attachment site of lateral collateral ligament and important landmark for reconstruction of this structure
- Proximal radius: primary role is to allow pronation and supination of the elbow
    - Radial head: Central depression that articulates with the capitellum, the radial head should always point at the capitellum on x-ray at all ranges of motion. There is a 240-degree rim of articular cartilage around the radial head that articulates with the

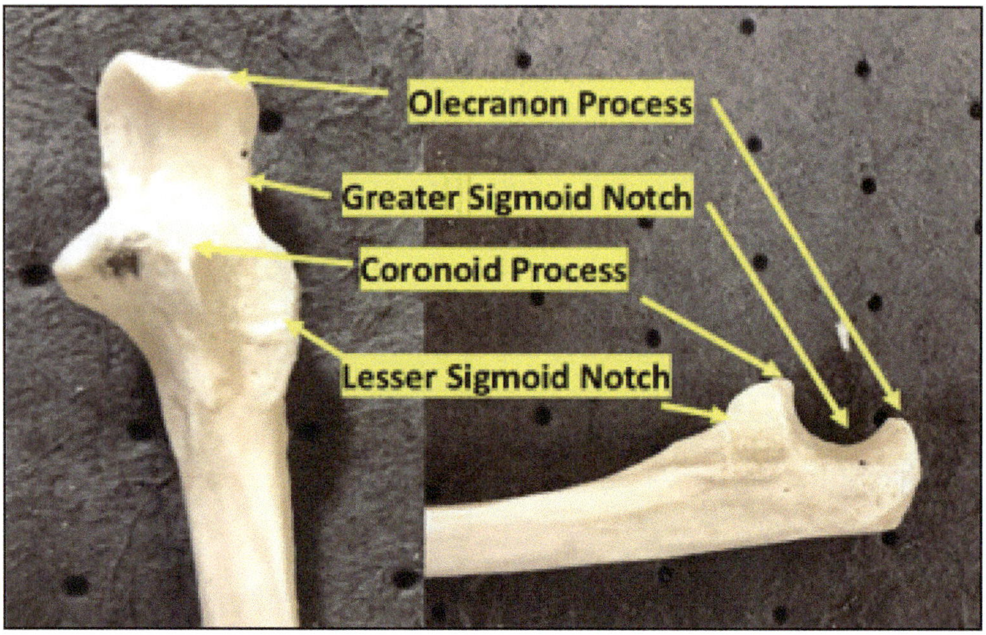

Figure 1-4. Osteology of the proximal ulna.

lesser sigmoid notch (proximal radioulnar joint); the remaining 120 degrees does not articulate and thus is a *safe zone* for hardware placement.

- The safe zone can be identified using distal radius landmarks such as the arc between the radial styloid and Lister tubercle.[4]

- Radial tuberosity: medial aspect of the proximal radius and serves as the attachment site of the distal biceps tendon
- Radial neck: distal to the radial head, transition point to the shaft, has 15 degrees of valgus angulation that should be taken into account during radial head replacement[3]

- Joint capsule and ligaments
  - The capsule surrounds the 3 joints, with thickenings medially and laterally, that create the collateral ligaments and provide static stabilization to the joint.
    - The maximum capacity of the capsule is approximately 25 to 30 mL and occurs at 80 degrees of flexion (Figures 1-5 and 1-6).[5]
  - Medial collateral ligament complex
    - Formed by the 3 bundles of the medial ulnar collateral ligament (Figure 1-7)
      - Anterior bundle: main restraint to valgus stress
      - Posterior bundle: may be released to gain more flexion in contracture without causing instability
      - Transverse ligament (ligament of Cooper/oblique bundle)
    - Medial ulnar collateral ligament originates on the medial epicondyle along with the flexor-pronator mass.
  - Lateral collateral ligament complex
    - Formed by multiple ligaments: radial collateral ligament; LUCL; annular ligament; accessory lateral collateral ligament (Figure 1-8)
    - Main restraint against varus stress and posterolateral rotatory instability[6] *Recommended reading for historical context and description of common pathology*

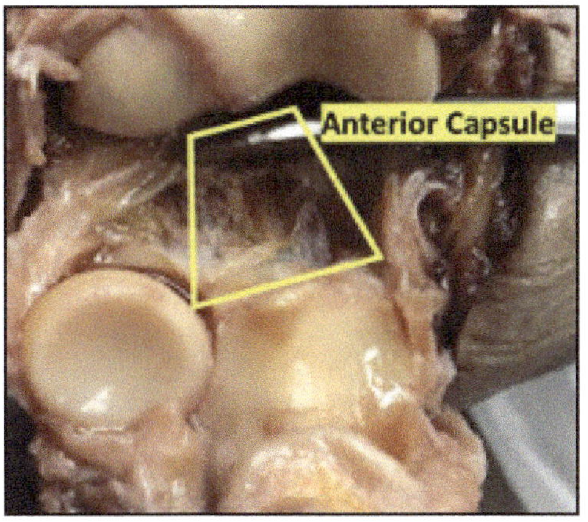

Figure 1-5. The anterior capsule attached to the coronoid process is demonstrated. Anterior to the capsule in the brachialis muscle, which protects the anterior neurovascular structures during surgical approaches to the capsule.

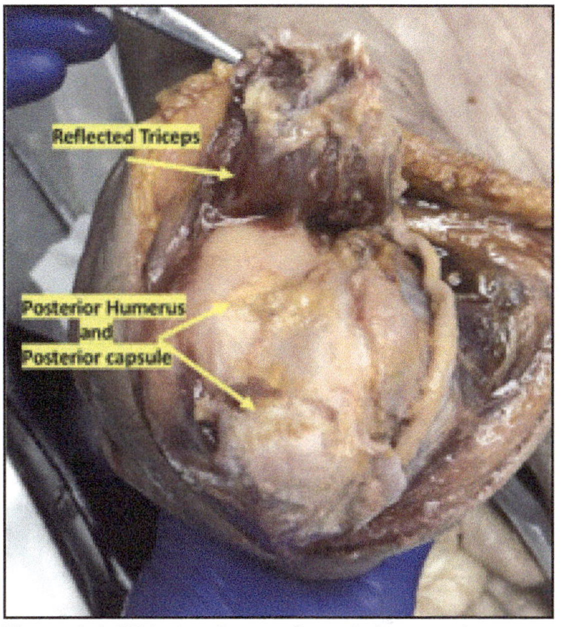

Figure 1-6. With the triceps reflected, the posterior aspect of the distal humerus and posterior capsule is demonstrated. The unroofed ulnar nerve is visualized on the right.

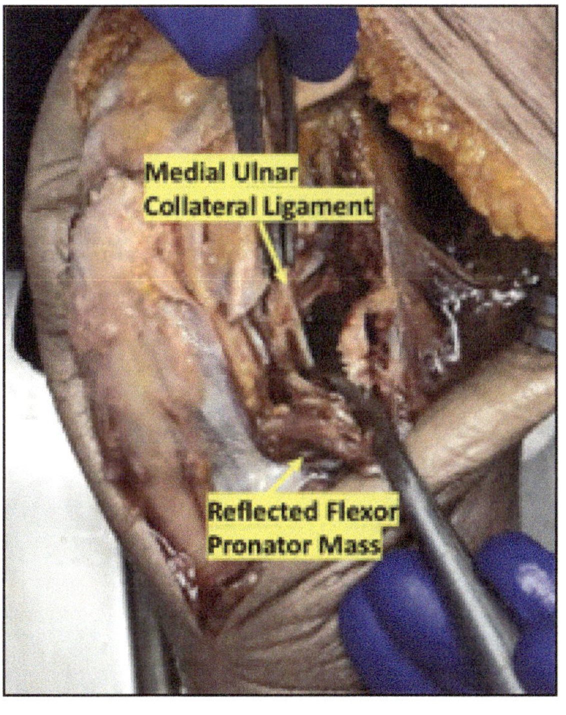

Figure 1-7. The flexor-pronator mass is reflected on the right side of the figure demonstrating the underlying medial capsule and medial collateral ligament complex. Note how closely associated the musculature is with the underlying capsule.

- Radial collateral ligament originates on the lateral epicondyle and attaches to the annular ligament
- LUCL originates on the lateral epicondyle, becomes confluent with the annular ligament, then inserts on the supinator crest

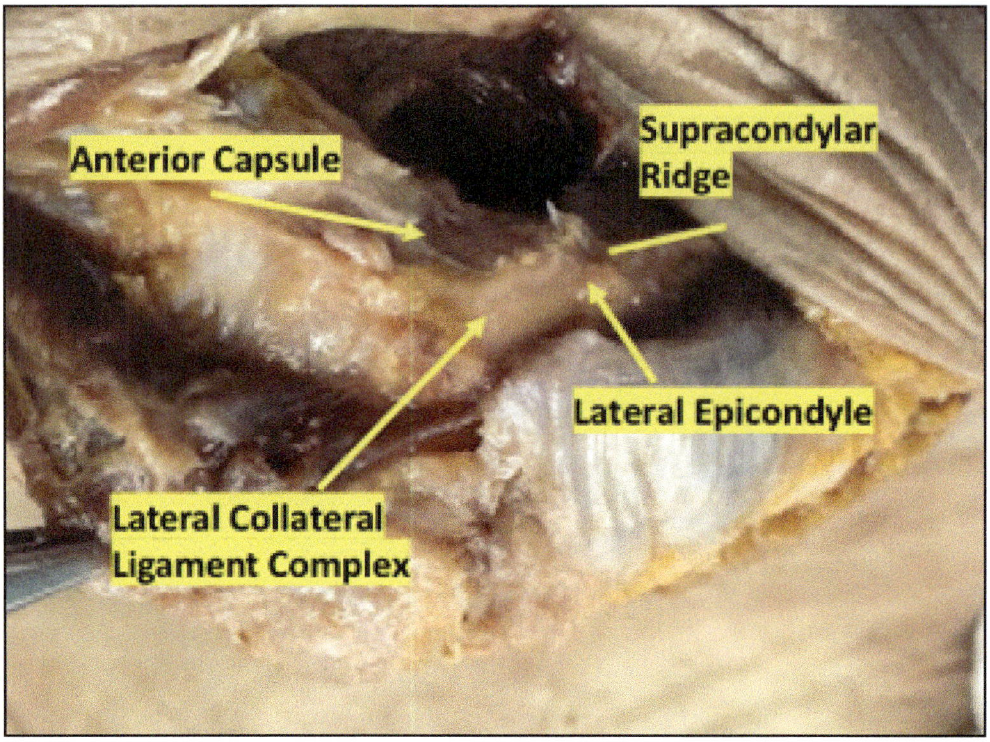

Figure 1-8. Deep portion of the lateral elbow. The humerus is to the right, and the forearm is to the left. The anterior capsule and lateral collateral ligament complex is demonstrated.

      - Annular ligament stabilizes the proximal radioulnar joint by wrapping around the radial head and inserting on the anterior and posterior borders of the radial notch
- Musculature
  - Four major muscle groups cross the elbow to provide flexion, extension, pronation, and supination.
  - Flexion
    - Primary flexors: brachialis; biceps brachii; BR (Figure 1-9)
      - Brachialis: musculocutaneous and radial nerve, brachial artery
      - Biceps brachii: musculocutaneous nerve, brachial artery
      - BR: radial nerve, radial recurrent artery
  - Extension
    - Primary extensors: triceps and anconeus (Figure 1-10)
      - Radial nerve and deep brachial artery
  - Pronation
    - Pronator teres: median nerve, radial and ulnar artery (Figure 1-11)
    - Pronator quadratus: anterior interosseous nerve and artery
  - Supination
    - Biceps brachii: musculocutaneous nerve, brachial artery
    - Supinator: radial nerve, radial recurrent artery
- Neurovasculature
  - Musculocutaneous nerve passes through the coracobrachialis and innervates the biceps and brachialis

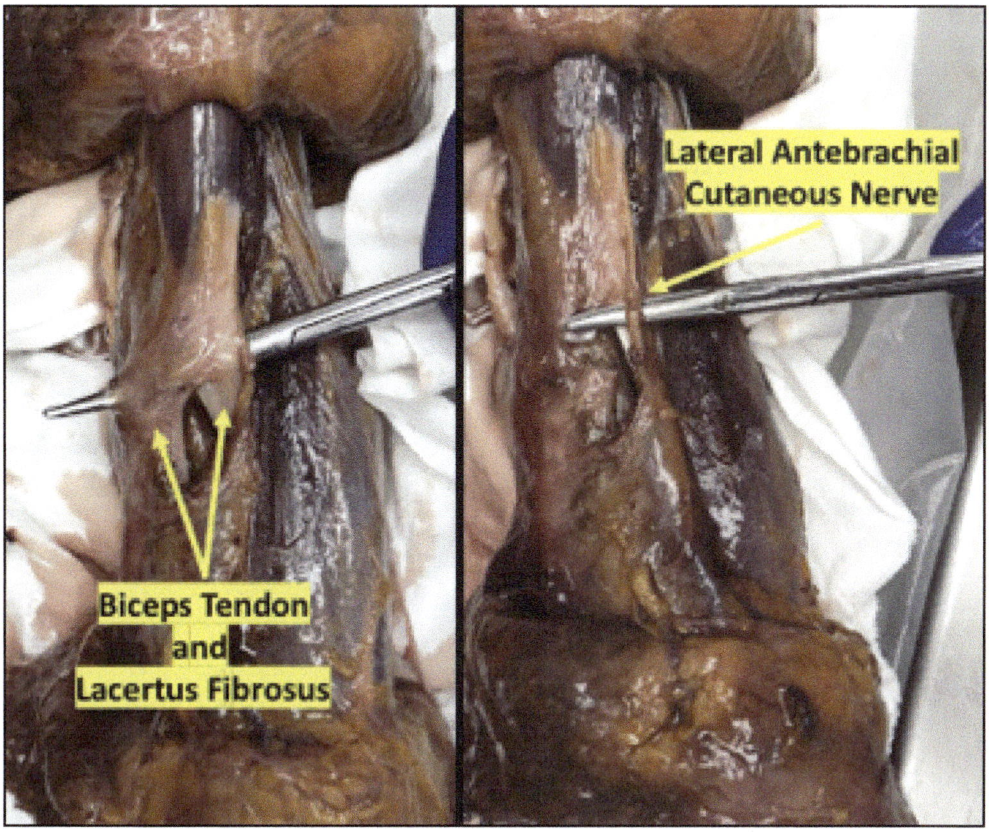

Figure 1-9. The anterior musculature of the elbow. The distal biceps tendon and lacertus fibrosus are demonstrated at left. At right, the lateral antebrachial cutaneous nerve is demonstrated lateral to the distal biceps tendon. This nerve is a continuation of the musculocutaneous nerve as it exits the biceps muscle.

    - The terminal branch is the lateral antebrachial cutaneous nerve, which must be identified and protected during exposure for distal biceps repair.
- The radial nerve passes from medial to lateral as it travels down the spiral groove of the humerus. It travels anterior to the lateral epicondyle to enter the forearm, dividing into the posterior interosseous nerve and superficial radial nerve. There are 5 main areas where the radial nerve may become compressed:
    - Lateral elbow joint at the radial head (osteoarthritis, fibrous bands, synovitis)
    - Arcade of anastomoses of the radial recurrent artery at the radial neck (leash of Henry; most common site of compression)
    - Fibrous proximal edge of the extensor carpi radialis brevis
    - Proximal edge of the supinator (arcade of Frohse)
    - Distal edge of the supinator
- The median nerve and the brachial artery share a similar path through the elbow to the forearm.
    - The median nerve travels medial to the brachialis with the brachial artery.
    - In those with a supracondylar process (present in 1% of the population), the nerve crosses this before crossing the ligament of Struthers.
    - The nerve then enters the antecubital fossa with the artery superficial to the brachialis, which will protect these structures for exposures of the anterior capsule or coronoid process.

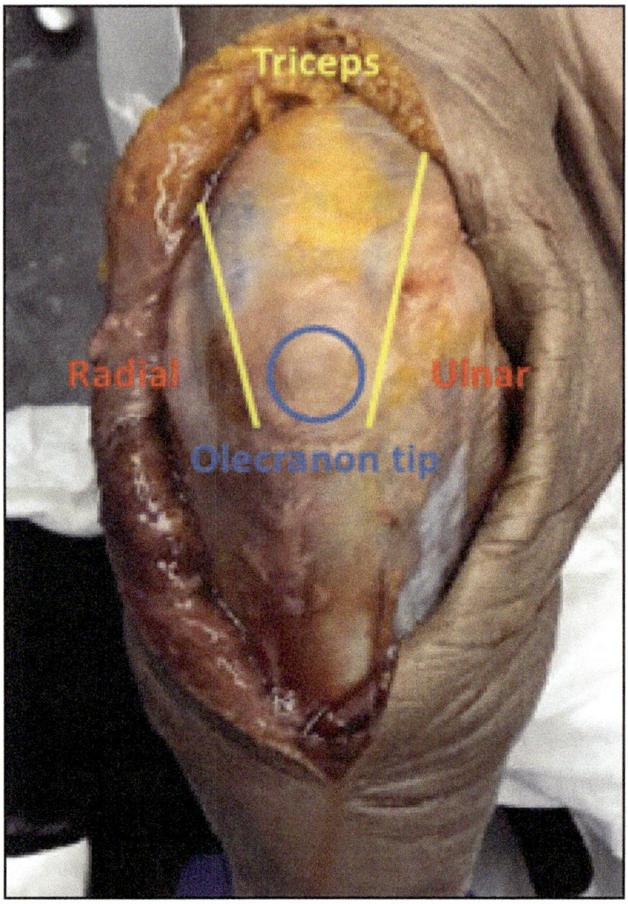

Figure 1-10. Superficial posterior elbow. The triceps muscle and its insertion to the olecranon process is demonstrated.

        - At the level of the antecubital fossa, from lateral to medial is the biceps tendon, the brachial artery, and the median nerve.
    - Both the nerve and the artery then pass beneath the bicipital aponeurosis and enter the forearm.
        - Brachial artery terminates into the radial artery and ulnar artery
        - The median nerve passes through the ulnar and humeral heads of the pronator teres, a possible site of compression.
- The ulnar nerve passes through the medial intermuscular septum at the level of the midarm and courses anterior to the medial head of the triceps. It then enters the cubital tunnel by traveling posterior and inferior to the medial epicondyle. Here the nerve may become compressed or inflamed because of subluxation. The nerve then travels between the ulnar and humeral heads of the flexor carpi ulnaris, another site of compression by the ligament of Osborne (Figure 1-12).

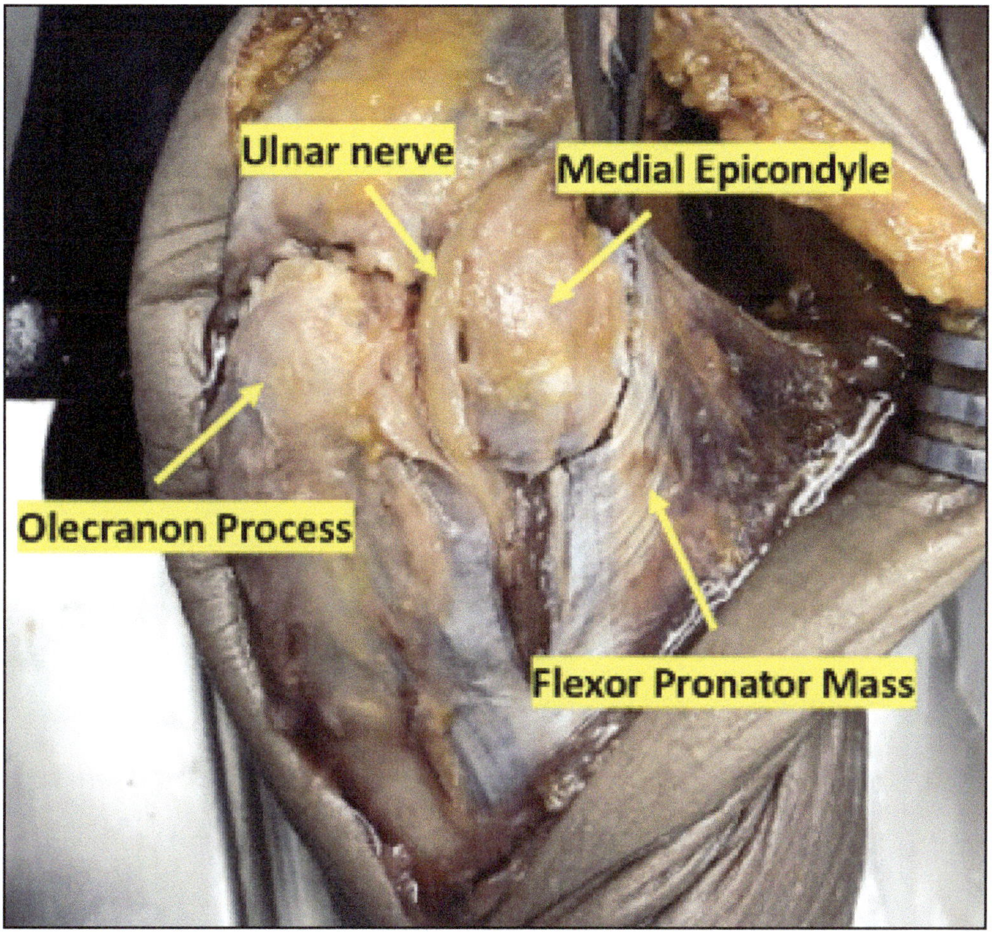

Figure 1-11. Superficial medial elbow. The flexor-pronator mass is shown with a split in the fascia used for medial elbow exposure. The ulnar nerve can be visualized traversing in the cubital tunnel and exiting into the flexor carpi ulnaris muscle.

Elbow Physical Examination

- Observation
  - Assess for any gross deformities of the elbow or any signs of trauma, including ecchymoses, lacerations, exposed bone, etc.
  - Measure the carrying angle of the elbow. The elbow should be extended, the forearm supinated, and the shoulder in neutral. The angle is formed by the long axis of the humerus and the long axis of the ulna. The normal range is 11 degrees to 14 degrees in men and 13 degrees to 16 degrees in women (Figure 1-13).
- Palpation
  - Palpate the "soft spot" at the infracondylar recess. Any fullness at this area is suggestive of joint effusion, synovial tissue proliferation, or radial head pathology.
    - The soft spot is the center of the triangle formed by the lateral portion of the olecranon process, the lateral epicondyle, and the radial head (Figure 1-14).
    - It is also the site used for joint aspiration or injection
  - Assess ulnar nerve for subluxation

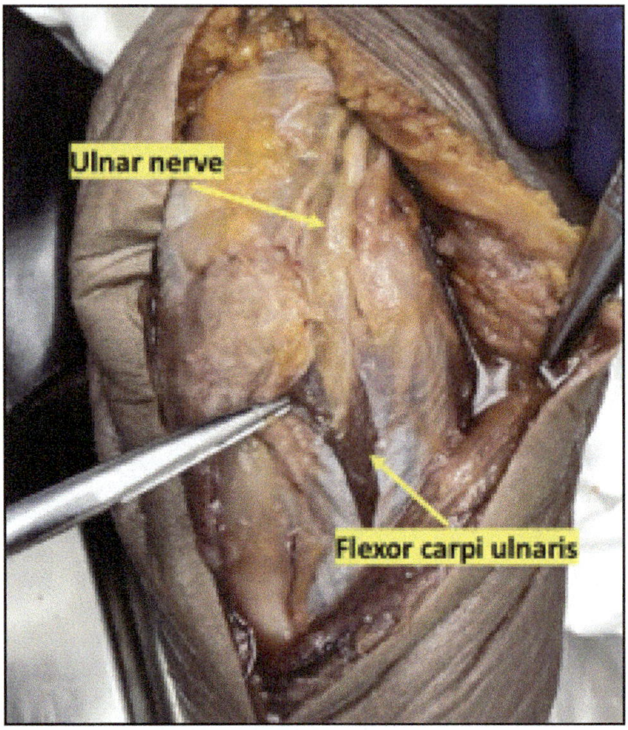

Figure 1-12. Ulnar nerve coursing through the cubital tunnel and exiting into the flexor carpi ulnaris muscle.

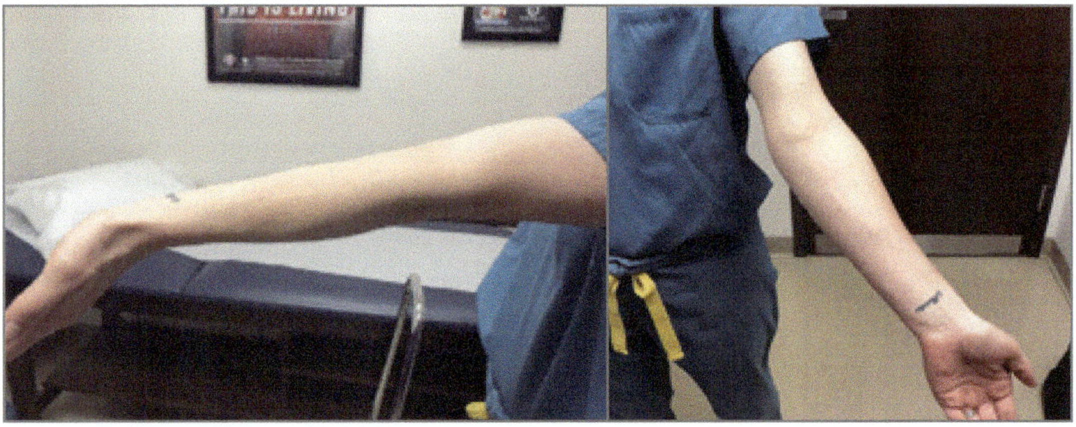

Figure 1-13. Full extension in this female patient demonstrates the hyperextension that may be observed as well as the increased carrying angle.

- Palpate the arcade of Frohse for posterior interosseous nerve (2 cm anterior, 3 cm distal to lateral epicondyle)
- The medial margin of the lacertus fibrosis can be palpated, in the setting of a distal biceps tendon rupture, this structure may become attenuated

• Neurological exam
  - C5: biceps reflex, elbow flexors, deltoid sensation
  - C6: BR reflex, wrist extensors, sensation to lateral forearm, thumb, index finger
  - C7: triceps reflex, elbow extensors, sensation to middle finger
  - C8: finger flexors, sensation to ring finger and small finger

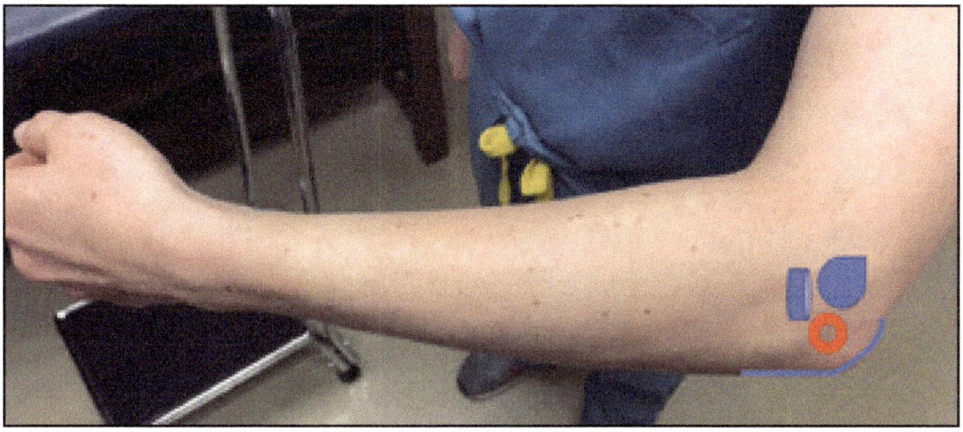

Figure 1-14. The marker notes the radial head, lateral distal humerus, and olecranon. The center of this spot is the location to feel fullness in the joint denoting an effusion and also the spot for an arthrocentesis of the joint.

  - T1: finger abductors; sensation to medial forearm
- Motor
  - Assess strength of flexion/extension and supination-pronation
  - Flexion best assessed with elbow flexed 90 degrees and forearm in neutral rotation; maximum elbow flexion strength occurs at 90 degrees
  - Pronation-supination strength best assessed with the elbow flexed 90 degrees and grasping the patient's wrist
- Range of motion (ROM)
  - Normal ROM: 0 degrees to 150 degrees flexion; 75 degrees pronation; 85 degrees supination (Figure 1-15)
  - Functional ROM: 30 degrees to 130 degrees; 50 degrees pronation; 50 degrees pronation
  - Loss of full extension is the first sign of elbow pathology; if the patient can fully extend in setting of trauma, x-rays are generally not warranted because of the low likelihood of injury.
- Provocative maneuvers
  - Mill's test: Lateral elbow pain with wrist extension against resistance with elbow extended, suggestive of lateral epicondylitis (Figure 1-16)
  - Pain with active pronation against resistance with elbow extended: suggestive of pronator syndrome
  - Tinel test: Tapping on ulnar nerve at level of elbow causing paresthesias in ulnar distribution; suggestive of cubital tunnel syndrome
  - Elbow flexion test: Hold elbow in full flexion for 1 minute; positive if produces paresthesias in ulnar distribution; suggestive of cubital tunnel syndrome
  - Milking maneuver: Valgus stress placed on flexed elbow, pain at the medial elbow is suggestive of ulnar collateral ligament injury (Figure 1-17)
    - Similar is moving valgus stress test performed with elbow flexion/extension[7]
  - Hook test: Palpation of the distal biceps tendon by hooking finger below tendon to test for integrity, an intact lacertus fibrosus may recreate a positive test[8] (Figure 1-18) *Recommended reading for development and validation of a ubiquitous diagnostic test*
  - Lateral pivot shift: Test for posterolateral rotatory instability. Patient is supine on table, shoulder abducted and externally rotated, the elbow is taken from an extended-supinated position to a flexed pronated position with valgus stress. A palpable reduction of the radial head is a positive test.[6]

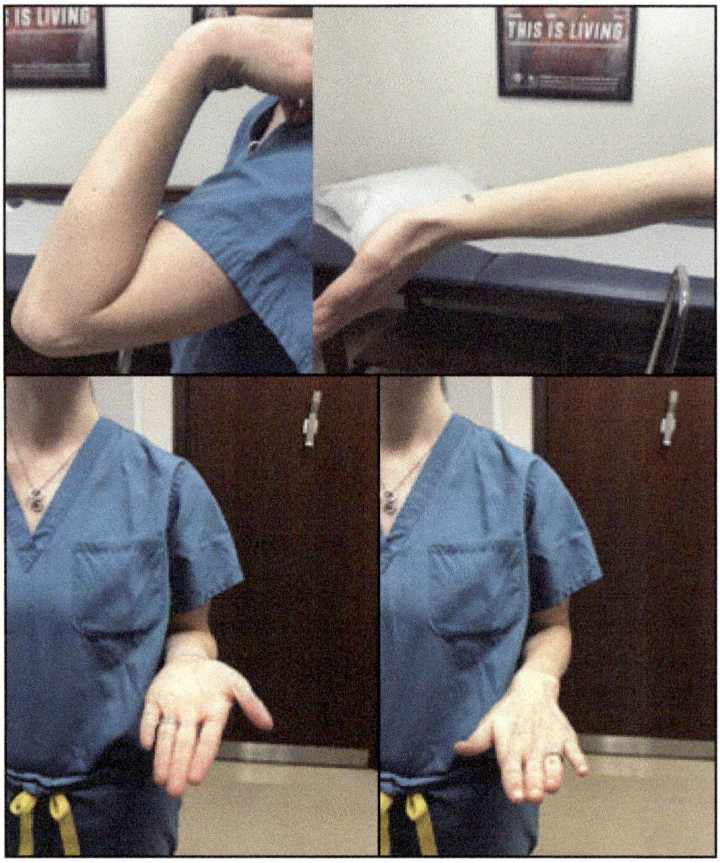

Figure 1-15. Normal ROM of the elbow in flexion, extension, pronation, and supination.

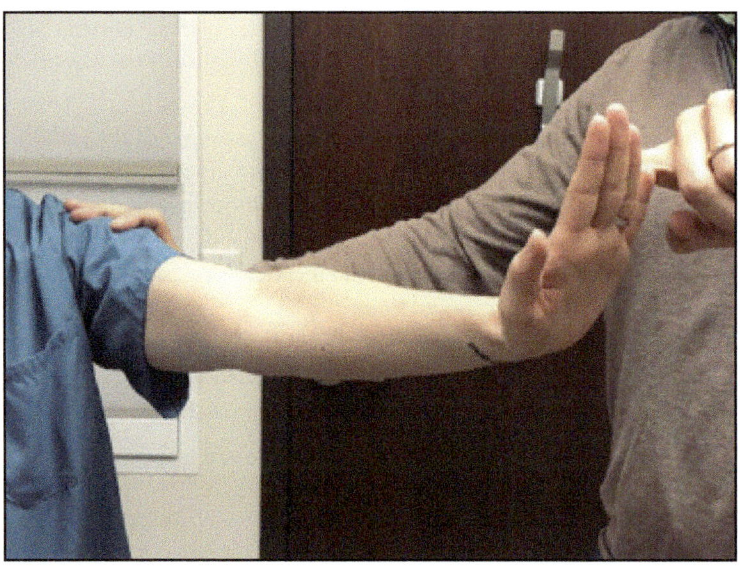

Figure 1-16. Mill's test. With the elbow extended and pronated, the long finger is extended against resistance. Pain over the lateral epicondyle is considered a positive exam for lateral epicondylitis.

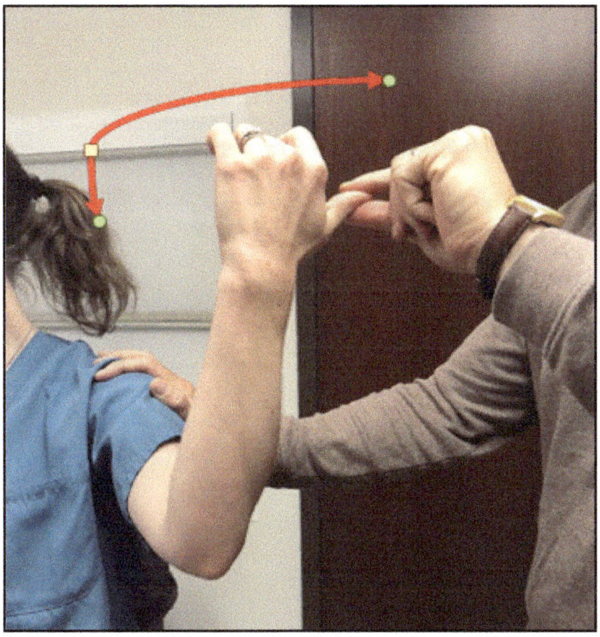

Figure 1-17. The milking maneuver and the moving valgus stress test are 2 maneuvers that place a valgus moment on the elbow and stress the medial ulnar collateral ligament.

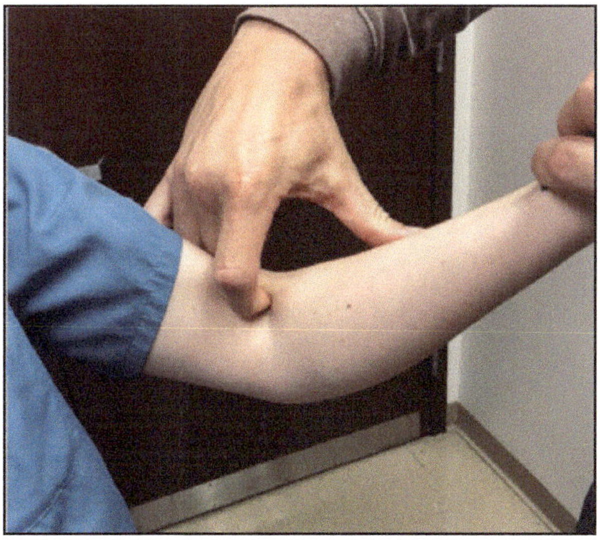

Figure 1-18. An index finger may be hooked under the distal biceps tendon to test for integrity and pain. An intact lacertus fibrosus may confuse the exam findings.

References

1. Nirsch RP. Etiology of tennis elbow. *J Sports Med.* 1975;3(5):261-263. doi:10.1177/036354657500300510.
2. Symeonides PP. The humerus supracondylar process syndrome. *Clin Orthop Relat Res.* 1972;82:141-143.
3. Acevedo DC, Paxton ES, Kukelyansky I, Abboud J, Ramsey M. Radial head arthroplasty: state of the art. *J Am Acad Orthop Surg.* 2014;22(10):633-642. doi:10.5435/JAAOS-22-10-633.
4. Smith GR, Hotchkiss RN. Radial head and neck fractures: anatomic guidelines for proper placement of internal fixation. *J Shoulder Elbow Surg.* 1996;5(2 pt 1):113-117. doi:10.1016/S1058-2746(96)80005-X.
5. O'Driscoll SW, Morrey BF, An KN. Intraarticular pressure and capacity of the elbow. *Arthroscopy.* 1990;6(2):100-103. doi:10.1016/0749-8063(90)90007-z.
6. O'Driscoll SW, Bell DF, Morrey BF. Posterolateral rotatory instability of the elbow. *J Bone Joint Surg Am.* 1991;73(3):440-446.
7. O'Driscoll SW, Lawton RL, Smith AM. The "moving valgus stress test" for medial collateral ligament tears of the elbow. *Am J Sports Med.* 2005;33(2):231-239. doi:10.1177/0363546504267804.
8. O'Driscoll SW, Goncalves LBJ, Dietz P. The hook test for distal biceps tendon avulsion. *Am J Sports Med.* 2007;35(11):1865-1869. doi:10.1177/0363546507305016.

2

Tendon Injuries

Jason S. Klein, MD and Joseph A. Abboud, MD

Triceps Tendon

Pathophysiology

- Most common mechanism of injury (MOI): sudden eccentric load to a contracting triceps muscle (eg, fall onto an outstretched arm)[1]
  - Associated injuries include radial head and wrist fractures.[2,3]
  - Less common mechanisms include traumatic injuries (lacerations and open fractures) and direct blows to the posterior elbow.
- Most common injury site: tendon-osseous insertion[3]
  - Other reports include avulsion injuries,[4] muscle belly rupture (due to fatigue failure),[5] or tears at the musculotendinous junction.[6,7]
- Predisposing conditions
  - Metabolic bone diseases (hyperparathyroidism and renal osteodystrophy)[8,9]
    - Increased osteoclastic bone resorption leads to weakening of the tendon's olecranon insertion.
  - Olecranon bursitis[10]
  - Marfan syndrome[11]
  - Osteogenesis imperfect[12]
  - Rheumatoid arthritis
  - Type 1 diabetes[7]
- Classification
  - There is no formal classification system.
  - Instead, these injuries are described by the following[13]:

Namdari S, Zmistowski B, Omid R, eds.
The Foundations of Shoulder and Elbow Surgery (pp 17-37).

    - MOI
    - Location of the tear (bone avulsion, tendinous insertion, muscle belly, musculotendinous junction, proximal origin)
    - Degree of tear (partial vs complete)
    - Integrity of the lateral expansion (intact vs torn)

Presentation and Diagnosis

- Demographics
  - Rare condition constituting less than 1% of all tendon ruptures[14]
  - Most common in the following:
    - Male-to-female ratio, 3:2
    - Fourth decade of life (range, adolescents postphyseal closure to eighth decade of life)[8,15]
    - Anabolic steroid use[16]
    - Bodybuilders and weightlifters[17]
    - History of local and/or systemic steroid use[16,18,19]
    - Associated disorders as described above
- Presentation
  - Patients may recall a popping sound or tearing sensation at the time of injury.
  - Patients report pain, swelling, and bruising along the posterior elbow.
  - Delayed presentation is common when some motion and strength is preserved.
  - Complaints of numbness or tingling in the ulnar nerve distribution, particularly when presents with a concomitant hematoma
- Physical examination
  - The diagnosis may be difficult to ascertain from physical exam alone depending on the size of the tear (partial vs full), the amount of swelling (depending on the acuity of the injury), or the patient's body habitus.[20]
  - In addition to tenderness to palpation over posterior aspect of the elbow, a palpable defect of the tendon proximal to the olecranon may (or may not) be appreciated.
  - Motion
    - Passive motion is usually preserved.
    - Some active extension may be present with complete ruptures but the inability to actively extend against resistance or gravity is pathognomonic for a complete rupture.
  - Adapted from Achilles ruptures, a positive modified Thompson squeeze test may confirm complete triceps rupture.[21,22]
    - A partially or fully intact tendon will extend against the resistance of gravity with squeeze of the arm, whereas a full disruption will not.
  - However, an intact lateral expansion may mask the common exam findings above in acute triceps ruptures. As a result, one must have a high index of suspicion to avoid misdiagnosis.[3]
- Diagnostic imaging
  - Standard radiographs (anteroposterior and lateral) of the elbow should be obtained. A fleck sign on the lateral radiograph is pathognomonic for an avulsion fracture or triceps rupture.[23]
  - Radiographs of the joints above and below (including the distal radius) should be evaluated for concomitant injuries.

- Advanced imaging will provide definitive diagnosis as well as localize the site and extent of the tear
  - Computed tomography scan of the elbow may be considered to exclude or assess for concomitant radial head, olecranon, coronoid, or distal humerus fractures.[6,24]
  - Magnetic resonance imaging (MRI) may be used for preoperative planning or in difficult cases in which it is difficult to determine whether the rupture is partial or complete and to localize the exact location of the tear.[25-27]
    - Sagittal views may be most useful.
    - Small, fluid-filled defects within the distal triceps tendon with edema along the surrounding subcutaneous tissues are consistent with a partial triceps rupture.[13]
    - Paratricipital edema with a large, fluid-filled gap between the tendon and olecranon process is consistent with a complete rupture.[27]
  - Ultrasound is operator dependent. However, in well-trained hands, the dynamic imaging modality is less expensive and yields similar data.[28]

Treatment

- The patient's function, medical status, and chronicity of the tear may guide treatment toward nonoperative or operative management. Therefore, all treatment decisions must be considered in the context of the patient's health and social factors.
  - Partial and/or complete tears in a debilitated older patient may be treated nonoperatively.[29]
- Anatomic factors also contribute to treatment decision making.
  - Tear location
    - Muscle belly tears tend to heal with scar tissue rather than newly regenerated muscle; however, outcomes are similar regardless of treatment.[13]
      - Direct suturing in complete muscle belly ruptures has been reported in young healthy athletes, but it is unknown whether the intervention allows for improved return to sports, strength, function, or long-term outcomes.[30]
    - Partial ruptures at tendon-osseous insertion often do not heal.[31]
  - Tear size
    - Partial tears
      - Tears comprising less than 50% of the tendon width can be treated nonsurgically with satisfactory results.[32]
      - Tears greater than 50% in an active individual may require surgical intervention,[18,29] unless comorbidities or functional status precludes such treatment.
    - Complete tears are usually treated operatively.[3,20,23]
  - Functional loss
    - Complete ruptures do not always translate to full loss of function and strength because of intact lateral triceps expansion that blends with the anconeus and antebrachial fascia.[29]
      - The degree of functional loss must be factored with the patient's functional goals to decide whether to intervene operatively.
- Nonsurgical
  - Indications
    - Incomplete tendon rupture should be treated initially with a trial of nonoperative management[33]
    - Partial or complete tears without significant weakness

        - Medical comorbidities or overall function preclude surgical intervention.
    - When indicated, splint immobilization may be employed for approximately 4 weeks at 30 degrees of flexion.[20,21,32,34]
    - Nonsurgical outcomes
        - Good return to preinjury level of function[18,21,35]
        - In partial tears or muscle belly tears, nonoperative management is not associated with acute muscle weakness, but can result in poor endurance during repetitive activity.[5,34]
        - In a study of 10 professional football players with partial triceps tears, Mair et al[18] noted that 6 healed with nonsurgical treatment and no signs of residual pain or weakness, whereas 3 required repair after the season for continued symptoms and 1 underwent repair after converting a partial to a complete rupture despite bracing.[18]
        - For athletes with partial tears, one study of professional football players reported full return to competition with brace use around 5 weeks postinjury.
        - Immediate return to competition prior to rest and rehabilitation may result in tear progression to complete rupture.[16-18]
- Operative
    - Indications
        - Acute, complete tears, particularly at the distal tendinous insertion in the setting of elbow extension weakness[29]
        - Failed nonoperative management
        - Relative indication: laborers; athletes; active individuals with more than 50% tendon tear
    - Techniques
        - Approach: posterior incision
        - Most techniques involve passing nonabsorbable suture through the tendon as a grasping stitch (eg, Bunnel or Krackow whipstitch) and reattaching the tendon to bone via bone tunnels[3,36-38] (Figure 2-1) or with suture anchors.[6,20]
            - The bony bed should be debrided and prepared to optimize soft-tissue repair to bone
            - A double-row construct has superior repair strength and is more accurate in recreating the native anatomic footprint compared to transosseous tunnels or traditional bone tunnels.[1]
        - In avulsion fractures off the olecranon, the fragment can be reduced and fixed with one the following:
            - A screw and washer technique
            - A tension band construct[21]
            - Fragment excision and primary reattachment of the tendon to bone via one of the techniques described previously
        - Repair at the myotendinous junction (if deemed operative) may be addressed with the V-Y triceps advancement technique augmented with an interwoven tendon autograft or allograft.[7]
            - Chronic retracted tears or revisions may require the use of one of the following to achieve repair[7,39-42]:
                - An anconeus slide
                - A forearm fascial flap turn-up
                - A triceps fascial flap turn-down
                - An allograft reconstruction/augmentation
    - Postoperative care

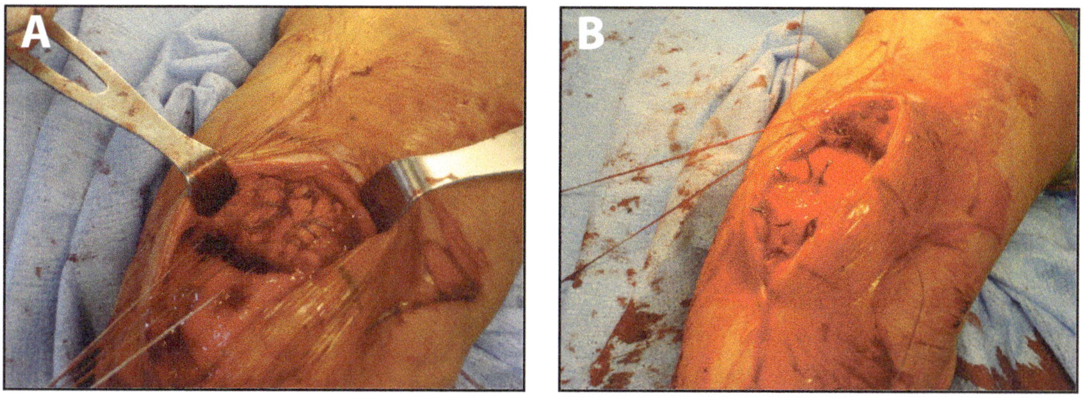

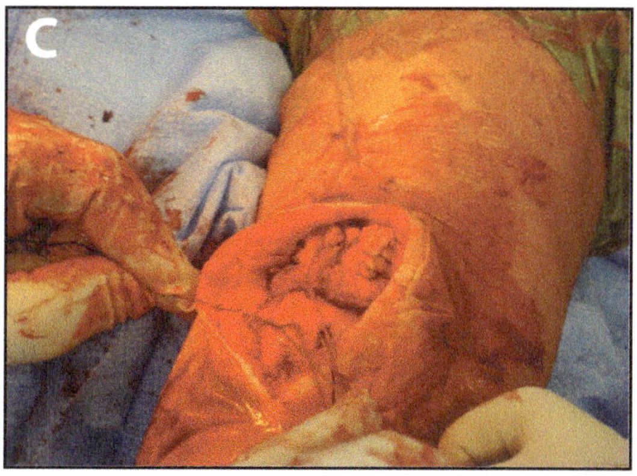

Figure 2-1. Triceps repair technique via bone tunnels. (A) Triceps is repaired with 3 sets of heavy, nonabsorbable sutures placed in a Krackow grasping fashion. (B) Sutures are passed via bone tunnels. (C) Near-final product as the tissue is reduced and tied over the bone tunnels.

    - In general, depending on the quality of the repair, the plan usually involves the following[3,30]:
        - A period of immobilization (splint or sling) approximately 7 to 10 days
        - Flexion block motion that increases weekly after splint discontinuation
        - Active extension starting around 6 weeks
        - Strengthening beginning around 12 weeks
        - Unrestricted activity around 4 to 6 months
  - Prognosis
    - Most acute primary repairs regain near full strength but may lose 5 to 10 degrees of full extension.
    - Repair and/or reconstruction for chronic cases also fare well.
        - However, the recovery process (including regaining strength) may take much longer (upward to 6 months to a year) for full improvement.
  - Complications
    - Retear, olecranon bursitis, weakness, decreased range of motion (ROM), and/or function, irritation from underlying internal structures that may require reoperation, flexion/extension contractures, poor wound healing, infection, ulnar nerve dysfunction

Distal Biceps Tendon

Pathophysiology

- MOI: Similar to the triceps, the injury is usually a result of a sudden eccentric load to a contracting biceps muscle with a supinated forearm position.[4,43]
- Most common injury site: tendon-osseous junction
- Hypovascularity of the tendon at the distal insertion, mechanical impingement[44] during ROM, and cubital "bursitis" predispose a patient to injury[45]
  - Other sites of failure
    - Bony avulsion from the radial tuberosity
    - Musculotendinous junction tear
      - Similar predisposing factors as mentioned in the triceps section
- Classification
  - Similar to triceps ruptures, there is no formal classification system. Injuries are routinely described with the following:
    - Tear size
      - Complete
      - Partial
    - Chronicity
      - Acute (less than 4 weeks)
      - Chronic (greater than 4 weeks)
    - Anatomic location
      - Tendinous/insertional
      - Musculotendinous junction
      - Intramuscular
  - Of note are the following:
    - The long head of the biceps inserts more proximal (and further from the center of rotation making it a more powerful forearm supinator)
    - The short head more distal (longer lever arm contributing more to elbow flexion)[46]

Presentation and Diagnosis

- Demographics
  - Affects men in their 40s and 60s and occurs in the dominant arm of most individuals[4,47-49]
  - Other risk factors include smoking, anabolic steroid use, and bodybuilding.[47,50,51]
- Presentation
  - Patients often describe a pop or sharp pain followed by ecchymosis and swelling in the antecubital fossa.
    - May describe a second episode of pain a few days later (completion of a partial to complete rupture, or secondary failure of the lacertus fibrosus)[52,53]
  - May describe pain and/or weakness with elbow flexion and supination
  - If presenting chronically, pain with activity is common
- Physical examination
  - Antecubital fossa swelling, ecchymosis

- Asymmetry, particularly after swelling has subsided
  - Accentuated with active flexion, during a palpable or visible defect may develop compared with the contralateral side
- Hook test when a distal biceps cannot be identified
  - When positive, the test is close to 100% sensitive and specific.[54]
  - A negative test with pain may suggest a partial tear.
- Biceps squeeze test
  - Similar to Thompson test for Achilles ruptures
  - Positive test when squeezing the biceps does not result in forearm supination
  - 96% sensitivity[55]
    - Beware of an intact lacertus fibrosis, which may mask the above exam findings consistent with a biceps rupture.
- Weakness with supination and elbow flexion[43]
- Partial tears may develop bursitis or peritendinosis, resulting in crepitance with forearm rotation or elbow flexion/extension.[52]
- Motion is usually preserved.

- Diagnostic imaging
  - Radiographs
    - May identify bony avulsion. Otherwise, advanced imaging necessary to confirm diagnosis if a distal biceps rupture is suspected.
    - Spurring sometimes present on the radial tuberosity, indicative of the degenerative process prior to rupture.[43,49]
  - Advanced imaging: may be useful to confirm rupture when history and examination is unclear (especially in context of a partial rupture or intact lacertus fibrosis) or to assist with preoperative planning in identifying zone of rupture, degree of retraction, and tendon quality
    - MRI
      - Conventional MRI plus a more recently described flexion, abduction, supination view has been shown effective in evaluating the distal biceps from the musculotendinous junction down to insertion on the radial tuberosity.[56]
        - For the flexion, abduction, supination view, the patient is positioned in the scanner with the shoulder abducted to 180 degrees over the head, elbow flexed 90 degrees around the head and forearm in supination
    - Ultrasound is operator dependent, but when performed by an experienced technician is a more cost-effective option that allows for improved understanding of partial tears given the dynamic nature of the study

Treatment

- General
  - Anatomic location, tear size (partial vs complete), hand dominance, profession, overall health status, and chronicity all play roles in management selection.
    - Surgical repair may be considered for intratendinous ruptures and insertional avulsions.
    - Intramuscular tears are predominantly managed nonoperatively.
    - Shared decision making should be employed, allowing the patient to make a decision in the context of his or her activity needs and goals.
- Nonsurgical

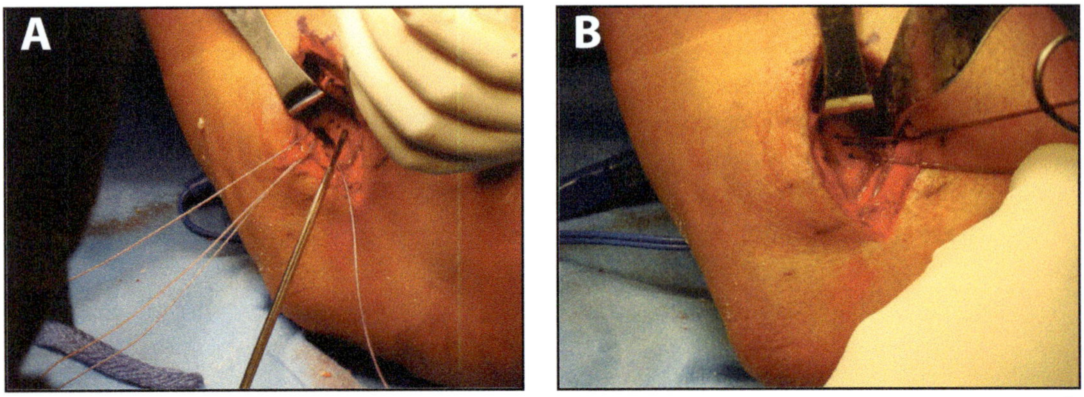

Figure 2-2. Trough and bone tunnel technique for distal biceps repair. (A) Placing bone tunnels adjacent to trough. (B) Sutures passed prior to securing the tendon repair with knot tying.

- Indications
  - Older, sedentary patients who do not require strength and endurance in forearm supination
  - Some partial tears less than 50% in size[57,58]
- Rehabilitation
  - Aims to obtain full ROM, strength, and pain relief
- Outcomes
  - Weakness: may see up to a 40% loss of supination strength, 15% to 30% loss of flexion strength, 86% decrease in supination endurance, and 15% decrease in grip strength[48,59]
  - Many develop concomitant cubital bursitis.
    - Many fail to improve clinically and ultimately go on to surgical repair.

- Operative
  - Indications
    - Acute complete tears
      - Surgical repair indicated as soon as possible before scar formation occurs
    - Chronic injuries or partial tears that have failed nonoperative management
      - May require graft augmentation, particularly if the tendon stump has retracted and scarred into the muscle belly
  - Techniques
    - One (anterior) vs 2-incision (Boyd-Anderson, Mayo [modified Boyd-Anderson]) technique
      - Early literature demonstrated higher rates of nerve injury or neuropraxia with the single-incision technique and higher rates of heterotopic ossification with the 2-incision technique.[60]
      - However, a more recent systematic review comparing the 2 showed minor differences, noting a slightly higher lateral antebrachial cutaneous nerve (LABCN) neuropraxia with the single-incision technique compared with a slightly higher risk of stiffness associated with the 2-incision technique.[61] *Recommended reading for comparison of 1- vs 2-incision technique*
    - Fixation types
      - Various techniques described including fixation with suture and bone tunnels (Figure 2-2), suture buttons, suture anchors, and transosseous screws.

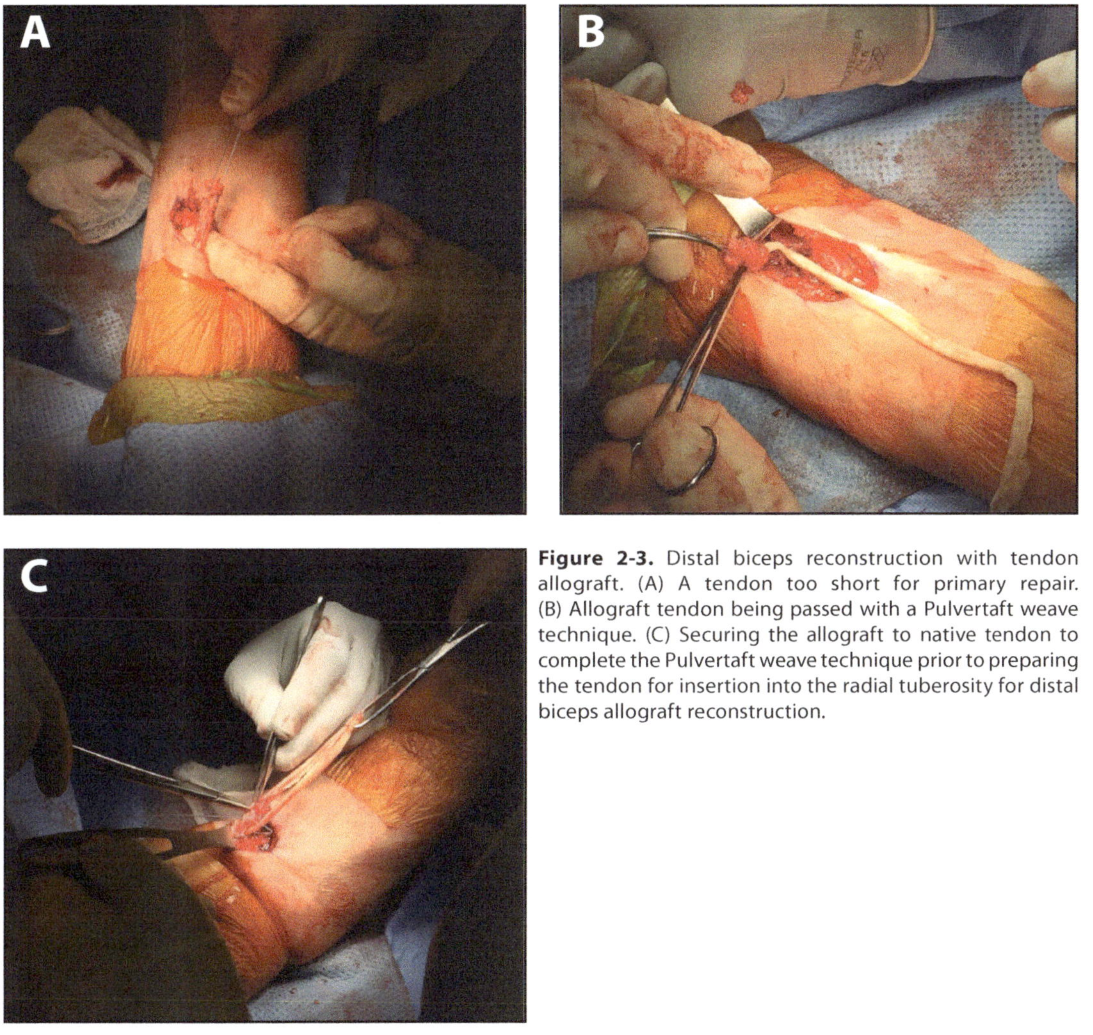

Figure 2-3. Distal biceps reconstruction with tendon allograft. (A) A tendon too short for primary repair. (B) Allograft tendon being passed with a Pulvertaft weave technique. (C) Securing the allograft to native tendon to complete the Pulvertaft weave technique prior to preparing the tendon for insertion into the radial tuberosity for distal biceps allograft reconstruction.

- Bone tunnels and suture-button techniques have been shown to have a smaller complication risk.[61]
- Late reconstruction
  - There are several reports in the literature regarding the use of autologous vs allograft tendon reconstruction[24,62-66] (Figure 2-3).
- Outcomes
  - Two-incision technique
    - Significant improvement in strength
      - Restoration strength approaches normal in flexion and supination 15 months following repair[59]
      - Restoration of full strength in dominant arm, but 20% to 30% loss if nondominant side involved[67]
  - EndoButton
    - Ninety-seven percent recovery of flexion and 82% return of supination strength, satisfactory return to preinjury activities and occupations[68]

- Complications (radioulnar synostosis, posterior interosseous nerve [PIN] neuropraxia, LABCN injury, superficial radial nerve injury, heterotopic ossification, rerupture, infection)
  - Increased risk of complication with delay to surgery[60]
  - Nerve injuries: usually transient
    - LABCN
      - Terminal branch of the musculocutaneous nerve
      - Runs along radial aspect of antecubital fossa in superficial fascia
      - Susceptible to iatrogenic injury during repair,[69] particularly with retraction during single-incision approach
    - PIN
      - Deep branch of the radial nerve
      - Course dorsally around the radial neck into the supinator muscle
      - Seen with single- and 2-incision approaches
        - At risk with fixation to the dorsal radial cortex or during the dorsal approach[70]
    - Median nerve
      - Injury with dissection or overtensioning of graft with lacertus fibrosis intact[71]
  - Ectopic bone formation
    - Reported both with single- and 2-incision techniques
      - More common with original Boyd-Anderson 2-incision technique with exposure along the periosteum of the proximal ulna
        - May be avoided with muscle-splitting Mayo approach
      - Indomethacin (75 mg) for up to 6 weeks postoperatively was found to significantly reduce (37% vs 1%) the incidence of radioulnar synostosis after distal biceps repair without any adverse events (including gastrointestinal bleeding and rerupture).[72]
      - Symptomatic heterotopic ossification or radioulnar synostosis may be addressed 9 to 12 months after initial fixation once it has matured.
  - Recurrent tear

Lateral Epicondylitis

Pathophysiology

- MOI
  - Overuse: commonly occurs with repetitive wrist extension and supination of the forearm with the elbow in near extension
- Epicondylitis is a misnomer: condition is secondary to degeneration, tendinosis, and microtears of the extensor tendon origin[73]
  - Microscopic evaluation: noninflammatory "angiofibroblastic tendinosis"[73]
    - Dysfunctional vascular and fibrous invasion and a disordered collagen scaffold with mucoid degeneration[73]
      - Consistent with repetitive microtearing and healing attempts[74]
    - Absence of acute or chronic inflammatory cells
  - Primarily involves the extensor carpi radialis brevis (ECRB) origin

- In 50% of cases, also involves the leading edge of the extensor digitorum communis origin
- Less commonly involved are the extensor carpi radialis longus (ECRL) or extensor carpi ulnaris tendon origins.

- Classification
  - No formal classification system
  - Nirschl described tendinosis phases of pain (phases I to VII) based on the spectrum of symptoms in relation to activity and sleep.[72]
  - Baker and colleagues described the arthroscopic appearance of the lateral capsule in lateral epicondylitis from type 1 (smooth capsule without irregularity) to type 3 (ruptured and retracted capsule with frayed extensor carpi radilis brevis visible).[75]
- Differential diagnosis
  - Cervical radiculopathy
  - Radial tunnel syndrome
    - PIN nerve compression: maximal tenderness 3 to 4 cm distal and anterior to the epicondyle over the mobile wad[76]
  - Intra-articular elbow disorder
    - Arthritis, radiocapitellar osteochondritis dissecans, loose bodies, posterolateral elbow plica, posterolateral elbow instability

Presentation and Diagnosis

- Demographics
  - Affects approximately 2% of the general population[77,78]
  - Affects men and women equally[79]
  - Most common in the fourth and fifth decades of life[73]
  - More commonly affects the dominant arm[80]
  - Common with tennis, racquetball, squash, fencing, and manual laborers who work in meat cutting, plumbing, carpentry, painting, raking, and mechanics.[81,82]
- Presentation
  - Pain at the lateral elbow, often radiating into the forearm
  - Made worse with repetitive wrist extension and supination activities
  - Inability to hold objects because of lateral elbow pain
- Physical examination
  - Tenderness to palpation over the extensor tendon origin around 2 to 5 mm distal and anterior to the lateral epicondyle[81]
  - Pain with resisted wrist extension
    - Absence of pain with wrist extension and presence of pain with thumb and finger extension or resisted supination may be more consistent with radial tunnel syndrome
    - The 2 syndromes may coexist in 5% of patients.[76]
  - Full active and passive elbow and forearm ROM
  - Possible pain limited wrist extension weakness
- Diagnostic imaging
  - Radiographs
    - Often normal

      - Twenty-two percent to 25% of patients may have calcific tendinitis in the soft tissue just distal to the lateral epicondyle.[73]
      - Evaluate for concomitant intra-articular pathology.
  - MRI
    - Evaluate for suspected intra-articular pathology or surrounding ligamentous structures.
    - Define the extent of tearing of the extensor origin.[83]
    - Less useful to follow response to treatment
  - Ultrasound
    - Identifies focal hypoechoic areas, intrasubstance tears, peritendinous fluid, and thickening of the common extensor origin[84]
    - Moderate sensitivity and variable specificity when evaluating extensor origin architecture[85,86]

Treatment

- Nonsurgical
  - Activity modification: first-line treatment for nearly all patients
    - Tennis: slower playing surfaces, more flexible racket, lower string tension, larger grip
      - Physical therapy: eccentric muscle training; stretching; ultrasound; other modalities[87]
      - Nonsteroidal anti-inflammatory drugs (NSAIDs): oral or topical
        - Although lateral epicondylitis is a noninflammatory condition, anti-inflammatories may relieve pain from associated synovitis or inflammation of surrounding supportive connective tissue.[88]
        - Mixed results in the literature regarding NSAID use vs placebo/other nonoperative measures.[89-93]
  - Counterforce bracing and cockup wrist splints reduce tension at extensor origin, lower extensor muscle activity and expansion. One randomized, controlled trial showed better pain relief with the wrist brace over the counterforce brace, but both were beneficial.[94]
  - Consider corticosteroid injections at site of maximal tenderness
    - Beware risk of lateral ulnar collateral ligament (UCL) rupture with resulting posterolateral rotatory instability after steroid injection and common extensor rupture[95,96]
    - Pain relief in 55% to 89% of patients, recurrence in 18% to 54%[97]
    - May provide earlier relief than other modalities but at long-term follow-up may be same or worse as other treatment groups[93,98]
  - Botulinum toxin injection and shock wave therapy
    - Newer treatment modalities: more long-term follow-up studies needed
    - Botulinum: paralysis of extensor apparatus providing time for tendinous healing in a less-tensioned environment
    - Extracorporeal shock waves are single-pulsed sonic waves that dissipate energy at the interface of 2 substances, but its exact mechanism of symptomatic relief for tennis elbow is not well understood.
- Operative
  - Indications
    - Persistent debilitating pain unresponsive to conservative measures described previously that have been tried for at least 6 months
    - Exclusion of other causes of lateral elbow or forearm pain
      - Techniques

- Arthroscopic: debridement and repair
    - No advantage over mini-open technique[88]
    - Risks: incomplete excision of pain-producing tendinosis, nerve injury, articular cartilage injury, increased cost (or time and instrument cost)[99]
        - Keeping debridement in line with the anterior half of the radial head prevents destabilization of the lateral elbow.[100]
- Mini-open
    - Tenex: ultrasound guided debridement of the diseased tendon with a Tenex handpiece through a 5-mm incision under local anesthesia
- Open
    - A 3-cm incision starting anterior and medial to the lateral epicondyle extending to just proximal to the joint line
    - Identify the interface between the ECRL (anteriorly) and the anterior edge of the extensor aponeurosis laterally; fascia is split in this interval
    - ECRL is elevated as a flap anteriorly to expose the underlying ECRB
    - Identify pathologic tissue often described as having a "gray hue" with the "Nirschl scratch test"[88] and excise pathologic tissue en bloc
    - The more distal nonpathologic ECRB and aponeurosis tendons if often still attached, obviating the need for "repair." If the debridement destabilizes the origin, repair is required.
    - Decorticate the lateral epicondyle that was exposed following pathologic ECRB tendon origin excision to encourage bleeding and formation of healthy fibrotendinous tissue. Role for anchor fixation to over-sew torn fibers may be beneficial (authors' preferred technique).
- Other options
    - Percutaneous release, ECRB lengthening, simultaneous decompression of radial nerve, percutaneous or endoscopic release
    - For chronic or recurrent cases, an anconeus flap can be used to provide coverage.[101]

- Postoperative care
    - If the extensor origin was not detached completely, early mobilization is allowed and encouraged.
        - If repair is required, consider splint or sling immobilization for 7 to 10 days.[102]
    - Counterforce support may be used until full strength and function returns (months).
    - Strengthening commences at 6 weeks.
    - Return to sports around approximately 8 to 12 weeks
- Results
    - Nonoperative management
        - Around 80% of patients report symptomatic improvement at 1 year.[77,98,103,104]
        - Twenty-six percent of patients have recurrence of symptoms and 40% have prolonged, persistent minor discomfort.[104]
        - Four percent to 11% of patients will ultimately require surgical intervention.[73,77,104-106]
            - Risk factors for nonoperative failure include the following:
                - Manual laborers; dominant arm involvement; higher baseline pain levels; longer duration of symptoms and poor coping mechanisms; presence of soft-tissue calcification[72,103]
    - Surgical management

- Mini-open lateral debridement: 97% of patients improve and 93% can expect full return to all preoperative activities[107]
  - However, one long-term follow-up study showed 40% had persistent pain at 6 weeks, 24% at 1 year, and 9% at 5 years postoperatively.[108]
- Arthroscopic management: Ninety-three to 100% of patients were better by 2 years postoperatively.[75,109,110]
  - However, only 62% to 80% of patients experienced complete elimination of lateral elbow pain.[110,111]
- Tenex
  - Positive early reports in the literature
    - 95% satisfaction, no complications, significant improvement in visual analog scale scores by 1 week, significant improvement disabilities of the arm, shoulder, and hand compulsory scores by 1 month, 95% tendon thickness reduction[112]
- Open vs arthroscopic
  - No statistically significant difference in outcomes at 6 months (approximately 70% good or excellent outcomes in each group).
  - Arthroscopic procedure allowed earlier return to work

- Complications
  - Iatrogenic posterolateral rotatory instability: excessive debridement may compromise lateral UCL
  - Neuroma of the posterior cutaneous nerve of the forearm
  - Reactive bone formation

Medial Epicondylitis

Pathophysiology

- MOI
  - Overuse: commonly occurs with repetitive eccentric loading of the common flexor tendons (CFTs) (which include the pronator teres, flexor carpi radialis [FCR], palmaris longus, flexor digitorum superficialis, and the flexor carpi ulnaris) that control wrist flexion and forearm pronation combined with valgus overload of the elbow[113]
    - Most commonly involve the pronator teres and FCR
  - Macroscopic tearing of the flexor-pronator origin identified in approximately 100% of cases that underwent surgical treatment[114]
- Classification
  - Morrey classification
    - Type I: isolated medial epicondylitis
    - Type II: medial epicondylitis combined with ulnar neuritis
      - A: minimal ulnar severity
      - B: moderate ulnar severity
- Differential diagnosis/associated conditions
  - Carpal tunnel
  - Cubital tunnel
  - Lateral epicondylitis

  - Rotator cuff tendinitis
  - Elbow UCL deficiency
  - Cervical radiculopathy

Presentation and Diagnosis

- Demographics
  - Rarer than lateral epicondylitis
    - Overall prevalence less than 1%, with increased rates in certain occupational settings[115-117]
  - Equally affects men and women[115-117]
  - Typically occurs in the fourth through sixth decades of life
  - Often seen in athletes playing golf, rowing, baseball or javelin, tennis, and in occupations subjected to repetitive valgus forces such as bricklaying, hammering, typing, and textile production[81]
- Presentation
  - Medial elbow pain
  - History of activities described previously
  - May complain of numbness, tingling, or shooting pain from elbow down to hand in ulnar nerve distribution
- Physical examination
  - Tenderness to palpation 5 to 10 mm distal and anterior to the medial epicondyle
  - May have overlying soft-tissue swelling, redness, or warmth
  - Resisted wrist flexion, forearm pronation, and forceful grip may elicit pain or appear weaker than the contralateral side[118]
  - Evaluate for concomitant injuries
    - Elbow UCL insufficiency (milking maneuver or moving valgus stress test)
    - Cubital or carpal tunnel (Tinel, 2-point discrimination, appropriate motor testing)
    - Lateral epicondylitis (see previous description)
    - Cervical radiculopathy
    - Shoulder pathology
- Diagnostic imaging
  - Radiographs
    - Usually normal
      - 25% may show evidence of calcification of the UCL or CFT (similar to lateral epicondylitis).[113]
  - MRI
    - Effective at identifying tendon disruption and other medial elbow pathology such as UCL injuries or osteochondral lesions
    - T2 sequencing may identify peritendinous edema, which is indicative of medial epicondylitis.[119]
  - Ultrasound
    - Evaluate for hypoechoic or anechoic areas consistent with focal tendon degeneration.
    - More than 90% sensitivity, specificity, and positive or negative predictive values in the hands of a musculoskeletal radiologist[120]

Treatment

- Nonsurgical
  - Mainstay, first-line treatment for medial epicondylitis
  - Activity modification: rest to allow tendon healing; avoid activities that require repetitive wrist flexion, pronation, and valgus stress across the elbow
    - If concomitant UCL injury, avoid throwing for 6 to 12 weeks.
    - Tennis: slower playing surfaces; more flexible racket; lower string tension; larger grip
    - Golfers: evaluate technique; avoid undue stress on the trail arm that is subjected to valgus forces during the swing
  - Ice and NSAIDs
    - Analgesic and vasoconstrictive effects
    - Decrease synovitis associated with medial epicondylitis[113]
  - Supportive orthoses (counterforce splints)/night splints
    - Similar to treatment of lateral epicondylitis
  - Extracorporeal shock waves
    - Electrical stimulation may promote angiogenesis, tendon healing, and analgesia.[121]
  - Steroid injection
  - Percutaneous needle injection trephination
    - Stimulate bleeding and tendon healing[122]
  - Physical therapy
    - Flexor-pronator mass stretching and strengthening once acute symptoms have resolved
- Operative
  - Indications
    - Recalcitrant medial epicondylitis more than 6 months
    - Elite athlete with definitive tear appreciable on MRI[113]
    - Concomitant medial elbow pathology that needs to be addressed surgically
  - Techniques
    - Arthroscopic debridement
      - Not widely used due to risk of ulnar nerve and UCL ligament iatrogenic injury[113]
      - Limited literature to support this technique
    - Open debridement
      - Incision over the medial epicondyle (avoid injury to medial antebrachial cutaneous nerve)
      - Dissect down to the common flexor-pronator tendon origin and medial epicondyle, identify the ulnar nerve for protection throughout the case, split interval between pronator teres and FCR to identify friable tissue below for debridement
      - Depending on the degree of involvement and resection, CFT repair may be required. Decortication of the medial epicondyle will facilitate healing. Prior to repair, inspect the UCL for concomitant injury.
    - Type II lesions require epicondylar debridement and ulnar nerve decompression vs submuscular transposition (rare) for types IIA and B lesions, respectively.[123]
  - Postoperative care
    - If no formal tendon repair or ulnar nerve transposition was required, early motion is encouraged.

- In more severe cases, immobilization via a sling or splint may be indicated for 10 to 14 days followed by active ROM and return to use with activities of daily living.
- Strengthening exercises may start approximately 6 to 8 weeks postoperatively.
- Return to full activity/sports usually occurs around 3 months postoperatively.

- Results
  - Open debridement resulted in 34/35 good or excellent results, with only 1 patient failing to return to preinjury athletic performance at 6-year follow-up.[114]
  - If moderate to severe ulnar nerve symptoms are present preoperatively, patient has a higher chance of poor results at final follow-up even with decompression ± ulnar nerve transposition.[124]
- Complications
  - Medial antebrachial cutaneous nerve and/or ulnar nerve injury, neuroma
  - Iatrogenic UCL injury with valgus instability
  - Incomplete resolution of pain or symptoms

References

1. Yeh PC, Stephens KT, Solovyova O, et al. The distal triceps tendon footprint and a biomechanical analysis of 3 repair techniques. *Am J Sports Med.* 2010;38(5):1025-1033. doi:10.1177/0363546509358319.
2. Preston FW, Adicoff A. Hyperparathyroidism with avulsion at three major tendons. Report of a case. *N Engl J Med.* 1962;266:968-971. doi:10.1056/NEJM196205102661903.
3. van Riet RP, Morrey BF, Ho E, O'Driscoll SW. Surgical treatment of distal triceps ruptures. *J Bone Joint Surg Am.* 2003;85(10):1961-1967. doi:10.2106/00004623-200310000-00015.
4. Baumann GI. Rupture of the biceps tendon. *J Bone Joint Surg.* 1934;16(4):966-967.
5. O'Driscoll SW. Intramuscular triceps rupture. *Can J Surg.* 1992;35(2):203-207.
6. Bach BR Jr, Warren RF, Wickiewicz TL. Triceps rupture. A case report and literature review. *Am J Sports Med.* 1987;15(3):285-289. doi:10.1177/036354658701500319.
7. Wagner JR, Cooney WP. Rupture of the triceps muscle at the musculotendinous junction: a case report. *J Hand Surg Am.* 1997;22(2):341-343. doi:10.1016/S0363-5023(97)80175-X.
8. Fery A, Sommelet J, Schmitt D, Lipp B. Avulsion bilaterale simultanée des tendons quadricipital et rotulien et rupture de tendon tricipital chez un hemodialiyse hypertparathyroidien. [Simultaneous bilateral avulsion of the quadriceps and Achilles tendons in 1 limb and of the patellar tendon in the other in a hyperparathyroid patient on chronic hemodialysis. In French.] *Rev Chri Ortho Reparatrice Appar Mot.* 1978;64(2):175-181.
9. Cirincione RJ, Baker BE. Tendon ruptures with secondary hyperparathyroidism. A case report. *J Bone Joint Surg Am.* 1975;57(6):852-853.
10. Clayton ML, Thirupathi RG. Rupture of the triceps tendon with olecranon bursitis: a case report with a new method of repair. *Clin Orthop Relat Res.* 1984;(184):183-185.
11. Schutt RC, Powell RL, Winter WG. Spontaneous ruptures of long tendons. Presented at: Annual Meeting of the American Academy of Orthopaedic Surgeons; January 25, 1982; New Orleans, LA.
12. Match RM, Corrylos EV. Bilateral avulsion fracture of the triceps tendon insertion from skiing with osteogenesis imperfecta tarda. A case report. *Am J Sports Med.* 1983;11(2):99-102. doi:10.1177/036354658301100210.
13. Yeh PC, Dodds SD, Smart LR, Mazzocca AD, Sethi PM. Distal triceps rupture. *J Am Acad Orthop Surg.* 2010;18(1):31-40. doi:10.5435/00124635-201001000-00005.
14. Anzel SH, Covey KW, Weiner AD, Lipscomb PR. Disruption of muscles and tendons: an analysis of 1,014 cases. *Surgery.* 1959;45(3):406-414.
15. Farrar EL III, Lippert FG III. Avulsion of the triceps tendon. *Clin Orthop Relat Res.* 1981;(161):242-246.
16. Sollender JL, Rayan GM, Barden GA. Triceps tendon rupture in weight lifters. *J Shoulder Elbow Surg.* 1998;7(2):151-153. doi:10.1016/S1058-2746(98)90227-0.
17. Duchow J, Kelm J, Kohn D. Acute ulnar nerve compression syndrome in a powerlifter with triceps tendon rupture—a case report. *Int J Sports Med.* 2000;21(4):308-310. doi:10.1055/s-2000-9468.
18. Mair SD, Isbell WM, Gill TJ, Schlegel TF, Hawkins RJ. Triceps tendon ruptures in professional football players. *Am J Sports Med.* 2004;32(2):431-434. doi:10.1177/0095399703258707.
19. Lambert MI, St Clair Gibson A, Noakes TD. Rupture of the triceps tendon associated with steroid injections. *Am J Sports Med.* 1995;23(6):778. doi:10.1177/036354659502300626.

20. Sharma SC, Singh R, Goel T, Singh H. Missed diagnosis of triceps tendon rupture: a case report and review of literature. *J Orthop Surg (Hong Kong)*. 2005;13(3):307-309. doi:10.1177/230949900501300317.
21. Viegas SF. Avulsion of the triceps tendon. *Orthop Rev*. 1990;19(6):533-536.
22. Bos CF, Nelissen RG, Bloem JL. Incomplete rupture of the tendon of triceps brachii. A case report. *Int Orthop*. 1994;18(5):273-275. doi:10.1007/bf00180224.
23. Pina A, Garcia I, Sabater M. Traumatic avulsion of the triceps brachii. *J Orthop Trauma*. 2002;16(4):273-276. doi:10.1097/00005131-200204000-00010.
24. Levy M, Goldberg I, Meir I. Fracture of the head of the radius with a tear or avulsion of the triceps tendon. A new syndrome? *J Bone Joint Surg Br*. 1982;64-B(1):70-72. doi:10.1302/0301-620X.64B1.7068723.
25. Kaempffe FA, Lerner RM. Ultrasound diagnosis of triceps tendon rupture. A report of 2 cases. *Clin Orthop Relat Res*. 1996;(332):138-142. doi:10.1097/00003086-199611000-00019.
26. Zionts LE, Vachon LA. Demonstration of avulsion of the triceps tendon in an adolescent by magnetic resonance imaging. *Am J Orthop (Belle Mead NJ)*. 1997;26(7):489-490.
27. Kijowski R, Tuite M, Sanford M. Magnetic resonance imaging of the elbow. Part II: abnormalities of the ligaments, tendons, and nerves. *Skeletal Radiol*. 2005;34(1):1-18. doi:10.1007/s00256-004-0854-y.
28. Popovic N, Ferrara MA, Daenen B, Georis P, Lemaire R. Imaging of overuse injury of the elbow in professional team handball players: a bilateral comparison using plain films, stress radiographs, ultrasound, and magnetic resonance imaging. *Int J Sports Med*. 2001;22(1):60-67. doi:10.1055/s-2001-11333.
29. Strauch RJ. Biceps and triceps injuries of the elbow. *Orthop Clin North Am*. 1999;30(1):95-107.
30. Singh RK, Pooley J. Complete rupture of the triceps brachii muscle. *Br J Sports Med*. 2002;36(6):467-469. doi:10.1136/bjsm.36.6.467.
31. Morrey B. Rupture of the triceps tendon. In: Morrey B, Sanchez-Sotelo J, eds. *The Elbow and its Disorders*. 4th ed. Philadelphia, PA: Saunders Elsevier; 2009:536-546.
32. Vidal AF, Drakos MC, Allen AA. Biceps tendon and triceps tendon injuries. *Clin Sports Med*. 2004;23(4):707-722. doi:10.1016/j.csm.2004.06.001.
33. Anderson KJ, LeCocq JF. Rupture of the triceps tendon. *J Bone Joint Surg Am*. 1957;39-A(2):444-446.
34. Harris PC, Atkinson D, Moorehead JD. Bilateral partial rupture of triceps tendon: case report and quantitative assessment of recovery. *Am J Sports Med*. 2004;32(3):787-792. doi:10.1177/0363546503258903.
35. Aso K, Torisu T. Muscle belly tear of the triceps. *Am J Sports Med*. 1984;12(6):485-487. doi: 10.1177/036354658401200614.
36. Tsourvakas S, Gouvalas K, Gimtsas C, Tsianas N, Founta P, Ameridis N. Bilateral and simultaneous rupture of the triceps tendons in chronic renal failure and secondary hyperparathyroidism. *Arch Orthop Trauma Surg*. 2004;124(4): 278-280. doi:10.1007/s00402-003-0628-3.
37. Langenhan R, Weihe R, Kohler G. Traumatic rupture of the triceps brachii tendon and ipsilateral Achilles tendon [in German]. *Unfallchirurg*. 2007;110(11):977-980. doi:10.1007/s00113-007-1282-y.
38. Esenyel CZ, Öztürk K, Ortak O, Kara AN. Rupture of the triceps brachii tendon: A case report [in Turkish]. *Acta Orthop Traumatol Turc*. 2003;37(2):178-181.
39. Sanchez-Sotelo J, Morrey BF. Surgical techniques for reconstruction of chronic insufficiency of the triceps. Rotation flap using anconeus and tendo achillis allograft. *J Bone Joint Surg Br*. 2002;84(8):1116-1120. doi:10.1302/0301-620x.84b8.12902.
40. Sai S, Fujii K, Chino H, Inoue J, Ishizaka J. Old rupture of the triceps tendon with unique pathology: a case report. *J Orthop Sci*. 2004;9(6):654-656. doi:10.1007/s00776-004-0820-5.
41. Dos Remedios C, Brosset T, Chantelot C, Fontaine C. Repair of a triceps tendon rupture using autogenous semi-tendinous and gracilis tendons. A case report and retrospective chart review [in French]. *Chir Main*. 2007;26:154-158. doi:10.1016/j.main.2007.05.006.
42. Weistroffer JK, Mills WJ, Shin AY. Recurrent rupture of the triceps tendon repaired with hamstring tendon autograft augmentation: a case report and repair technique. *J Shoulder Elbow Surg*. 2003;12(2):193-196. doi:10.1067/mse.2003.15.
43. Dobbie RP. Avulsion of the lower biceps brachii tendon: analysis of fifty-one previously reported cases. *Am J Surg*. 1941;51(3):661-683. doi:10.1016/S0002-9610(41)90203-9.
44. Seiler JG III, Parker LM, Chamberland PD, Sherbourne GM, Carpenter WA. The distal biceps tendon. Two potential mechanisms involved in its rupture: arterial supply and mechanical impingement. *J Shoulder Elbow Surg*. 1995;4(3):149-156.
45. Karanjia ND, Stiles PJ. Cubital bursitis. *J Bone Joint Surg Br*. 1988;70(5):832-833.
46. Eames MH, Bain GI, Fogg QA, van Riet RP. Distal biceps tendon anatomy: a cadaveric study. *J Bone Joint Surg Am*. 2007;89(5):1044-1049. doi:10.2106/JBJS.D.02992.
47. Safran MR, Graham SM. Distal biceps tendon ruptures: incidence, demographics, and the effect of smoking. *Clin Orthop Relat Res*. 2002;(404):275-283.
48. Baker BE, Bierwagen D. Rupture of the distal tendon of the biceps brachii. Operative versus non-operative treatment. *J Bone Joint Surg Am*. 1985;67(3):414-417.
49. Postacchini F, Puddu G. Subcutaneous rupture of the distal biceps brachii tendon; a report on seven cases. *J Sports Med Phys Fitness*. 1975;15(2):81-90.

50. D'Alessandro DF, Shields CL Jr, Tibone JE, Chandler RW. Repair of distal biceps tendon ruptures in athletes. *Am J Sports Med.* 1993;21(1):114-119. doi:10.1177/036354659302100119.
51. Visuri T, Lindholm H. Bilateral distal biceps tendon avulsions with use of anabolic steroids. *Med Sci Sports Exerc.* 1994;26(8):941-944.
52. Bourne MH, Morrey BF. Partial rupture of the distal biceps tendon. *Clin Orthop Relat Res.* 1991;(271):143-148.
53. Boyd HB, Anderson MD. A method for reinsertion of the distal biceps brachii tendon. *J Bone Joint Surg.* 1961;43(7):1041-1043.
54. Patterson RW, Sharma J, Lawton JN, Evans PJ. Distal biceps tendon reconstruction with tendoachilles allograft: a modification of the EndoButton technique utilizing an ACL reconstruction system. *J Hand Surg Am.* 2009;34(3):545-552. doi:10.1016/j.jhsa.2008.12.019.
55. Ruland RT, Dunbar RP, Bowen JD. The biceps squeeze test for diagnosis of distal biceps tendon ruptures. *Clin Orthop Relat Res.* 2005;(437):128-131. doi:10.1097/01.blo.0000167668.18444.f5.
56. Giuffrè BM, Moss MJ. Optimal positioning for MRI of the distal biceps brachii tendon: flexed abducted supinated view. *AJR Am J Roentgenol.* 2004;182(4):944-946. doi:10.2214/ajr.182.4.1820944.
57. Dürr HR, Stäbler A, Pfahler M, Matzko M, Refior HJ. Partial rupture of the distal biceps tendon. *Clin Orthop Relat Res.* 2000;(374):195-200. doi:10.1097/00003086-200005000-00018.
58. Vardakas DG, Musgrave DS, Varitimidis SE, Goebel F, Sotereanos DG. Partial rupture of the distal biceps tendon. *J Shoulder Elbow Surg.* 2001;10(4):377-379. doi:10.1067/mse.2001.116518.
59. Morrey BF, Askew LJ, An KN, Dobyns JH. Rupture of the distal tendon of the biceps brachii. A biomechanical study. *J Bone Joint Surg Am.* 1985;67(3):418-421.
60. Kelly EW, Morrey BF, O'Driscoll SW. Complications of repair of the distal biceps tendon with the modified two-incision technique. *J Bone Joint Surg Am.* 2000;82(11):1575-1581. doi:10.2106/00004623-200011000-00010.
61. Watson JN, Moretti VM, Schwindel L, Hutchinson MR. Repair techniques for acute distal biceps tendon ruptures: a systematic review. *J Bone Joint Surg Am.* 2014;96(24):2086-2090. doi:10.2106/JBJS.M.00481.
62. Hallam P, Bain GI. Repair of chronic distal biceps tendon ruptures using autologous hamstring grafts and the EndoButton. *J Shoulder Elbow Surg.* 2004;13(6):648-651. doi:10.1016/S1058274604000771.
63. Hovelius L, Josefsson G. Rupture of the distal biceps tendon. Report of five cases. *Acta Orthop Scand.* 1977;48(3):280-282. doi:10.3109/17453677708988769.
64. Rantanen J, Orava S. Rupture of the distal biceps tendon. A report of 19 patients treated with anatomic reinsertion, and a meta-analysis of 147 cases found in the literature. *Am J Sports Med.* 1999;27(2):128-132. doi:10.1177/03635465990270020201.
65. Sanchez-Sotelo J, Morrey BF, Adams RA, O'Driscoll SW. Reconstruction of chronic ruptures of the distal biceps tendon with use of an Achilles tendon allograft. *J Bone Joint Surg Am.* 2002;84(6):999-1005. doi:10.2106/00004623-200206000-00015.
66. Wiley WB, Noble J, Dunlaney TD, Bell RH, Noble DD. Late reconstruction of chronic distal biceps tendon ruptures with a semitendinosus autograft technique. *J Shoulder Elbow Surg.* 2006;15(4):440-444. doi:10.1016/j.jse.2005.08.018.
67. Agins HJ, Chess JL, Hokstra DV, Teitge RA. Rupture of the distal insertion of the biceps brachii tendon. *Clin Orthop Relat Res.* 1988;(234):34-38.
68. Greenberg JA, Fernandez JJ, Wang T, Turner C. EndoButton-assisted repair of distal biceps tendon ruptures. *J Shoulder Elbow Surg.* 2003;12(5):484-190. doi:10.1016/S1058274603001733.
69. Chiavaras MM, Jacobson JA, Billone L, Lawton JM, Lawton J. Sonography of the lateral antebrachial cutaneous nerve with magnetic resonance imaging and anatomic correlation. *J Ultrasound Med.* 2014;33(8):1475-1483. doi:10.7863/ultra.33.8.1475.
70. Lawton JN, Cameron-Donaldson M, Blazar PE, Moore JR. Anatomic considerations regarding the posterior interosseous nerve at the elbow. *J Shoulder Elbow Surg.* 2007;16(4):502-507. doi:10.1016/j.jse.2006.09.004.
71. Bain G, Prem H, Heptinstall R, Verhellen R, Paix D. Repair of distal biceps tendon rupture: A new technique using the EndoButton. *J Shoulder Elbow Surg.* 2000;9(2):120-126.
72. Costopoulos CL, Abboud JA, Ramsey ML, et al. The use of indomethacin in the prevention of postoperative radioulnar synostosis after distal biceps repair. *J Shoulder Elbow Surg.* 2017;26(2):295-298. doi:10.1016/j.jse.2016.11.011.
73. Nirschl RP. Elbow tendinosis/tennis elbow. *Clin Sports Med.* 1992;11(4):851-870.
74. Kraushaar BS, Nirschl RP. Tendinosis of the elbow (tennis elbow). Clinical features and findings of histological, immunohistochemical, and electron microscopy studies. *J Bone Joint Surg Am.* 1999;81(2):259-278.
75. Baker CL Jr, Murphy KP, Gottlob CA, Curd DT. Arthroscopic classification and treatment of lateral epicondylitis: two-year clinical results. *J Shoulder Elbow Surg.* 2000;9(6):475-482. doi:10.1067/mse.2000.108533.
76. Werner CO. Lateral elbow pain and posterior interosseous nerve entrapment. *Acta Orthop Scand Suppl.* 1979;174:1-62.
77. Verhaar JA. Tennis elbow. Anatomical, epidemiological and therapeutic aspects. *Int Orthop.* 1994;18(5):263-267. doi:10.1007/bf00180221.
78. Allander E. Prevalence, incidence, and remission rates of some common rheumatic diseases or syndromes. *Scand J Rheumatol.* 1974;3(3):145-153. doi:10.3109/03009747409097141.

79. Gruchow HW, Pelletier D. An epidemiologic study of tennis elbow. Incidence, recurrence, and effectiveness of prevention strategies. *Am J Sports Med.* 1979;7(4):234-238. doi:10.1177/036354657900700405.
80. Nirschl RP, Alvarado GJ. Tennis elbow tendinosis. In: Morrey B, Sanchez-Sotelo J, eds. *The Elbow and its Disorders.* 4th ed. Philadelphia, PA: Saunders Elsevier; 2009:626-638.
81. Jobe FW, Ciccotti MG. Lateral and medial epicondylitis of the elbow. *J Am Acad Orthop Surg.* 1994;2(1):1-8.
82. Haahr JP, Andersen JH. Physical and psychosocial risk factors for lateral epicondylitis: a population based case-referent study. *Occup Environ Med.* 2003;60(5):322-329. doi:10.1136/oem.60.5.322.
83. Potter HG, Hannafin JA, Morwessel RM, DiCarlo EF, O'Brien SJ, Altchek DW. Lateral epicondylitis: correlation of MR imaging, surgical, and histopathologic findings. *Radiology.* 1995;196(1):43-46. doi:10.1148/radiology.196.1.7784585.
84. Connell D, Burke F, Coombes P, et al. Sonographic examination of lateral epicondylitis. *AJR Am J Roentgenol.* 2001;176(3):777-782. doi:10.2214/ajr.176.3.1760777.
85. Miller TT, Shapiro MA, Schultz E, Kalish PE. Comparison of sonography and MRI for diagnosing epicondylitis. *J Clin Ultrasound.* 2002;30(4):193-202. doi:10.1002/jcu.10063.
86. Levin D, Nazarian LN, Miller TT, et al. Lateral epicondylitis of the elbow: US findings. *Radiology.* 2005;237(1):230-234. doi:10.1148/radiol.2371040784.
87. Martinez-Silvestrini JA, Newcomer KL, Gay RE, Schaefer MP, Kortebein P, Arendt KW. Chronic lateral epicondylitis: comparative effectiveness of a home exercise program including stretching alone versus stretching supplemented with eccentric or concentric strengthening. *J Hand Ther.* 2005;18(4):411-419; quiz 420. doi:10.1197/j.jht.2005.07.007.
88. Nirschl RP, Ashman ES. Tennis elbow tendinosis (epicondylitis). *Instr Course Lect.* 2004;53:587-598.
89. Burnham R, Gregg R, Healy P, Steadward R. The effectiveness of topical diclofenac for lateral epicondylitis. *Clin J Sports Med.* 1998;8(2):78-81.
90. Burton AK. A comparative trial of forearm strap and topical anti-inflammatory as adjuncts to manipulative therapy in tennis elbow. *Man Med.* 1988;3(4):141-143.
91. Labelle H, Guibert R. Efficacy of diclofenac in lateral epicondylitis of the elbow also treated with immobilization. The University of Montreal Orthopaedic Research Group. *Arch Fam Med.* 1997;6(3):257-262.
92. Hay EM, Paterson SM, Lewis M, Hosie G, Croft P. Pragmatic randomized controlled trial of local corticosteroid injection and naproxen for treatment of lateral epicondylitis of elbow in primary care. *BMJ.* 1999;319(7215):964-968. doi:10.1136/bmj.319.7215.964.
93. Stull PA, Jokl P. Comparison of diflunisal and naproxen in the treatment of tennis elbow. *Clin Ther.* 1986;9(suppl C):62-66.
94. Garg R, Adamson GJ, Dawson PA, Shankwiler JA, Pink MM. A prospective randomized study comparing forearm strap brace versus a wrist splint for the treatment of lateral epicondylitis. *J Shoulder Elbow Surg.* 2010;19(4):508-512. doi:10.1016/j.jse.2009.12.015.
95. Smith AG, Kosygan K, Williams H, Newman RJ. Common extensor tendon rupture following corticosteroid injection for lateral tendinosis of the elbow. *Br J Sports Med.* 1999;33(6):423-425; discussion 424-425. doi:10.1136/bjsm.33.6.423.
96. Kalainov DM, Cohen MS. Posterolateral rotatory instability of the elbow in association with lateral epicondylitis. *J Bone Joint Surg Am.* 2005;87(5):1120-1125. doi:10.2106/JBJS.D.02293.
97. Price R, Sinclair H, Heinrich I, Gibson T. Local injection treatment of tennis elbow—hydrocortisone, triamcinolone and lignocaine compared. *Br J Rheumatol.* 1991;30(1):39-44. doi:10.1093/rheumatology/30.1.39.
98. Smidt N, van der Windt DA, Assendelft WJ, Devillé WL, Korthals-de Bos IB, Bouter LM. Corticosteroid injections, physiotherapy, or a wait-and see policy for lateral epicondylitis: a randomised controlled trial. *Lancet.* 2002;359(9307):657-662. doi:10.1016/S0140-6736(02)07811-X.
99. Cummins CA. Lateral epicondylitis: in vivo assessment of arthroscopic debridement and correlation with patient outcomes. *Am J Sports Med.* 2006;34(9):1486-1491. doi:10.1177/0363546506288016.
100. Sodha S, Nagda SH, Sennett BJ. Heterotopic ossification in a throwing athlete after elbow arthroscopy. *Arthroscopy.* 2006;22(7):802.e1-e3. doi:10.1016/j.arthro.2005.05.035.
101. Luchetti R, Atzei A, Brunelli F, FairplayT. Anconeus muscle transposition for chronic lateral epicondylitis, recurrences, and complications. *Tech Hand Up Extrem Surg.* 2005;9(2):105-112.
102. Rosenberg N, Henderson I. Surgical treatment of resistant lateral epicondylitis: Follow-up study of 19 patients after excision, release and repair of proximal common extensor tendon origin. *Arch Orthop Trauma Surg.* 2002;122(9-10):514-517. doi:10.1007/s00402-002-0421-8.
103. Haahr JP, Andersen JH. Prognostic factors in lateral epicondylitis: a randomized trial with one-year follow-up in 266 new cases treated with minimal occupational intervention or the usual approach in general practice. *Rheumatology (Oxford).* 2003;42(10):1216-1225. doi:10.1093/rheumatology/keg360.
104. Binder AI, Hazleman BL. Lateral humeral epicondylitis—a study of natural history and the effect of conservative therapy. *Br J Rheumatol.* 1983;22(2):73-76. doi:10.1093/rheumatology/22.2.73.
105. Boyd HB, McLeod AC Jr. Tennis elbow. *J Bone Joint Surg Am.* 1973;55(6):1183-1187.
106. Coonrad RW, Hooper WR. Tennis elbow: its course, natural history, conservative and surgical management. *J Bone Joint Surg Am.* 1973;55(6):1177-1182.

107. Dunn JH, Kim JJ, Davis L, Nirschl RP. Ten- to 14-year follow-up of the Nirschl surgical technique for lateral epicondylitis. *Am J Sports Med.* 2008;36(2):261-266. doi:10.1177/0363546507308932.
108. Verhaar J, Walenkamp G, Kester A, van Mameren H, van der Linden T. Lateral extensor release for tennis elbow. A prospective long-term follow-up study. *J Bone Joint Surg Am.* 1993;75:1034-1043. doi:10.2106/00004623-199307000-00010.
109. Owens BD, Murphy KP, Kuklo TR. Arthroscopic release for lateral epicondylitis. *Arthroscopy.* 2001;17(6):582-587. doi:10.1053/jars.2001.20098.
110. Mullett H, Sprague M, Brown G, Hausman M. Arthroscopic treatment of lateral epicondylitis: clinical and cadaveric studies. *Clin Orthop Relat Res.* 2005;439:123-128. doi:10.1097/01.blo.0000176143.08886.fe.
111. Baker CL Jr, Murphy KP, Gottlob CA, Curd DT. Arthroscopic classification and treatment of lateral epicondylitis: two-year clinical results. *J Shoulder Elbow Surg.* 2000;9(6):475-482. doi:10.1067/mse.2000.108533.
112. Koh JS, Mohan PC, Howe TS, et al. Fasciotomy and surgical tenotomy for recalcitrant lateral elbow tendinopathy: early clinical experience with a novel device for minimally invasive percutaneous microresection. *Am J Sports Med.* 2013;41(3):636-644. doi:10.1177/0363546512470625.
113. Ciccotti MG, Ramani MN. Medial epicondylitis. *Tech Hand Up Extrem Surg.* 2003;7(4):190-196.
114. Vangsness CT Jr, Jobe FW: Surgical treatment of medial epicondylitis. Results in 35 elbows. *J Bone Joint Surg Br.* 1991;73(3):409-411.
115. Shiri R, Viikari-Juntura E, Varonen H, Heliövaara M. Prevalence and determinants of lateral and medial epicondylitis: a population study. *Am J Epidemiol.* 2006;164(11):1065-1074. doi:10.1093/aje/kwj325.
116. Descatha A, Leclerc A, Chastang JF, Roquelaure Y; Study Group on Repetitive Work. Medial epicondylitis in occupational settings: prevalence, incidence and associated risk factors. *J Occup Environ Med.* 2003;45(9):993-1001. doi:10.1097/01.jom.0000085888.37273.d9.
117. Wolf JM, Mountcastle S, Burks R, Sturdivant RX, Owens BD. Epidemiology of lateral and medial epicondylitis in a military population. *Mil Med.* 2010;175(5):336-339. doi:10.7205/milmed-d-09-00086.
118. Pienimäki T, Siira P, Vanharanta H. Widespread pain in chronic epicondylitis. *Eur J Pain.* 2011;15(9):921-927. doi:10.1016/j.ejpain.2011.04.002.
119. Kijowski R, De Smet AA. Magnetic resonance imaging findings in patients with medial epicondylitis. *Skeletal Radiol.* 2005;34(4):196-202. doi:10.1007/s00256-005-0896-9.
120. Park GY, Lee SM, Lee MY. Diagnostic value of ultrasonography for clinical medial epicondylitis. *Arch Phys Med Rehabil.* 2008;89(4):738-742. doi:10.1016/j.apmr.2007.09.048.
121. Sems A, Dimeff R, Iannotti JP. Extracorporeal shock wave therapy in the treatment of chronic tendinopathies. *J Am Acad Orthop Surg.* 2006;14(4): 195-204.
122. Suresh SP, Ali KE, Jones H, Connell DA. Medial epicondylitis: is ultrasound guided autologous blood injection an effective treatment? *Br J Sports Med.* 2006;40(11):935-939; discussion 939. doi:10.1136/bjsm.2006.029983.
123. Gabel GT. Medial epicondylitis. In: Morrey B, Sanchez-Sotelo J, eds. *The Elbow and Its Disorders.* 4th ed. Philadelphia, PA: Saunders Elsevier; 2009:643-657.
124. Gabel GT, Morrey BF. Operative treatment of medical epicondylitis. Influence of concomitant ulnar neuropathy at the elbow. *J Bone Joint Surg Am.* 1995;77(7):1065-1069. doi:10.2106/00004623-199507000-00013.

3

Elbow Instability

Jason L. Codding, MD and Alexander W. Aleem, MD

- Functional anatomy
  - Bony anatomy
    - Comprises the ulnohumeral, radiocapitellar, and proximal radioulnar joints
    - With the elbow extended and axially loaded, 40% of joint stress crosses the ulnohumeral joint and 60% crosses the radiocapitellar joint.
    - The greatest force across the radiocapitellar joint is with the elbow in full extension, where the muscles have poor mechanical advantage.
    - As serial portions of the coronoid are removed, the elbow becomes progressively more unstable.[1]
  - Primary static stabilizers
    - Ulnohumeral joint
      - Highly constrained, with 180 degrees of articulation between the trochlea and the proximal ulna
      - Coronoid process acts as an anterior buttress and also serves as the attachment site for the medial collateral ligament (MCL). Therefore, it is important not only in resisting valgus forces, but also varus moments.
      - Up to 50% of the olecranon can be resected without affecting elbow stability.[2]
    - Collaterals (Figure 3-1)
      - Specialized thickening of the medial and lateral capsule[3,4] *Recommended reading for historical context*
      - Medial ulnar collateral ligaments
        - Anterior band (most important)
          - Originates from anterior portion of medial epicondyle[5]
          - Inserts on sublime tubercle of the coronoid base
          - Isometric through range of motion (ROM)

Namdari S, Zmistowski B, Omid R, eds.
The Foundations of Shoulder and Elbow Surgery (pp 39-55).

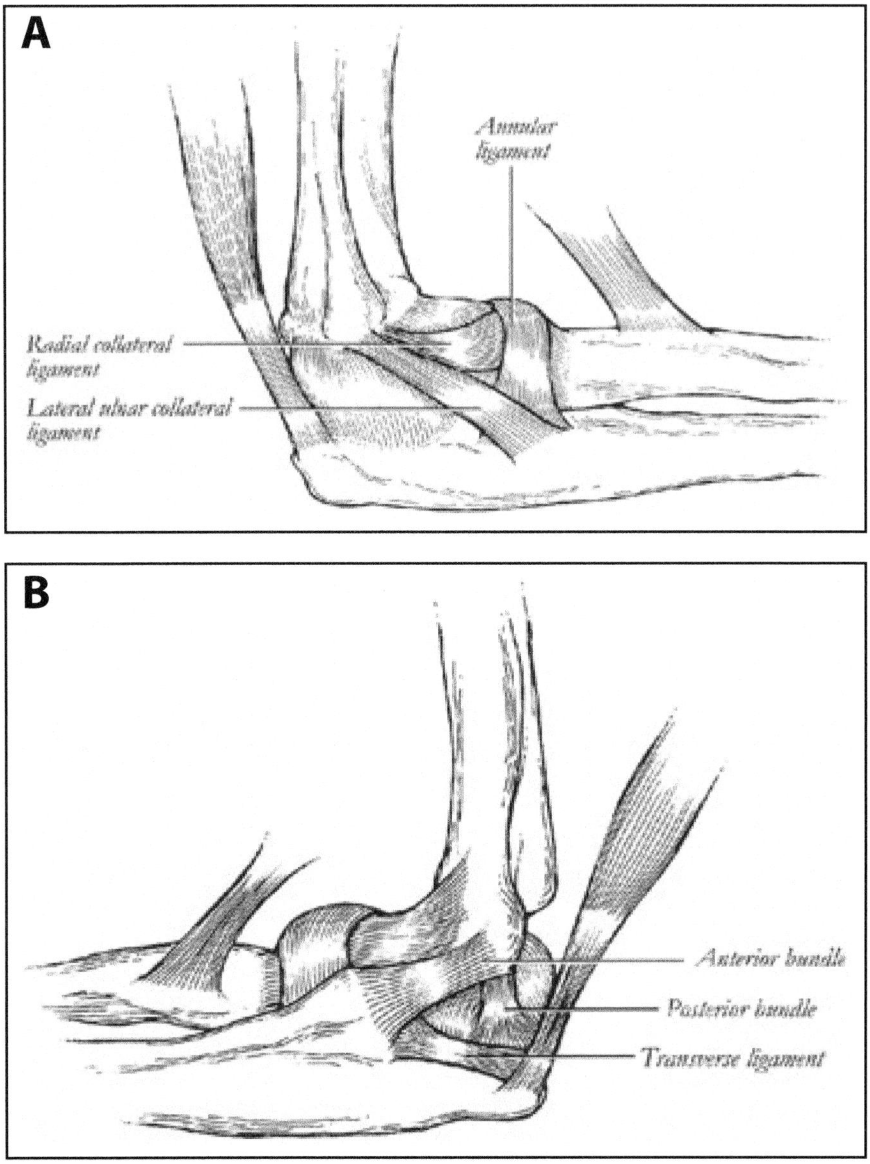

Figure 3-1. Key ligaments of the (A) lateral and (B) medial elbow. (Reprinted with permission from Armstrong AD, King GJW, Yamaguchi K. Total elbow arthroplasty design. In: Williams GR, Yamaguchi K, Ramsey ML, Galatz LM, eds. *Shoulder and Elbow Arthroplasty.* Philadelphia, PA: Lippincott Williams & Wilkins; 2005:303.)

      - › Anterior bundle: primary constraint to valgus forces and tight in extension
      - › Posterior bundle: tight in flexion
  - Posterior band and transverse ligament
    - Subtle thickenings of the capsule
- Lateral ulnar collateral ligament (LUCL) complex
  - Components function as one structure
  - Both radial collateral ligament and LUCL must be cut to produce instability.[6,7]

- Radial collateral ligament
  - Origin near axis of flexion
  - Uniformly taut throughout normal ROM
- LUCL
  - Primary lateral stabilizer
  - Prevents posterolateral subluxation of the radial head
  - Originates from lateral epicondyle just anterior to common extensor origin
  - Inserts on the crista supinatorum of the ulna
  - Blends with fibers of annular ligament distally
  - Not isometric: loose in extension and tight in flexion
  - There is no perfect isometric point but the most isometric point is the center of rotation, which is 2 mm proximal to center of capitellum.[8]
  - Injury most commonly occurs at its origin at the lateral epicondyle (bare spot).
- Annular ligament
  - Originates and inserts on the anterior and posterior margins of the lesser sigmoid notch
  - Maintains the radial head in contact with the ulna
  - Anterior portion taut in supination
  - Posterior portion taut in extremes of pronation
- Accessory lateral collateral ligament (LCL)
  - Proximally, the fibers bend with the inferior margin of the annular ligament.
  - Helps stabilize annular ligament during varus stress

- Secondary static stabilizers
  - Radiocapitellar joint (radial head)
    - Secondary stabilizer of the MCL to valgus stress. Also acts as an anterior buttress to posterolateral rotatory subluxation.
    - With an incompetent MCL or coronoid injury, the radial head will act as a primary stabilizer to valgus stress.
    - As little as 25% of radial head resection causes subluxation at 70 degrees of flexion.
    - At least 50% of the coronoid is necessary for stability if the radial head is removed.
  - Capsule
    - Volume of elbow joint space is 35 to 40 mL.[9]
    - Greatest stabilizing effect when elbow extended
      - Oblique and transverse bands of anterior capsule taut in extension and lax in flexion
  - Flexor and extensor tendons[10]
- Dynamic stabilizers
  - Biceps, brachialis, and triceps stabilize the trochlea in the semilunar notch.
  - The flexor and extensor masses dynamically stabilize the medial and lateral sides of the joint, respectively.
  - Anconeus is active with resisted pronation and supination as well as varus and valgus motion.

        - Major dynamic restraint to varus and posterolateral rotatory instability (PLRI)
        - Flexor carpi ulnaris is a primary dynamic contributor to valgus stability, and flexor digitorum superficialis is a secondary stabilizer.[11]
        - The intermuscular septum between the extensor digitorum communis and extensor digiti quinti adds an additional unyielding restraint to subluxation of the lateral aspect of the elbow. This septum tightens when the forearm is in supination.
        - Of all of the extensors, the stout fascial band of the extensor carpi ulnaris has the best mechanical advantage in resisting rotatory instability because of its course. It originates on the most inferior aspect of the lateral epicondyle and inserts onto the ulna approximately 5 cm distal to the center of the radial head.[12-14]
    - Biomechanical considerations
        - Normal elbow ROM is 0 degrees to 150 degrees. Forearm rotation averages 75 degrees to 80 degrees of pronation and 80 degrees to 85 degrees of supination.
        - In elbow flexion and extension, the center of rotation is in line with the anterior cortex of the distal humerus.
        - Valgus forces are resisted by the anterior band of the MCL (70%) and the radiocapitellar joint.
        - In extension, the anterior capsule provides 70% of the soft-tissue restraint to joint distraction.
        - At 90 degrees of flexion, the MCL provides the soft-tissue restraint to joint distraction.
        - Varus forces are resisted by the LCL and ulnohumeral joint when the coronoid is intact.
        - Forearm pronation tightens the anconeus and lateral structures.[15]
            - If the LCL complex is disrupted but the MCL is intact, the elbow may be more stable in pronation.[13]
            - LCL-deficient elbows should be rehabilitated by performing flexion and extension exercise with the forearm pronated in the supine position with the arm overhead.
        - Forearm supination tightens the medial structures.[15]
            - If the MCL is disrupted but the LCL is intact, the elbow may be more stable in supination.[16]
        - An incompetent LUCL is associated with subluxation and recurrent dislocation, whereas an attenuated MCL is associated with valgus instability but not recurrent dislocation.
- Soft-tissue instability
    - Valgus elbow instability
        - Typically seen in overhead athletes
        - Can also be the result of trauma (simple elbow dislocation or associated with a radial head fracture)
        - During the acceleration phase of throwing, the elbow reaches a high angular velocity, placing significant tensile stress on the MCL.
        - The elbow displays increased varus/valgus laxity with forearm pronation, particularly in patients with a deficient MCL. This may be a risk factor that puts pitchers at risk for MCL injury.
        - Valgus extension overload syndrome
            - Tensile stress along the medial side and shear stress in the posterior compartment (posteromedial tip of the olecranon and olecranon fossa) with compression of the lateral side of the radiocapitellar joint
            - Osteophyte formation on the medial aspect of the olecranon tip and olecranon fossa

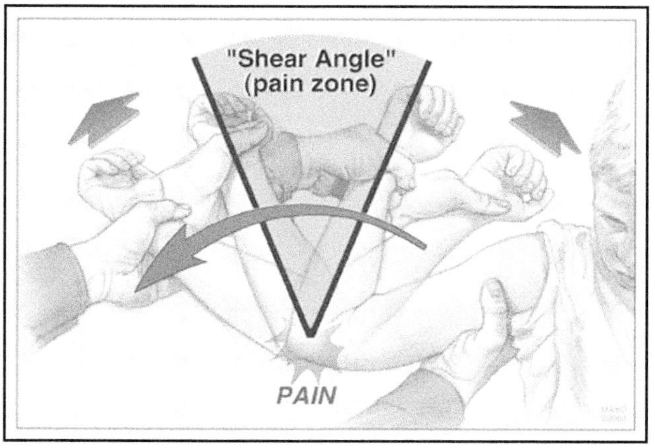

Figure 3-2. Moving valgus stress test. (Reprinted with permission from O'Driscoll SWM, Lawton RL, Smith AM. The "moving valgus stress test" for medial collateral ligament tears of the elbow. *Am J Sports Med.* 2005;33[2]:231-239. doi:10.1177/0363546504267804.)

  - In professional baseball players who underwent olecranon debridement for valgus extension overload syndrome, 25% developed valgus instability and eventually required MCL reconstruction.[17]
  - Sequential partial resection of the posteromedial aspect of the olecranon causes increased elbow valgus angulation. Aggressive olecranon resection to treat posteromedial impingement places the MCL at risk of injury.[18,19]
  - Subtle valgus instability may lead to symptomatic posteromedial impingement. Patients with posteromedial impingement pain should be evaluated for MCL injuries.[20]
- Athletes may describe a "popping" sound. Pain during late-cocking and early acceleration.
- Physical examination
  - Point tenderness over sublime tubercle or medial epicondyle
  - Tested by flexing the elbow between 20 and 30 degrees to unlock the olecranon from the fossa while applying valgus stress
  - Milking maneuver: examiner pulls on the thumb to create a valgus stress while the forearm is supinated and the elbow flexed beyond 90 degrees
  - Moving valgus stress test (Figure 3-2): Valgus stress is applied to the elbow until the shoulder reaches its limit of external rotation. The elbow is then flexed and extended with the torque held constant, and is positive if there is pain over the MCL and is most intense between 70 to 120 degrees.[21]
    - Most sensitive and specific test for diagnosing a partial tear
- Imaging
  - Valgus stress x-rays may show gapping medially.[22]
  - Magnetic resonance imaging (MRI) arthrogram is more sensitive than MRI for evaluation of an isolated MCL tear.
  - Ultrasound allows for dynamic evaluation.[23]
- When symptomatic and unstable, may be treated with MCL reconstruction

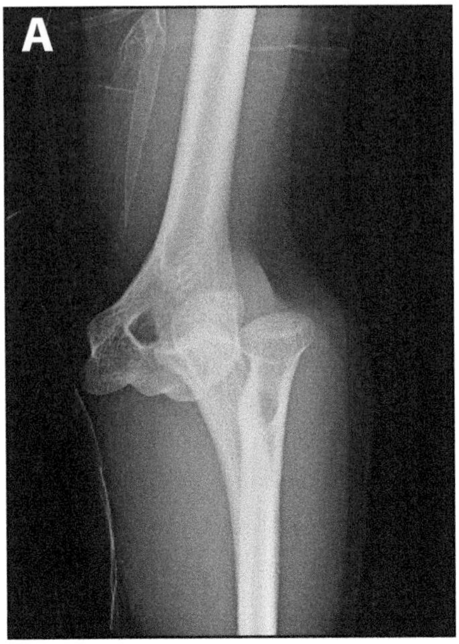

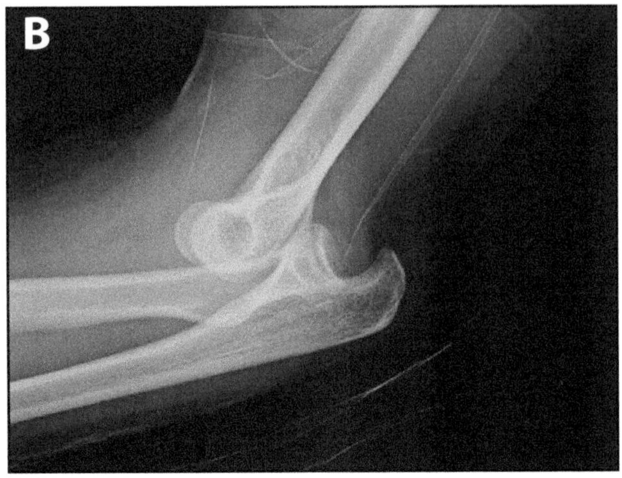

Figure 3-3. (A) Anteroposterior and (B) lateral radiographs of a simple elbow dislocation.

- Long-term follow-up studies after a simple elbow dislocation found that 15% to 35% of patients had chronic valgus instability, and 50% of these patients had elbow arthrosis.[24-26]

- Elbow dislocations
  - 90% are posterior or posterolateral
    - Anterior dislocations are rare in adult patients and are usually part of an olecranon fracture-dislocation.
  - Simple elbow dislocations
    - Dislocations without significant associated fractures (Figures 3-3)
    - During a simple dislocation event, an axial force travels through the elbow as it flexes, the humerus internally rotates around the elbow, resulting in a valgus moment because the mechanical axis passes through the lateral elbow.
    - Stages of simple elbow dislocation: "Horii circle" (Figure 3-4)
      - Disruption occurs from lateral to medial.
      - Stage 1: LUCL disruption
      - Stage 2: soft-tissue tearing anteriorly and posteriorly, resulting in subluxation and perching of the trochlea on the coronoid
      - Stage 3A: all soft tissues torn including the posterior band of the MCL but the anterior band of the MCL is intact
      - Stage 3B: anterior band of the MCL is torn and complete elbow dislocation occurs
    - Both the MCL and LCL were found to be disrupted in acutely dislocated elbows explored surgically,[10] *Recommended reading for historical context* with the LCL typically avulsing off the humeral origin.[27]
    - Treatment
      - Closed reduction is performed, and treatment is then dictated by the stability of the joint.

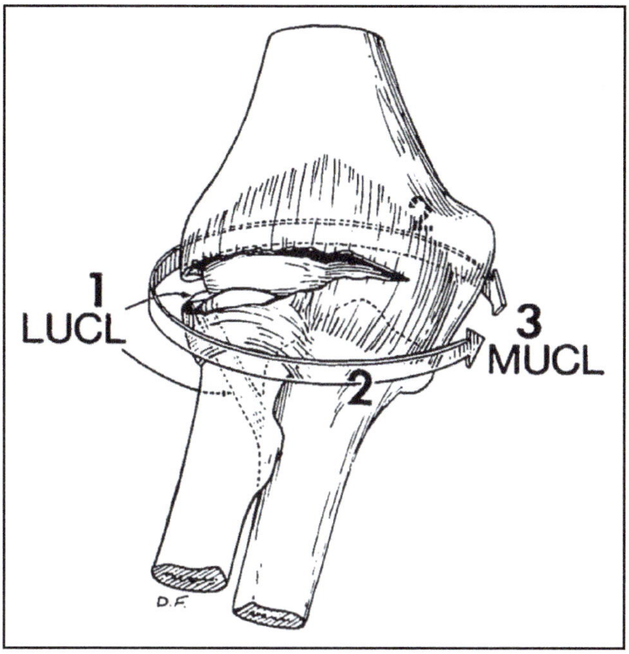

Figure 3-4. Stages of simple elbow dislocation (Horii circle). Abbreviation: MUCL, medial ulnar collateral ligament. (Reprinted with permission from O'Driscoll SW, Morrey BF, Korinek S, An KN. Elbow subluxation and dislocation. A spectrum of instability. *Clin Orthop Relat Res.* 1992;[280]:186-197.)

        - Widening of the ulnohumeral joint may indicate the presence of an entrapped osteochondral fragment or entrapped soft tissue, both of which require surgical intervention.
        - Static widening of the ulnohumeral joint measured from the trochlear sulcus to the olecranon greater than or equal to 4 mm on the lateral radiograph is known as the "drop sign," which may be suggestive of elbow instability, especially if it persists at follow-up.[28]
        - Dynamic stress views with the forearm in pronation, neutral, and supination should be obtained under fluoroscopy to determine stability.
        - If the elbow is stable and concentric after reduction, treatment consists of sling and early ROM.
        - If the elbow is unstable but concentric, immobilize at 90 degrees of flexion for 5 to 7 days then transition to a hinged ROM brace with appropriate extension block for 3 to 4 weeks.
        - Active ROM allows for compressive stability due to muscle contraction, whereas passive ROM can accentuate instability.
        - Repeat radiographs should be obtained weekly for 3 to 4 weeks in cases that are unstable but concentric.
        - Recurrent dislocations can be successfully treated by reconstructions of the LCL complex alone, without reconstruction of the MCL, suggesting that the LCL injury is the essential lesion.[10]
- Complex elbow dislocations (see following)
    - Dislocations associated with fractures of the radial head and/or coronoid (Figure 3-5)
- PLRI
    - Most common pattern of elbow instability
    - Due to LUCL and MCL disruption[29] *Recommended reading for historical context*

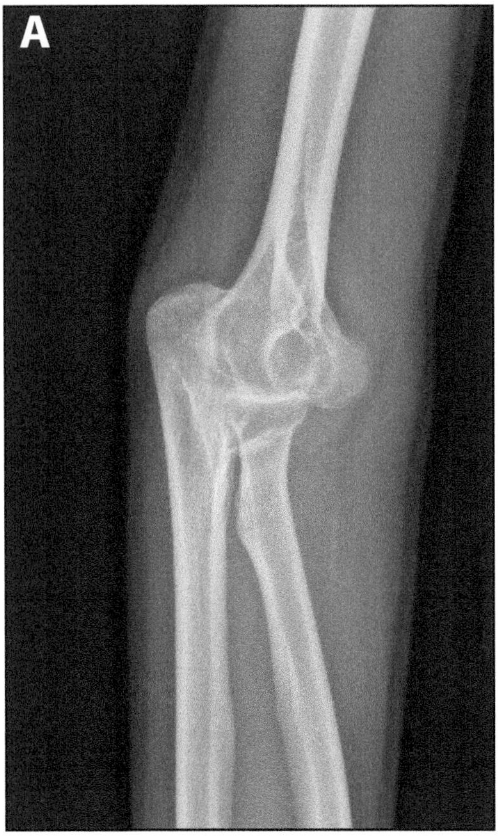

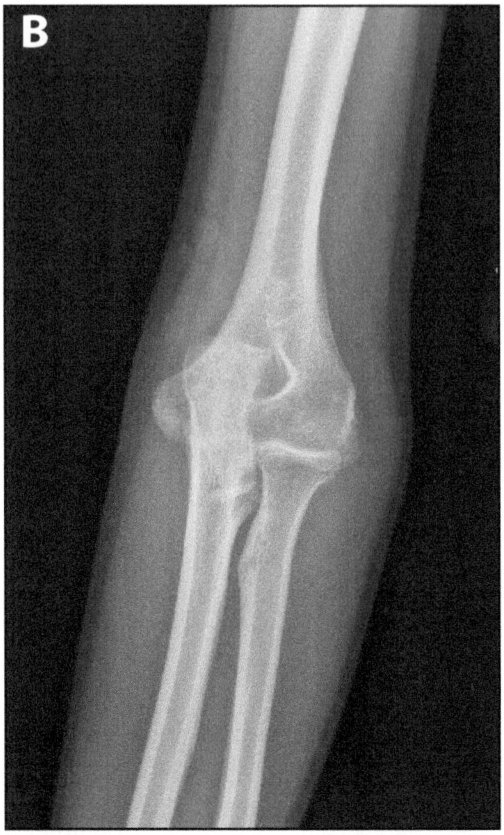

Figure 3-5. (A) Lateral, (B) anteroposterior, and (C) oblique radiographs of a complex elbow dislocation. Note the posterior dislocation of the ulna and radius, as well as the presence of a coronoid fracture.

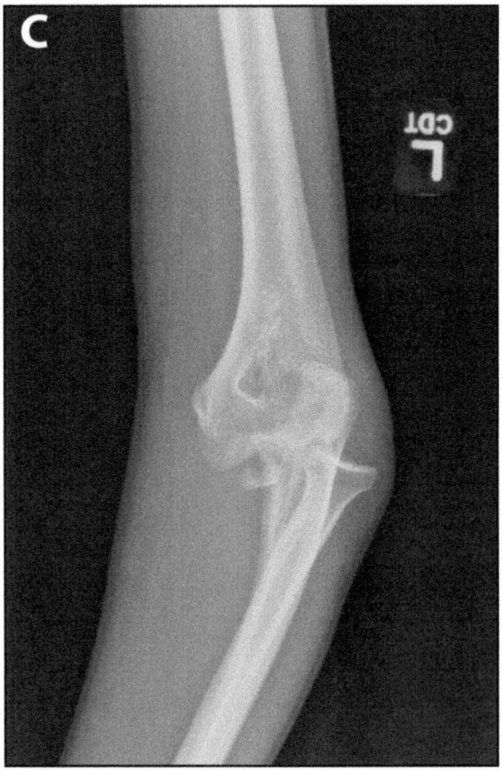

- Results from trauma (fall or elbow dislocation), iatrogenic injuries (aggressive lateral epicondyle release or steroid injections) or long-standing cubitus varus from supracondylar humerus malunion
- Laxity of the LUCL complex allows posterior subluxation of the radial head around the capitellum with the forearm supinated and elbow extended.
- Patients describe painful catching, clicking, or locking during extension or weight-bearing.
- Physical examination
  - Lateral pivot shift test: With the patient supine with the extremity positioned overhead, the forearm is held and supinated with valgus stress with a slight compressive force applied as the elbow is brought from flexed to extended position, causing the radial head to subluxate posterolaterally at about 30 degrees. This typically results in apprehension by the patient.
  - Posterolateral rotatory drawer test: The arm is held in a similar overhead position. The lateral side of the forearm is rotated away from the humerus, pivoting around the MCL behind the radial head.
  - Chair/push-up test: Symptoms reproduced when the patient attempts to stand from a seated position with shoulders abducted and pushes up with the forearms in full supination.
- Imaging
  - Anteroposterior and lateral elbow radiographs may demonstrate a drop sign with widening of the ulnohumeral joint.[30]
  - Though the utility of MRI is controversial, significant disruption of the LUCL from the humeral attachment may be obvious (Figure 3-6).
  - Dynamic fluoroscopy or ultrasonography performed with a posterolateral rotatory force applied may be useful adjuncts if the diagnosis of PLRI is unclear from exam or static imaging.[31]
- Reconstruction is the preferred treatment for symptomatic PLRI.
  - The ligament and posterolateral capsule is imbricated along with reconstruction of the ulnar part of the LCL.
  - The isometric point is at the center of the capitellum, which is distal to the lateral epicondyle.
  - To keep the graft tensioned with the elbow extended, the burr hole should be drilled slightly posterior and proximal to the isometric point.
  - Results are more predictable in those whose primary symptom was instability rather than pain, and whose injury was due to trauma rather than iatrogenic.[32]
- Forearm immobilized in pronation after LUCL reconstruction

- Fracture-associated instability
  - Coronoid fractures
    - Presence of a coronoid tip fracture is pathognomonic for elbow subluxation or dislocation; it is a shear fracture
    - Fractures involving greater than 50% of the coronoid tend to displace posteriorly even if the collateral ligaments are intact.
    - Classification
      - Regan-Morrey
        - Type 1: shear fracture of the tip
        - Type 2: fracture involving less than 50%

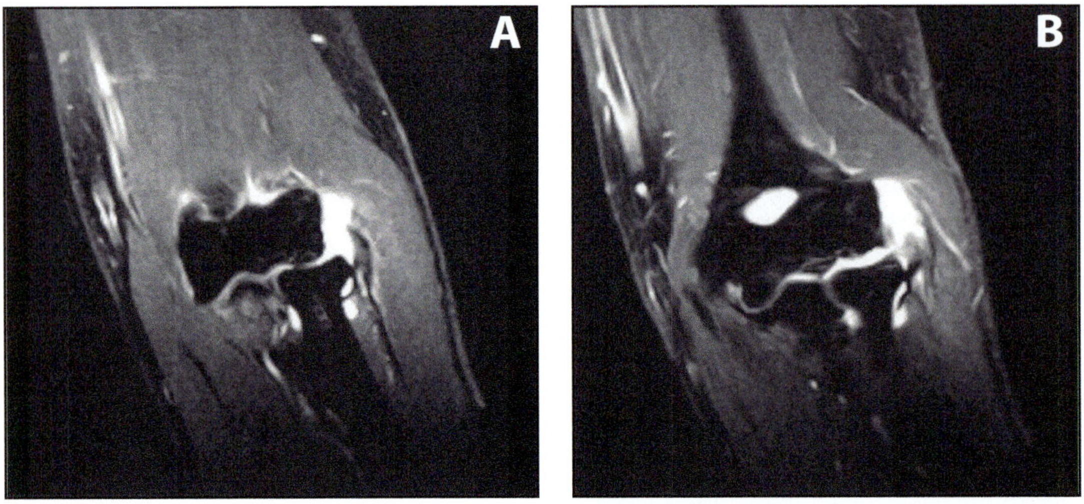

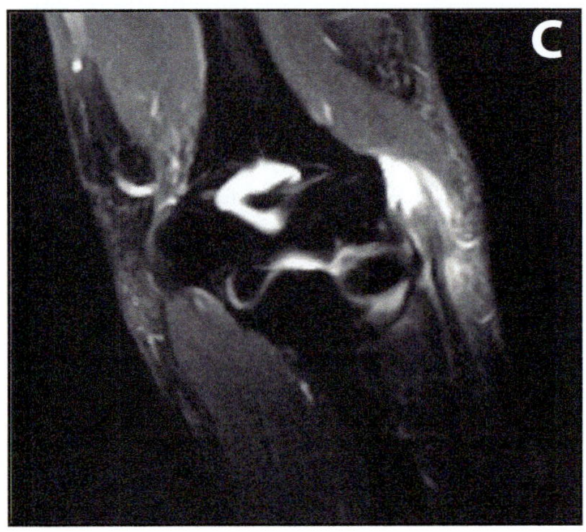

Figure 3-6. (A through C) T2-weighted elbow coronal magnetic resonance images demonstrating complete disruption of the LUCL from its humeral attachment. This "bare spot" is demonstrated in a patient with PLRI.

    - Type 3: fracture involving greater than 50% (thus involving the anterior band of the MCL; Figure 3-7)
  - O'Driscoll classification[33] *Recommended reading for understanding classification*
    - Type 1: tip fracture
      - Fracture line does not extend medially past the sublime tubercle or into the body.
      - Result of an elbow subluxation or dislocation via a posterolateral rotatory displacement of the ulna under the trochlea.
      - Mechanism involves outstretched hand with valgus and supination moments applied to the ulna as it flexes on the humerus during axial loading.
      - The LCL is disrupted in virtually all instances, although the MCL can remain at least partially intact.
      - Be cautious to accurately test elbow stability when associated with a radial head fracture.
      - Need for fixation of type 1 fractures in the setting of a radial head fracture is controversial.

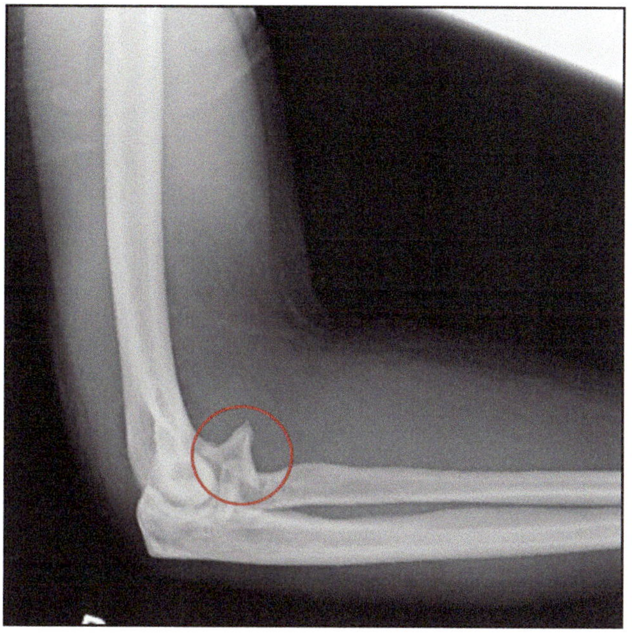

Figure 3-7. Lateral elbow radiograph of a Regan-Morrey type 3 coronoid fracture, involving greater than 50% of the coronoid.

- Can be fixed from the lateral approach, working past a radial head fracture. Arthroscopic-assisted fixation using an anterior cruciate ligament guide and retrograde screws has also been described.[34]

- Type 2: anteromedial fragment
  - Fracture line exits the medial cortex in the anterior half of the sublime tubercle in the anterior portion of the anterior bundle of the MCL
  - Extends laterally just medial to the tip of the coronoid
    - Subtype 1 is an anteromedial rim coronoid fracture without tip or sublime tubercle involvement.
    - Subtype 2 involves the tip of the coronoid.
    - Subtype 3 involves the sublime tubercle.
  - Mechanism of injury is varus/posteromedial rotation with axial loading. Coronoid is fractured via a shearing mechanism.
  - Collateral ligaments are disrupted and the radial head can be fractured
  - The medial trochlea articulates with the small coronoid fragment, but not the majority of the ulna, which leads to point loading and high stress at the medial trochlea articular surface.
  - Can lead to posteromedial rotatory instability of the elbow
- Type 3: base
  - Involving the coronoid body with greater than 50% of height
  - Usually comminuted
  - May result in a single fragment if part of an olecranon fracture-dislocation
  - Extent of soft-tissue disruption is often less than that with tip fractures

- Posteromedial rotatory instability
  - Characterized as either an anteromedial coronoid fracture or a comminuted coronoid fracture with disruption of the LCL complex without a radial head fracture (Figure 3-8)

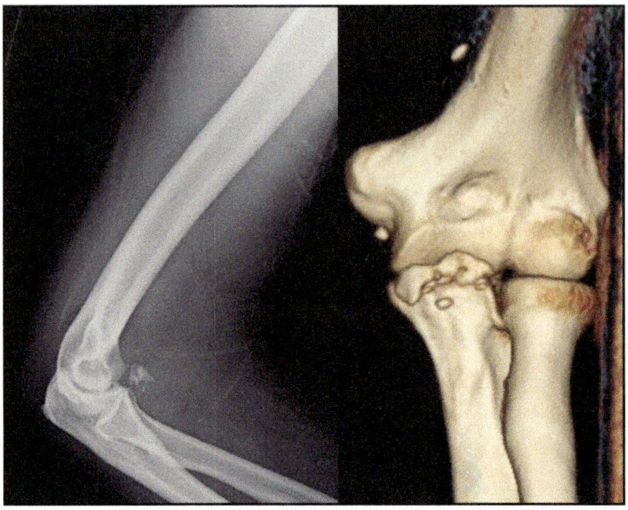

Figure 3-8. Lateral elbow radiograph and coronal elbow 3-dimensional reconstruction demonstrating a comminuted coronoid fracture without a concomitant radial head fracture in the setting of posteromedial rotatory instability.

- There is an obligatory fracture or deficiency of the anteromedial coronoid and the posterior bundle of the MCL is disrupted
- Occurs under flexion and abduction torque at the shoulder while the elbow is flexed under axial load, causing the elbow to go into varus
- Subtle findings on radiographs
    - On an anteroposterior radiograph the ulnohumeral joint appears asymmetric and the radiohumeral joint may be widened.
    - On a lateral radiograph the depressed medial coronoid fragment causes a double-subchondral density termed the "double-crescent sign" and is pathognomonic for an anteromedial coronoid facet fracture.[35]
    - Computed tomography imaging will show incongruity of the joint.
- Be wary of the "isolated" coronoid fracture because this may represent an unstable elbow with concomitant LCL injury.
- The ulnar nerve is prone to compression because of swelling due to the torn posterior band of the MCL.
- Failure to treat these operatively leads to rapid onset of post-traumatic arthritis due to chronic instability.[36] *Recommended reading for importance in change of practice*
- Internal fixation should be considered for anteromedial subtype 2 fractures greater than 2.5 mm, depending on whether the soft-tissue restraints remain intact.[37]
- Anteromedial subtype 1 fractures can be treated with LCL repair alone, and subtypes 2 and 3 should be addressed with a buttress plate.[38]

- Radial head fractures
    - Displaced fractures are frequently associated with ligamentous injury, including the interosseous membrane (Essex-Lopresti lesion).[39,40]
    - The anterior one-third of the radial head is most often fractured by the radial head subluxating posteriorly, rather than inherent weakness in this area as once previously thought.
    - With coronoid or MCL deficiency the radial head is crucial for stability, therefore the radial head should be fixed or replaced whenever possible because this is a secondary stabilizer to valgus stress.[41]

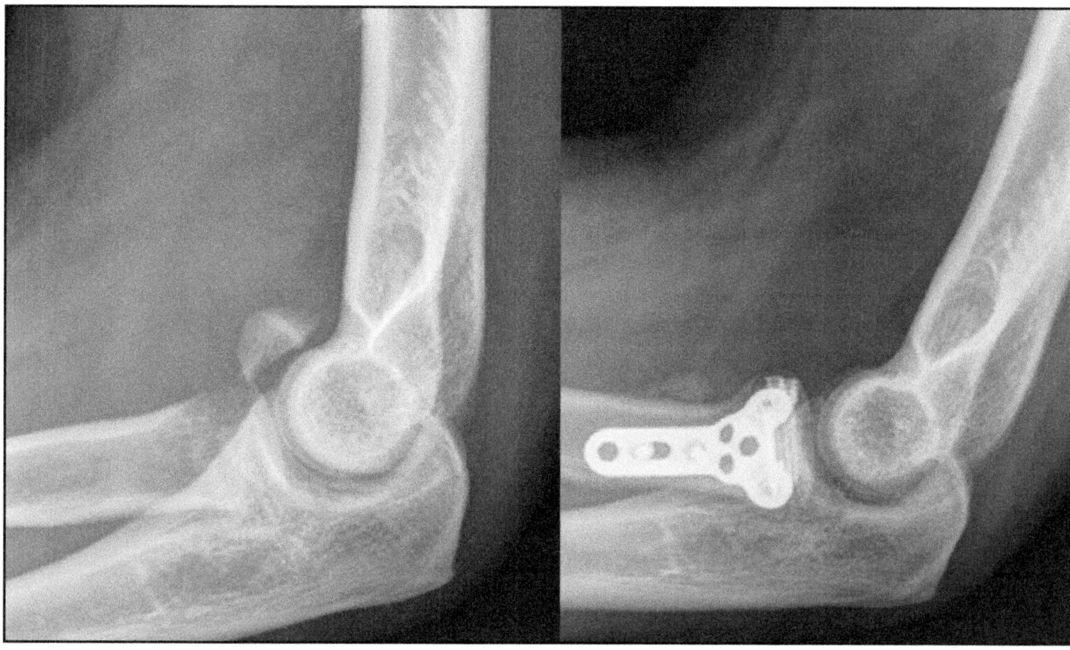

Figure 3-9. Preoperative and postoperative lateral elbow radiograph demonstrating a Mason type 2 radial head fracture treated with open reduction internal fixation.

- With a radial head fracture associated with a dislocation, the LCL is typically avulsed from its origin and needs to be addressed surgically. The MCL is sometimes disrupted, but rarely needs to be addressed because it uncommonly causes persistent instability.[42]
- Classification
  - Mason
    - Type 1: nondisplaced (or less than 2 mm displaced); fat pad may be the only sign of fracture
    - Type 2: displaced (greater than 2 mm) with involvement of more than 30% that is reconstructible with open reduction internal fixation, and is more than just a marginal lip fracture (Figure 3-9)
    - Type 3: comminuted fracture that is unreconstructible and requires either excision or replacement
    - Type 4: type 3 fracture with elbow dislocation
  - Morrey modified the Mason classification by including fractures of the radial neck
- Treatment
  - Minimally displaced fractures with no mechanical block to motion or associated ligamentous injury can be treated nonoperatively with early ROM.
  - Open reduction internal fixation of a complex radial head fracture involving more than 3 articular fragments may lead to early failure.[43]
  - If associated with a ligamentous injury or unstable coronoid fractures, the radial head must be fixed or replaced to restore stability.

- Terrible triad
  - Elbow dislocation with radial head and coronoid fractures, as well as LCL disruption (Figure 3-10)

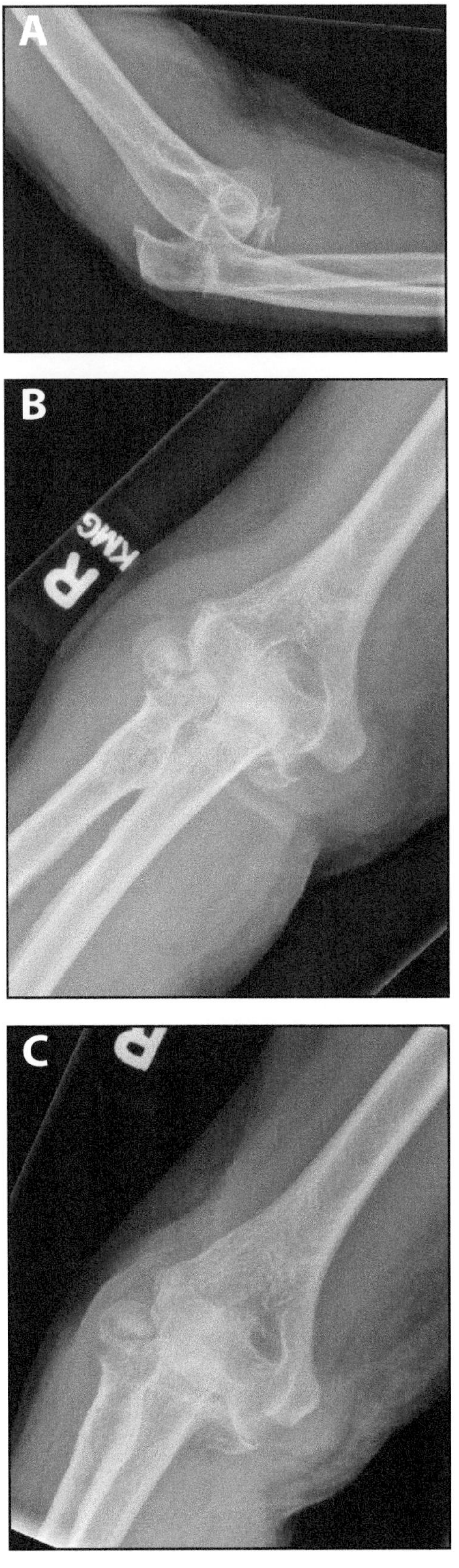

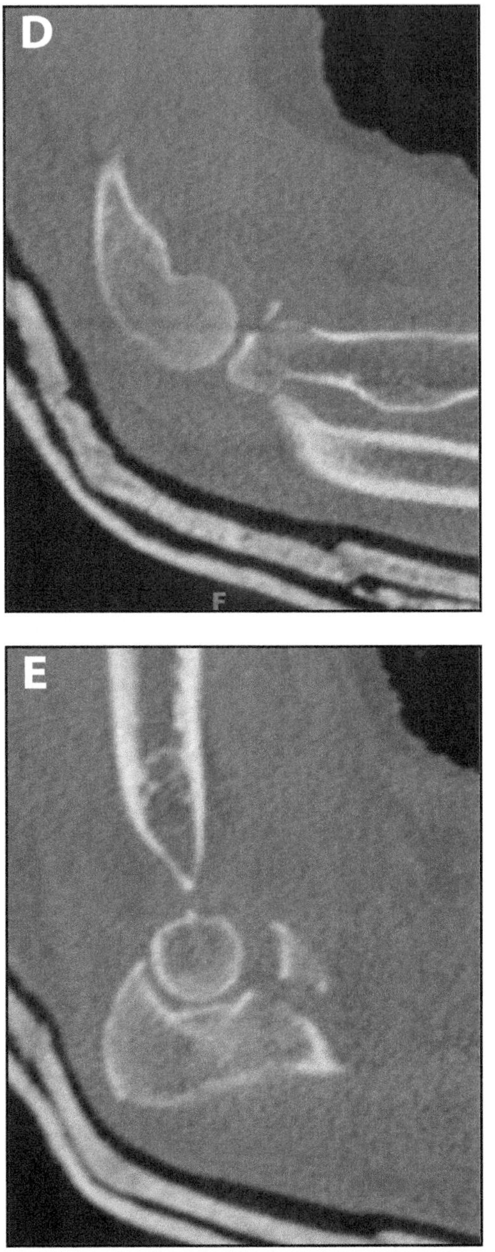

Figure 3-10. (A) Lateral, (B) anteroposterior, and (C) oblique radiographs demonstrate a terrible triad fracture-dislocation, with posterior dislocation of the radius and ulna, and displaced fractures of the radial head and coronoid process. Sagittal computed tomography scan images reveal the (D) radial head and (E) coronoid process fractures in more detail.

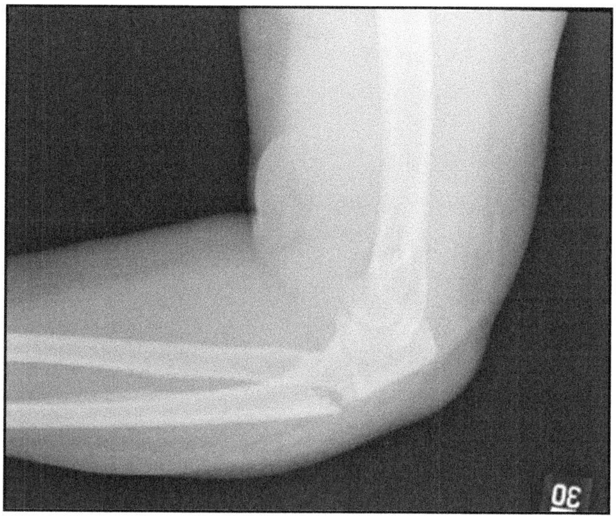

Figure 3-11. Lateral elbow radiograph demonstrating a Monteggia fracture-dislocation. Note the radial head dislocation, proximal ulna fracture, and disruption of the proximal radioulnar joint.

        - The MCL is also usually disrupted, although the anterior bundle of the MCL may remain intact.
        - Elbow stability is dependent on the size and location of the coronoid fragment, the amount of radial head comminution, and the extend of ligamentous injury.[44]
        - The radial head is an important constraint to valgus forces.
            - Radial head excision in an LCL-deficient elbow worsens instability, therefore the radial head should be fixed or replaced in addition to reconstruction of the LCL.[41]
        - The anterior capsule is usually still attached to the coronoid piece and must be considered, even if the coronoid piece is small.
        - The standard surgical approach includes fixation of the coronoid fracture and anterior capsule, addressing the radial head fracture, and then LCL complex repair. If the elbow remains unstable, the MCL is repaired or reconstructed. If still unstable, an external fixator is placed.[45,46]
        - Nonoperative treatment can be considered in patients with a concentric joint, a radial head fracture that does not cause a mechanical block, a small coronoid fracture, and a stable arc of motion to a minimum of 30 degrees of extension.[47]
    - Olecranon fracture-dislocations
        - Complex fracture of the proximal ulna, dislocation and/or fracture of the radial head, and fracture of the coronoid
        - Proximal radioulnar joint relationship remains intact, thus distinguishing it from a Monteggia fracture-dislocation
        - Elbow stability is typically restored after reduction and fixation of the proximal ulna.
    - Monteggia fracture-dislocation (Figure 3-11)
        - Characterized by radial head dislocation, proximal ulna fracture, and disruption of the proximal radioulnar joint[48]
            - Radial head is fractured in two-thirds of injuries
            - LCL may be injured but MCL is typically spared
    - Delayed treatment of elbow instability
        - Assess nerve function. The ulnar nerve must be identified at the beginning of the dissection.
        - The thickened capsule must be excised both anteriorly and posteriorly.

- Identify and preserve the remnants of the LCL complex.
- Clean and reduce the fracture fragments and, if needed, replace the radial head.
- An osteotomy of the ulna may be needed if unable to achieve ulnohumeral reduction easily
- Use fluoroscopic imaging to determine stability and the need for an external fixator.
- If the elbow is unstable at the end of fixation and reconstruction of the ligaments, place an external fixator (static or dynamic)

References

1. Fern SE, Owen JR, Ordyna NJ, Wayne JS, Boardman ND. Complex varus elbow instability: a terrible triad model. *J Shoulder Elbow Surg.* 2009;18(2):269-274. doi:10.1016/j.jse.2008.10.022.
2. An KN, Morrey BF, Chao EY. The effect of partial removal of proximal ulna on elbow constraint. *Clin Orthop.* 1986;(209):270-279. doi:10.1097/00003086-198608000-00041.
3. Regan WD, Korinek SL, Morrey BF, An KN. Biomechanical study of ligaments around the elbow joint. *Clin Orthop.* 1991;(271):170-179.
4. Morrey BF, Tanaka S, An KN. Valgus stability of the elbow. A definition of primary and secondary constraints. *Clin Orthop.* 1991;(265):187-195.
5. O'Driscoll SW, Jaloszynski R, Morrey BF, An KN. Origin of the medial ulnar collateral ligament. *J Hand Surg.* 1992;17(1):164-168. doi:10.1016/0363-5023(92)90135-C.
6. Dunning CE, Zarzour ZD, Patterson SD, Johnson JA, King GJ. Ligamentous stabilizers against posterolateral rotatory instability of the elbow. *J Bone Joint Surg Am.* 2001;83-A(12):1823-1828. doi:10.2106/00004623-200112000-00009.
7. McAdams TR, Masters GW, Srivastava S. The effect of arthroscopic sectioning of the lateral ligament complex of the elbow on posterolateral rotatory stability. *J Shoulder Elbow Surg.* 2005;14(3):298-301. doi:10.1016/j.jse.2004.08.003.
8. Moritomo H, Murase T, Arimitsu S, Oka K, Yoshikawa H, Sugamoto K. The in vivo isometric point of the lateral ligament of the elbow. *J Bone Joint Surg Am.* 2007;89(9):2011-2017. doi:10.2106/JBJS.F.00868.
9. Van Den Broek M, Van Riet R. Intra-articular capacity of the elbow joint. *Clin Anat.* 2017;30(6):795-798. doi:10.1002/ca.22915.
10. Josefsson PO, Gentz CF, Johnell O, Wendeberg B. Surgical versus non-surgical treatment of ligamentous injuries following dislocation of the elbow joint. A prospective randomized study. *J Bone Joint Surg Am.* 1987;69(4):605-608. doi:10.2106/00004623-198769040-00018.
11. Park MC, Ahmad CS. Dynamic contributions of the flexor-pronator mass to elbow valgus stability. *J Bone Joint Surg Am.* 2004;86-A(10):2268-2274. doi:10.2106/00004623-200410000-00020.
12. Ring D, Jupiter JB. Fracture-dislocation of the elbow. *J Bone Joint Surg Am.* 1998;80(4):566-580.
13. Dunning CE, Zarzour ZD, Patterson SD, Johnson JA, King GJ. Muscle forces and pronation stabilize the lateral ligament deficient elbow. *Clin Orthop Relat Res.* 2001;(388):118-124. doi:10.1097/00003086-200107000-00018.
14. Funk DA, An KN, Morrey BF, Daube JR. Electromyographic analysis of muscles across the elbow joint. *J Orthop Res.* 1987;5(4):529-538. doi:10.1002/jor.1100050408.
15. Seiber K, Gupta R, McGarry MH, Safran MR, Lee TQ. The role of the elbow musculature, forearm rotation, and elbow flexion in elbow stability: an in vitro study. *J Shoulder Elbow Surg.* 2009;18(2):260-268. doi:10.1016/j.jse.2008.08.004.
16. Armstrong AD, Dunning CE, Faber KJ, Duck TR, Johnson JA, King GJ. Rehabilitation of the medial collateral ligament-deficient elbow: an in vitro biomechanical study. *J Hand Surg.* 2000;25(6):1051-1057. doi:10.1053/jhsu.2000.17819.
17. Andrews JR, Timmerman LA. Outcome of elbow surgery in professional baseball players. *Am J Sports Med.* 1995;23(4):407-413. doi:10.1177/036354659502300406.
18. Kamineni S, Hirahara H, Pomianowski S, et al. Partial posteromedial olecranon resection: a kinematic study. *J Bone Joint Surg Am.* 2003;85-A(6):1005-1011. doi:10.2106/00004623-200306000-00004.
19. Kamineni S, ElAttrache NS, O'Driscoll SW, et al. Medial collateral ligament strain with partial posteromedial olecranon resection. A biomechanical study. *J Bone Joint Surg Am.* 2004;86-A(11):2424-2430. doi:10.2106/00004623-200411000-00010.
20. Ahmad CS, Park MC, Elattrache NS. Elbow medial ulnar collateral ligament insufficiency alters posteromedial olecranon contact. *Am J Sports Med.* 2004;32(7):1607-1612. doi:10.1177/0363546503263149.
21. O'Driscoll SWM, Lawton RL, Smith AM. The "moving valgus stress test" for medial collateral ligament tears of the elbow. *Am J Sports Med.* 2005;33(2):231-239. doi:10.1177/0363546504267804.

22. Hariri S, Safran MR. Ulnar collateral ligament injury in the overhead athlete. *Clin Sports Med.* 2010;29(4):619-644. doi:10.1016/j.csm.2010.06.007.
23. Tagliafico AS, Bignotti B, Martinoli C. Elbow US: anatomy, variants, and scanning technique. *Radiology.* 2015;275(3):636-650. doi:10.1148/radiol.2015141950.
24. Eygendaal D, Verdegaal SH, Obermann WR, van Vugt AB, Pöll RG, Rozing PM. Posterolateral dislocation of the elbow joint. Relationship to medial instability. *J Bone Joint Surg Am.* 2000;82(4):555-560.
25. Josefsson PO, Johnell O, Gentz CF. Long-term sequelae of simple dislocation of the elbow. *J Bone Joint Surg Am.* 1984;66(6):927-930. doi:10.2106/00004623-198466060-00014.
26. Mehlhoff TL, Noble PC, Bennett JB, Tullos HS. Simple dislocation of the elbow in the adult. Results after closed treatment. *J Bone Joint Surg Am.* 1988;70(2):244-249. doi:10.1016/S0196-0644(88)80585-7.
27. McKee MD, Schemitsch EH, Sala MJ, O'Driscoll SW. The pathoanatomy of lateral ligamentous disruption in complex elbow instability. *J Shoulder Elbow Surg.* 2003;12(4):391-396. doi:10.1016/mse.2003.S1058274603000272.
28. Coonrad RW, Roush TF, Major NM, Basamania CJ. The drop sign, a radiographic warning sign of elbow instability. *J Shoulder Elbow Surg.* 2005;14(3):312-317. doi:10.1016/j.jse.2004.09.002.
29. O'Driscoll SW, Bell DF, Morrey BF. Posterolateral rotatory instability of the elbow. *J Bone Joint Surg Am.* 1991;73(3):440-446.
30. Anakwenze OA, Kancherla VK, Iyengar J, Ahmad CS, Levine WN. Posterolateral rotatory instability of the elbow. *Am J Sports Med.* 2014;42(2):485-491. doi:10.1177/0363546513494579.
31. Camp CL, Smith J, O'Driscoll SW. Posterolateral rotatory instability of the elbow: part II. Supplementary examination and dynamic imaging techniques. *Arthrosc Tech.* 2017;6(2):e407-e411. doi:10.1016/j.eats.2016.10.012
32. Sanchez-Sotelo J, Morrey BF, O'Driscoll SW. Ligamentous repair and reconstruction for posterolateral rotatory instability of the elbow. *J Bone Joint Surg Br.* 2005;87-B(1):54-61. doi:10.1302/0301-620X.87B1.15096.
33. O'Driscoll SW, Jupiter JB, Cohen MS, Ring D, McKee MD. Difficult elbow fractures: pearls and pitfalls. *Instr Course Lect.* 2003;52:113-134.
34. Adams JE, Merten SM, Steinmann SP. Arthroscopic-assisted treatment of coronoid fractures. *Arthroscopy.* 2007;23(10):1060-1065. doi:10.1016/j.arthro.2007.05.017.
35. Sanchez-Sotelo J, O'Driscoll SW, Morrey BF. Medial oblique compression fracture of the coronoid process of the ulna. *J Shoulder Elbow Surg.* 2005;14(1):60-64. doi:10.1016/j.jse.2004.04.012.
36. Doornberg JN, Ring DC. Fracture of the anteromedial facet of the coronoid process. *J Bone Joint Surg Am.* 2006;88(10):2216-2224. doi:10.2106/JBJS.E.01127.
37. Pollock JW, Brownhill J, Ferreira L, McDonald CP, Johnson J, King G. The effect of anteromedial facet fractures of the coronoid and lateral collateral ligament injury on elbow stability and kinematics. *J Bone Joint Surg Am.* 2009;91(6):1448-1458. doi:10.2106/JBJS.H.00222.
38. Park SM, Lee JS, Jung JY, Kim JY, Song KS. How should anteromedial coronoid facet fracture be managed? A surgical strategy based on O'Driscoll classification and ligament injury. *J Shoulder Elbow Surg.* 2015;24(1):74-82. doi:10.1016/j.jse.2014.07.010.
39. Davidson PA, Moseley JB Jr, Tullos HS. Radial head fracture. A potentially complex injury. *Clin Orthop Relat Res.* 1993;(297):224-230.
40. van Riet RP, Morrey BF. Documentation of associated injuries occurring with radial head fracture. *Clin Orthop Relat Res.* 2008;466(1):130-134. doi:10.1007/s11999-007-0064-8.
41. Schneeberger AG, Sadowski MM, Jacob HA. Coronoid process and radial head as posterolateral rotatory stabilizers of the elbow. *J Bone Joint Surg Am.* 2004;86-A(5):975-982. doi:10.2106/00004623-200405000-00013.
42. Forthman C, Henket M, Ring DC. Elbow dislocation with intra-articular fracture: the results of operative treatment without repair of the medial collateral ligament. *J Hand Surg.* 2007;32(8):1200-1209. doi:10.1016/j.jhsa.2007.06.019.
43. Ring D, Quintero J, Jupiter JB. Open reduction and internal fixation of fractures of the radial head. *J Bone Joint Surg Am.* 2002;84-A(10):1811-1815. doi:10.2106/00004623-200210000-00011.
44. Doornberg JN, Ring D. Coronoid fracture patterns. *J Hand Surg.* 2006;31(1):45-52. doi:10.1016/j.jhsa.2005.08.014.
45. Pugh DM, Wild LM, Schemitsch EH, King GJ, McKee MD. Standard surgical protocol to treat elbow dislocations with radial head and coronoid fractures. *J Bone Joint Surg Am.* 2004;86-A(6):1122-1130. doi:10.2106/00004623-200406000-00002.
46. Gupta A, Barei D, Khwaja A, Beingessner D. Single-staged treatment using a standardized protocol results in functional motion in the majority of patients with a terrible triad elbow injury. *Clin Orthop Relat Res.* 2014;472(7):2075-2083. doi:10.1007/s11999-014-3475-3.
47. Chan K, MacDermid JC, Faber KJ, King GJ, Athwal GS. Can we treat select terrible triad injuries nonoperatively? *Clin Orthop Relat Res.* 2014;472(7):2092-2099. doi:10.1007/s11999-014-3518-9.
48. Ring D, Jupiter JB, Simpson NS. Monteggia fractures in adults. *J Bone Joint Surg Am.* 1998;80(12):1733-1744. doi:10.2106/00004623-199812000-00003.

4

Neuropathies of the Upper Extremity

Talia Chapman, MD and Asif Ilyas, MD, FACS

Median Neuropathies

- Anatomy of the median nerve
  - Has contributions from C5 to T1 spinal nerve roots
  - Formed from medial and lateral cords of brachial plexus
  - Runs between biceps brachii and brachialis muscles
  - Passes under ligament of Struthers (anatomic variant that extends from the supracondylar process to the medial epicondyle)
  - At the elbow, passes under the bicipital aponeurosis (lacertus fibrosus) and into the antecubital fossa
  - The median nerve is medial to the biceps tendon and brachial artery.
  - Passes between the 2 heads of pronator teres (PT) into the forearm
  - In the forearm, travels between the flexor digitorum superficialis (FDS) and profundus (FDP)
    - Distal to the elbow, the median nerve innervates the PT, FDS, palmaris longus, and flexor carpi radialis
  - Anterior interosseous nerve (AIN) branches just below the elbow, approximately 4 cm distal to the medial epicondyle
  - The AIN runs distally between the FDP and flexor pollicis longus (FPL) along the anterior interosseous membrane.
    - The AIN innervates the pronator quadratus, FDP (index and middle), FPL, and the volar wrist capsule.

Namdari S, Zmistowski B, Omid R, eds.
The Foundations of Shoulder and Elbow Surgery (pp 57-75).

Pronator Syndrome

- Pathophysiology
  - Initially described in 1951 by Seyffarth.[1]
  - Proximal median nerve dysfunction due to compression at a number of possible sites[2,3] (see Johnson et al)[3] *Recommended reading for sites of compression and outcomes*
    - Two heads of the PT muscle
    - Ligament of Struthers
    - Lacertus fibrosus[4]
    - Accessory head of the FPL (Gantzer muscle)[5]
  - Incidence is rare and not well established.
- Diagnosis
  - Symptoms
    - Similar symptoms to carpal tunnel syndrome (CTS)
      - Numbness/paresthesias in radial 3 digits[1-3]
    - Numbness/paresthesias in the distribution of the palmar cutaneous branch of the median nerve
    - Pain in the medial and volar forearm
  - Physical examination
    - Must distinguish from CTS
      - CTS maneuvers should not be positive (ie, negative Tinel sign at the wrist, negative Phalen maneuver).
    - Pronator compression test[6,7]
      - Apply pressure to proximal and lateral edge of the PT muscle.
      - Positive test reproduces pain and paresthesias within 30 seconds of compression
    - Resisted pronation-supination with reproduction of symptoms
      - To determine whether the site of compression is at the lacertus fibrosus
    - Resisted flexion of the proximal interphalangeal (IP) joint of middle finger
      - May cause reproduction of symptoms if nerve is compressed by the heads of the FDS
    - Positive Tinel sign over the proximal volar forearm
  - Diagnostic studies
    - Electromyography (EMG)/nerve conduction velocity (NCV)
      - Unclear whether nerve studies aid in diagnosis
      - Many studies report normal nerve testing in pronator syndrome.[7,8]
      - Conduction delay and denervation may be evident in PT, FDS, and FDP.
      - Also, helpful to rule out other sites of compression (eg, CTS or cervical radiculopathy)
- Treatment
  - Nonoperative management has limited evidence and consists of the following:
    - Local injection of steroids in PT muscle[9]
    - Immobilization/activity modification
    - Anti-inflammatories
    - Forearm flexors stretching
  - Operative management
    - No consensus on optimal surgical technique[10,11]
      - Complete decompression of the median nerve in the forearm

      - Longitudinal vs oblique vs S-shaped incision
      - Endoscopic-assisted[12] vs minimal decompression of lacertus fibrosus[4] vs minimally invasive decompression of PT fascia[8]
      - Authors recommend longitudinal incision with identification and decompression of the median nerve under the lacertus fibrosus, followed by its release distally across the PT.
    - Outcomes
      - Nine percent to 30% have no improvement after surgical intervention.[7,13]

Anterior Interosseous Nerve Syndrome

- Pathophysiology
  - Unclear etiology with typically a self-limited natural history
  - Potential nerve compression at sites similar to pronator syndrome and along the interosseous membrane
  - Sustained AIN palsy, or a self-limited AIN neuritis
    - Self-limited AIN neuritis is more common than a sustained AIN palsy.[14-16]
- Diagnosis
  - Symptoms
    - Vague forearm pain
    - Dysfunction of the AIN-innervated muscles (FPL, FDP to index and middle), resulting in painless weakness with pinch and grip
    - Absence of sensory deficits
  - Physical examination
    - Weakness to thumb IP flexion and index and middle distal IP flexion
    - Kiloh-Nevin sign
      - Unable to make "OK" sign (inability to flex IP of thumb and distal IP of index finger)
  - Diagnostic studies
    - EMG/NCV
      - Helpful to rule out other lesions
      - Affected muscles may exhibit denervation.[14]
- Treatment
  - Nonoperative management
    - Controversial because natural history is not well defined
    - Prolonged period of observation is recommended because there is a high rate of spontaneous resolution of symptoms even after 1 year of symptoms.[15,16]
    - Repeat EMG/NCV to evaluate for recovery.
  - Operative management[17] *Recommended reading for pathophysiology and surgical outcomes*
    - Considered with a known compressive lesion or after failed nonoperative treatment
    - Approach similar to pronator syndrome
      - Exploration and decompression of the median nerve proximal to the PT, and distal decompression of the median nerve and its AIN branch

Ulnar Neuropathy

- Anatomy of the ulnar nerve
    - The ulnar nerve arises from the medial cord of the brachial plexus (C8, T1).
    - Runs along the medial side of the brachial artery in the anterior compartment of the proximal aspect of the arm
    - Pierces the medial intermuscular septum and it passes under the arcade of Struthers
    - Passes posterior to the medial epicondyle of the humerus and enters the cubital tunnel
    - Cubital tunnel is formed by the olecranon process inferiorly, the medial epicondyle superiorly, the elbow joint capsule and posterior bundle of the medial collateral ligament anteriorly, and the ligament of Osborne posteriorly (see Figure 1-12 in Chapter 1).
    - The nerve exits the cubital tunnel to enter the forearm between the superficial and deep heads of the flexor carpi ulnaris (FCU) muscle.
    - Cross-sectional area of the tunnel decreases significantly with elbow flexion.[18]

Cubital Tunnel Syndrome: Compression of the Ulnar Nerve at the Elbow

- Pathophysiology
    - Epidemiology
        - Ulnar nerve compression at the elbow is the second most common nerve entrapment of the upper extremity, after CTS.
        - An estimated annual incidence of 19 to 25 cases per 100,000 people[19-22]
        - McGowan classification[23] *Recommended reading for historical context and understanding of classification*
            - Grade 1: purely subjective symptoms and mild hypoesthesia
            - Grade 2: sensory loss and weakness of intrinsic hand muscles, with or without slight wasting
            - Grade 3: severe sensorimotor deficit
    - Risk factors
        - Prolonged flexed posture of the elbow or repetitive flexion
        - Ulnar nerve instability/subluxation
        - Cubitus valgus
        - Hypoplastic trochlea
        - Elbow trauma
    - Sites of compression[24]
        - Most commonly between the 2 heads of the FCU[25]
        - Arcade of Struthers
        - Ligament of Osborne (cubital tunnel)
        - Medial intermuscular septum
        - Medial head of triceps
        - Mass effect from joint swelling or ganglia, anconeus epitrochlearis, osteophytes, or hardware
- Diagnosis
    - Symptoms

    - Paresthesias of small finger, ulnar half of ring finger, and dorsal ulnar hand
    - Weakened grip and pinch of the hand
    - Altered dexterity of the hand
    - Exacerbated with excessive flexion or nighttime symptoms.
  - Physical examination
    - Decreased sensation in ulnar nerve distribution
    - Decreased intrinsic strength of the hand (ie, weak finger abduction)
    - Interosseous, first webspace, and hypothenar atrophy
    - Ring and small finger clawing
    - Froment sign
      - Patient attempts a key pinch and exhibits obligate thumb IP joint flexion as the FPL (AIN innervated) attempts to compensate for weakness of the adductor pollicis (ulnar nerve innervated)
    - Wartenberg sign
      - The small finger sits in abduction and cannot be actively adducted as a result of weakness in the ulnar innervated third palmar interosseous muscle and abducts as a result of the ulnar insertion of the extensor digiti quinti (EDQ)
    - Jeanne sign
      - Extensor pollicis longus (EPL) hyperextends the metacarpophalangeal joint while the patient attempts to adduct the thumb during a key pinch
    - Tinel sign over cubital tunnel
      - Nerve percussion at the retrocondylar groove
    - Elbow flexion test
      - The elbow is held in full flexion and the wrist is extended; a positive test reproduces paresthesia and pain[26]
    - Palpate for ulnar nerve subluxation over the medial epicondyle as elbow flexes and extends[27]
  - Diagnostic studies
    - EMG/NCV
      - Conduction velocities less than 50 m per second across the elbow are diagnostic
      - Decrease of greater than 20% of conduction velocity between the symptomatic and asymptomatic sides may be diagnostic[28]
      - Drop of more than 10 m per second across a measured interval around the elbow
      - Denervation of the first dorsal interosseous and FCU muscles
- Treatment
  - Nonoperative management[29-31]
    - Indicated for mild cases without active denervation or muscle wasting
    - Activity modification, nonsteroidal anti-inflammatory drugs, nighttime elbow extension splinting, and nerve gliding therapy
  - Operative management
    - Indicated for advanced cases and/or cases with active denervation or muscle wasting
    - In situ decompression (Figure 4-1)
      - Decompresses the ulnar nerve without moving it
      - Ligament of Osborne and the superficial and deep fascia of the FCU are released distally, whereas the fascia between the medial triceps and medial intermuscular

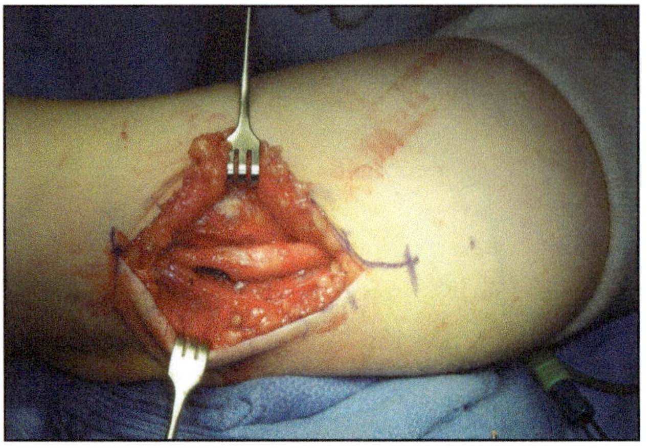

Figure 4-1. Ulnar neuropathy at the elbow following in situ release within the cubital tunnel. Note the bulbous nature of the ulnar nerve proximal to the cubital tunnel and narrower diameter distally highlighting significant compression of the ulnar nerve.

septum is released proximally through a limited incision centered behind the medial epicondyle

- Open vs endoscopic with similar rates of neurologic recovery and satisfaction[32]
- Outcomes of in situ decompression equivalent to ulnar nerve transposition[33,34]
- However, in the context of a hypermobile nerve preoperatively or postoperatively, most experts recommend transposition

- Medial epicondylectomy
  - First described in 1950s by King and Morgan[35]
  - Complete epicondylectomy may result in elbow instability.
  - Limited epicondylectomy with concomitant in situ ulnar nerve decompression
    - Decompress the ulnar nerve and then perform an oblique osteotomy of the medial epicondyle, taking care to preserve the insertion of the medial collateral ligament and repair the periosteum to prevent perineural scarring[36]
- Anterior transposition
  - Relieves both nerve compression and tension by moving the ulnar nerve anterior to the ulnohumeral axis
  - Several techniques of transposition exist following decompression and medial intermuscular septum excision.
    - Submuscular
      - The nerve is placed beneath the flexor-pronator mass after decompression and transposition.
    - Intramuscular
      - The nerve is transposed within the flexor-pronator mass.
    - Subcutaneous
      - The nerve is secured superficial to the flexor-pronator mass with subcutaneous tissue or with a fascial sling.
  - No significant outcome differences between techniques.[37,38]

Radial Neuropathies

- Anatomy of the radial nerve
    - Contributions from C5 to T1
    - Posterior divisions of the upper, middle, and lower trunks contribute to the posterior cord.
        - Radial nerve arises from the posterior cord
    - Leaves the axilla through the triangular interval
    - Courses along the spiral groove of the humerus between lateral and medial heads of triceps
    - Passes through lateral intermuscular septum 8 to 10 cm above the elbow
    - Crosses the elbow and runs between brachialis and brachioradialis
    - Bifurcates into superficial and deep branch
    - Superficial branch is sensory and continues beneath brachioradialis into the forearm
    - Deep branch becomes posterior interosseous nerve (PIN) and passes through the radial tunnel into the supinator
        - Roof: brachioradialis muscle
        - Floor: capsule of radiocapitellar joint
        - Medially: biceps tendon and brachialis
        - Laterally: extensor carpi radialis longus (ECRL) and brevis, brachioradialis
        - Distally: arcade of Frohse (proximal edge of supinator)
    - PIN exits supinator and divides into medial and lateral branches and traverses along the posterior interosseous membrane
        - Medial PIN branch innervates the extensor digitorum communis (EDC), EDQ, extensor carpi ulnaris, and supinator
        - Lateral PIN branch innervates the abductor pollicis longus, extensor pollicis brevis, EPL, and extensor indicis proprius
        - Radial nerve innervates brachioradialis, ECRL, and extensor carpi radialis brevis (ECRB)

Radial Tunnel Syndrome

- Pathophysiology
    - Radial neuropathy is rare: 1 to 3 cases per 100,000 people[22]
    - First described in 1972 in cases of resistant lateral epicondylitis[39] *Recommended reading for historical context*
    - Compression of the radial nerve and PIN within the radial tunnel with pain only (no motor or sensory dysfunction)
    - Many potential sites of compression
        - Fibrous bands anterior to radiocapitellar joint
        - Radial recurrent vessels (leash of Henry)
        - Medial edge of ECRB
        - Arcade of Frohse at proximal supinator (most frequent site of entrapment)
        - Distal margin of supinator
- Diagnosis
    - Symptoms
        - Pain at the site of entrapment in the mobile wad of the forearm (3 to 5 cm distal to lateral epicondyle)[40]

        - No motor weakness of PIN-innervated muscles
        - No sensory changes
        - No pain over the lateral epicondyle
    - Physical examination
        - Resisted long finger extension reproduces pain in the radial tunnel
        - Resisted supination test reproduces pain in the radial tunnel[41]
        - Passive pronation with wrist flexion reproduces pain due to increasing pressure inside radial tunnel
        - Radial tunnel injection test with local anesthetic
            - Test is positive if injection relieves pain while causing a temporary PIN palsy
    - Diagnostic studies
        - Magnetic resonance imaging (MRI)
            - Usually negative
            - May show muscle changes in PIN-innervated muscles
            - May show other causes of entrapment (masses, fractures, synovitis)
        - EMG/NCV
            - Usually normal
            - May elucidate other sites of compression
- Treatment
    - Nonoperative management[39,41]
        - Activity modification
        - Splinting
        - Anti-inflammatories
        - Steroid injection[42,43]
        - Physical therapy
        - Avoid tennis elbow braces
    - Operative management
        - Decompress the radial nerve and PIN in the radial tunnel.
            - Release arcade of Frohse
            - Release distal edge of supinator
            - Release fibrous bands superficial to the radiocapitellar joint
        - Dorsal approach
            - Between EDC and ECRB (leash of Henry)
            - Transmuscular splitting of brachioradialis
            - Between brachioradialis and ECRL
        - Volar approach
            - Between brachioradialis and brachialis
        - Outcome variables
            - Approximately 70% to 90% relief with decompression[42,44]
            - Outcomes worse with coexisting lateral epicondylitis, concomitant nerve compression syndromes, or workers compensation patients[45]

Posterior Interosseous Nerve Syndrome

- Pathophysiology
  - Incidence is rare: 264 cases reported over 50 years[46]
  - Differentiated from radial tunnel syndrome by the presence of motor weakness
  - Etiology
    - Mechanical: compressive force on the nerve
      - Compression within the radial tunnel
      - Mass effect from lipomas, ganglions, adhesions, rheumatoid synovium, or cysts
    - Nonmechanical: intrinsic inflammatory reaction within the nerve
      - Parsonage-Turner syndrome
        - Viral-induced neuritis
        - May be associated with systemic illnesses
      - Spontaneous "hourglass" constriction[47,48]
        - May be associated with torsion of nerve fascicles
        - Weak association with vasculitic disorders
        - Hypoperfusion of nerve causing intrafascicular edema with subsequent healing with segmental fibrosis and constriction
- Diagnosis
  - Symptoms
    - Spontaneous weakness of thumb and finger extension
    - Preserved wrist extension with radial deviation due to intact ECRL/ECRB function
    - Pain over lateral forearm within the mobile wad may or may not be present.
  - Physical examination
    - Weakness of extensor carpi ulnaris, EDQ, EDC if medial branch is affected
    - Weakness of abductor pollicis longus, extensor pollicis brevis, EPL, and extensor indicis proprius if lateral branch is affected
    - If the entire PIN proximal to bifurcation is affected, then all muscle groups could be weak.
    - Normal wrist extension unless ECRB is innervated by the PIN, then wrist extension will result in radial deviation due to intact ECRL
    - Sensation is generally intact.
  - Diagnostic studies
    - MRI to assess for space-occupying lesions
    - EMG/NCV may confirm diagnosis and provide prognostic information on reinnervation of the nerve.[49,50]
      - Slowed conduction velocity
      - Prolonged distal latency
      - Reduced amplitude
      - Fibrillations; positive sharp waves; decreased recruitment
- Treatment
  - Nonoperative management
    - Generally, a period of observation of at least 6 weeks prior to surgical exploration is indicated,[51] consisting of the following:
      - Activity modification

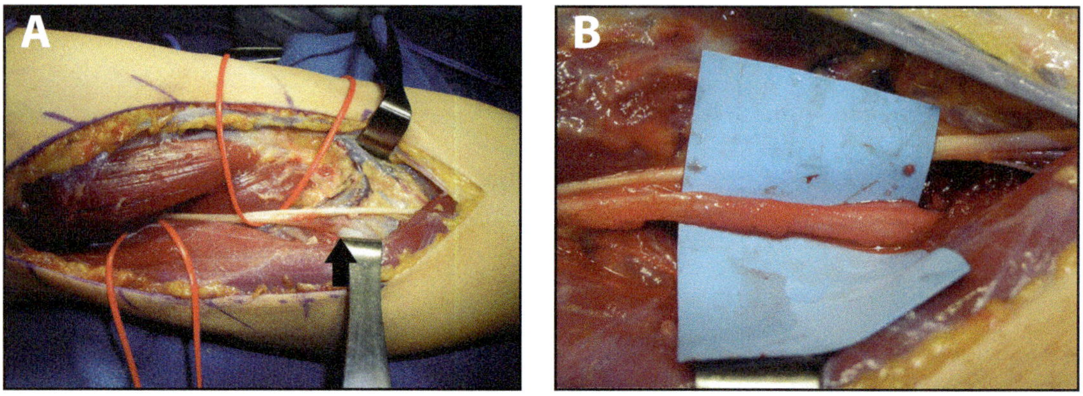

Figure 4-2. Release of the radial nerve across the elbow, with bifurcation of the PIN from the radial sensory nerve. (A) Postbifurcation. Note the PIN diving deep under the proximal edge of the supinator (black arrow) with edema surrounding the PIN. (B) Postrelease. Note the PIN decompressed with increased diameter and improved appearance.

- Splinting
- Physical therapy

- If the cause is thought to be neuralgic amyotrophy, the period of observation may be extended.
  - Cases due to neuralgic amyotrophy do well with nonoperative management.[52]
    - There is 90% recovery by 3 years in those showing signs of recovery within the first month.
    - There is 70% recovery by 3 years in those showing no spontaneous recovery within the first month.
- Operative management
  - Indications
    - Progressive motor weakness
    - Failed nonoperative management
  - Neurolysis of the PIN from takeoff from the radial nerve through the supinator
  - Anterior approach to the PIN (Figure 4-2)
    - Oblique incision starting proximal to the elbow crease extending along the lateral border of the biceps and extending distally along the medial border of the brachioradialis
    - The lateral antebrachial cutaneous nerve is identified and retracted
    - The radial nerve is identified proximal to the elbow crease between the brachialis and brachioradialis
    - The radial nerve dissected distally, where superficial and deep branches are encountered
    - The radial tunnel is surgically released
  - Posterior approach to PIN
    - An incision is made in the groove between the mobile wad and the rest of the extensors.
    - Interval between EDC and ECRB
    - The PIN is identified as it emerges from the supinator and is released under direct visualization.
  - Lateral approach to PIN

      - Curvilinear incision along lateral elbow
      - Brachioradialis retracted laterally to expose proximal PIN and retracted medially to expose distal PIN
    - Outcomes
      - In cases of mechanical compression, good outcomes after surgical decompression[52]
      - In nonmechanical, viral, or inflammatory cases, results are more variable and dependent on extent of interfascicular scarring[51,52]

Proximal Neuropathies

Suprascapular Nerve

- Anatomy
  - Peripheral nerve with mixed motor and sensory from upper trunk of the brachial plexus
  - Mostly C5 with contributions from C4 and C6
  - Leaves the trunk 3 cm above the clavicle, passes deep to trapezius and omohyoid muscles
  - Passes within the suprascapular notch underneath the transverse scapular ligament
  - Innervates supraspinatus muscle within the supraspinatus fossa and provides sensory branches to the glenohumeral and acromioclavicular joints
  - Traverses the spinoglenoid notch at the lateral edge of the scapular spine and passes into the infraspinatus fossa to innervate infraspinatus
- Pathophysiology
  - May be entrapped at the level of the suprascapular notch or at the spinoglenoid notch
    - Compression at the spinoglenoid notch is often caused by a cyst associated with a labral tear.
  - More commonly compressed in the suprascapular notch
  - Trauma
    - After shoulder dislocation, may be associated with additional neuropathies
  - Atraumatic
    - Associated with repetitive cross-body adduction of the arm
    - Gymnasts, weight lifters, pitchers, tennis players, linemen, volleyball players[53,54]
- Diagnosis
  - Symptoms
    - Entrapment at suprascapular notch
      - Shoulder pain: deep and throbbing at the superior border of scapula with extension toward the shoulder and occasional radiation down the arm[55]
      - Shoulder weakness in abduction and external rotation
    - Entrapment at spinoglenoid notch
      - Painless shoulder external rotation weakness[53]
    - Differential diagnosis
      - Rotator cuff tendinitis/tears
      - Shoulder impingement
      - Adhesive capsulitis
      - Cervical radiculopathy
      - Neuralgic amyotrophy

- Physical examination
  - Weakness and atrophy of supraspinatus (abduction) and infraspinatus (external rotation) or infraspinatus only depending on the site of entrapment
  - Tenderness over scapular notch
- Diagnostic studies
  - MRI of the shoulder
    - Evaluate for spinoglenoid notch cyst associated with superior labral anterior posterior lesions.
    - Evaluate for rotator cuff pathology.
    - Evaluate the extent of muscle atrophy.
  - EMG/NCV[56]
    - Evaluate for atrophy of supraspinatus and infraspinatus.
    - Exclude cervical radiculopathy or brachial plexopathy.
    - Supraspinatus motor latency upper limit 3.7 ms
    - Infraspinatus motor latency upper limit 4.3 ms[57]

- Treatment
  - Nonoperative management
    - Avoidance of causative repetitive motion
    - Physical therapy for range of motion and scapular stabilization
    - Outcomes: good with nonoperative management[54]
  - Operative management
    - Surgical exploration with resection of the transverse scapular ligament and neurolysis
    - Indicated with failure of nonoperative treatment
    - Indicated when a ganglion cyst is present at the spinoglenoid notch
    - Outcomes: approximately 85% improvement in pain and function after decompression after failed nonoperative management[58]

Axillary Nerve: Quadrilateral Space Syndrome

- Anatomy
  - Mixed motor and sensory nerve
  - Innervates deltoid and teres minor and provides sensation to lateral shoulder
  - Terminal branch of posterior cord of brachial plexus
  - C5 to C6 fibers
  - Travels along anterior surface of subscapularis
  - Leaves the axilla through the quadrilateral space
    - Roof: teres minor
    - Floor: teres major
    - Lateral: neck of humerus
    - Medial: long head to triceps
  - Bifurcation into anterior and posterior branches
    - Anterior: travels with posterior circumflex humeral artery and innervates middle and anterior deltoid
    - Posterior: innervates teres minor and forms the upper lateral brachial cutaneous nerve which innervates the skin over the deltoid

- Pathophysiology
  - Traumatic
    - Dislocation of the shoulder[59]
    - Humeral fracture
    - May be associated with brachial plexopathy
  - Quadrilateral space syndrome
    - Compression of the posterior humeral circumflex artery or axillary nerve[60]
    - First described by Cahill and Palmer in 1983[61]
    - Etiology
      - Fibrous bands[62]
      - Space-occupying lesions
        - Paralabral cysts; bony fragments; lipomas
      - Muscle hypertrophy[61]
    - Epidemiology[63]
      - Most commonly seen in patients 20 to 40 years old
      - Most common in dominant shoulder
      - Occurs more often in men than in women
      - Overhead athletes
- Diagnosis
  - Symptoms
    - Patch of sensory loss over the lateral shoulder
    - Weakness in shoulder abduction
    - Poorly localized shoulder pain
    - Aggravated with abduction and external rotation of shoulder
  - Physical examination
    - Decreased sensation over the lateral shoulder
    - Weakness and atrophy of deltoid muscle
    - Tenderness over quadrilateral space
    - Lidocaine injection test
      - Disappearance of pain with injection of local anesthetic
  - Differential diagnoses
    - Radiculopathy
    - Brachial plexopathy
    - Neuralgic amyotrophy
    - Suprascapular neuropathy
    - Rotator cuff tear
  - Diagnostic studies
    - Plain radiographs
    - MRI
      - Evaluate for space-occupying lesions.
      - Evaluate for muscle atrophy.
    - EMG/NCV
      - Often negative because of the dynamic nature of quadrilateral space syndrome

            - May show decreased amplitude of axillary nerve and teres minor or deltoid muscle denervation
        - Computed tomography or MRI angiogram
            - May reveal posterior circumflex humeral artery occlusion or thrombosis[60]
- Treatment
    - Nonoperative management
        - Anti-inflammatory medications; activity modification; physical therapy
        - Outcomes generally good: reports of complete resolution of symptoms[64]
    - Operative management
        - Indicated for space-occupying lesions or failure of conservative treatment after 6 months
        - Open surgical decompression has been described in overhead athletes[65]
        - May perform concomitant arthroscopy to address intra-articular pathology
        - Outcomes generally good: most with complete relief of symptoms after decompression[65]

Thoracic Outlet Syndrome (TOS)

- Pathophysiology
    - First described in 1956 by Peet et al[66]
    - Compression of the neurovascular bundles as it passes through the thoracic outlet (interval from the supraclavicular fossa to the axilla that passes between the clavicle and the first rib)
        - Contains 3 structures that may be compressed: subclavian artery; subclavian vein; brachial plexus
        - Compression may occur at 3 places
            - Interscalene triangle
            - Costoclavicular space
            - Retropectoralis minor space
    - Paget-Schroetter syndrome
        - Thoracic outlet syndrome (TOS) with compression of subclavian vein in an athlete due to scalene hypertrophy
    - Epidemiology
        - More frequent in women than men
        - Usually occurs in the third and fourth decades[67]
        - May be preceded by a traumatic injury or repetitive activity[68]
- Diagnosis
    - Symptoms
        - Vascular
            - Arterial ischemia
            - Raynaud phenomenon
            - Cold intolerance[69]
        - Neurologic
            - Swelling of upper extremity
            - Pain and paresthesias in the shoulder, arm, and hand in nonradicular distribution
            - Occipital headache
        - Worsened by overhead position of arms

        - Symptoms are vague and poorly defined[70]
    - Physical examination[71]
        - Adson test
            - Extension of the arm with the neck extended and turned toward the affected side may result in loss of radial pulse or reproduction of symptoms with inhalation
        - Roos test
            - Hands repeatedly opened and closed while holding them overhead for 1 minute can reproduce symptoms
        - Wright test
            - Abduction and external rotation with the neck rotated away leads to loss of pulse and reproduction of symptoms
        - A blood pressure difference of 20 mmHg between the upper extremities is a significant but rare finding of vascular TOS.[68]
    - Differential diagnoses
        - Radiculopathy
        - Brachial plexopathy
        - Neuralgic amyotrophy
        - Fibromyalgia
    - Diagnostic studies
        - Radiographs
            - Cervical spine to rule out cervical rib
            - Chest to rule out Pancoast tumor
        - EMG/NCV are usually equivocal
        - Intramuscular anterior scalene block may be a diagnostic test with temporary benefit due to reduced muscle spasm compressing the thoracic outlet[67]
        - Angiography
            - If etiology is vascular, will show compression or aneurysm
- Treatment
    - Nonoperative management
        - First line of treatment
        - Activity modification
        - Physical therapy: posture; shoulder girdle strengthening
        - Outcomes variable with good results in some series: 50% to 70% of patients with improvement[72]
    - Operative management
        - Indicated for failure to respond to nonsurgical management
        - Transaxillary approach[73]
            - Most common approach
            - Allows more complete exposure of first rib
            - More cosmetic scar
            - No retraction of neurovascular structures necessary for first rib removal
            - Risk of iatrogenic brachial plexus injury
        - Supraclavicular approach[74]
            - Allows better exposure of the middle and upper trunks, neck of the first rib, and anterior and middle scalene muscles

- May also allow effective first rib resection
- Allows vascular reconstruction
- Retraction of brachial plexus and vascular structure necessary for complete first rib removal

- Posterior approach[75]
  - Favored for recurrent TOS and in cases of prior anterior neck surgery
  - May allow better exposure of proximal elements of the brachial plexus
  - Requires extensive muscle dissection that can lead to postoperative shoulder dysfunction
  - Risk of injury to the long thoracic, dorsal scapular, and accessory nerves

References

1. Seyffarth H. Primary myoses in the M. pronator teres as cause of lesion of the N. medianus (the pronator syndrome). *Acta Psychiatr Neurol Scand Suppl.* 1951;74:251-254.
2. Fuss FK, Wurzl GH. Median nerve entrapment. Pronator teres syndrome. Surgical anatomy and correlation with symptom patterns. *Surg Radiol Anat.* 1990;12(4):267-271. doi:10.1007/bf01623702.
3. Johnson RK, Spinner M, Shrewsbury MM. Median nerve entrapment syndrome in the proximal forearm. *J Hand Surg Am.* 1979;4(1):48-51. doi:10.1016/s0363-5023(79)80104-5.
4. Seitz WH, Matsuoka H, McAdoo J, Sherman G, Stickney DP. Acute compression of the median nerve at the elbow by the lacertus fibrosus. *J Shoulder Elbow Surg.* 2007;16(1):91-94. doi:10.1016/j.jse.2006.04.005.
5. al-Qattan MM. Gantzer's muscle. An anatomical study of the accessory head of the flexor pollicis longus muscle. *J Hand Surg Br.* 1996;21(2):269-270. doi:10.1016/s0266-7681(96)80114-8.
6. Gainor BJ. The pronator compression test revisited. A forgotten physical sign. *Orthop Rev.* 1990;19(10):888-892.
7. Hartz CR, Linscheid RL, Gramse RR, Daube JR. The pronator teres syndrome: compressive neuropathy of the median nerve. *J Bone Joint Surg Am.* 1981;63(6):885-890.
8. Zancolli ER III, Zancolli EP IV, Perrotto CJ. New mini-invasive decompression for pronator teres syndrome. *J Hand Surg Am.* 2012;37(8):1706-1710. doi:10.1016/j.jhsa.2012.05.033.
9. Morris HH, Peters BH. Pronator syndrome: clinical and electrophysiological features in seven cases. *J Neurol Neurosurg Psychiatry.* 1976;39(5):461-464. doi:10.1136/jnnp.39.5.461.
10. Eid N, Ito Y, Otsuki Y. Median nerve decompression at lacertus tunnel: possible complications. *Hand N Y.* 2013;8(2):246-247. doi:10.1007/s11552-013-9525-6.
11. Tsai TM, Syed SA. A transverse skin incision approach for decompression of pronator teres syndrome. *J Hand Surg Br.* 1994;19(1):40-42. doi:10.1016/0266-7681(94)90047-7.
12. Lee AK, Khorsandi M, Nurbhai N, Dang J, Fitzmaurice M, Herron KA. Endoscopically assisted decompression for pronator syndrome. *J Hand Surg Am.* 2012;37(6):1173-1179. doi:10.1016/j.jhsa.2012.02.023.
13. Olehnik WK, Manske PR, Szerzinski J. Median nerve compression in the proximal forearm. *J Hand Surg Am.* 1994;19(1):121-126. doi:10.1016/0363-5023(94)90235-6.
14. Seror P. Anterior interosseous nerve lesions. Clinical and electrophysiological features. *J Bone Joint Surg Br.* 1996;78-B(2):238-241. doi:10.1302/0301-620X.78B2.0780238.
15. Seki M, Nakamura H, Kono H. Neurolysis is not required for young patients with a spontaneous palsy of the anterior interosseous nerve: retrospective analysis of cases managed non-operatively. *J Bone Joint Surg Br.* 2006;88(12):1606-1609. doi:10.1302/0301-620X.88B12.17700.
16. Miller-Breslow A, Terrono A, Millender LH. Nonoperative treatment of anterior interosseous nerve paralysis. *J Hand Surg Am.* 1990;15(3):493-496. doi:10.1016/0363-5023(90)90069-4.
17. Stern MB. The anterior interosseous nerve syndrome (the Kiloh-Nevin syndrome). Report and follow-up study of three cases. *Clin Orthop Relat Res.* 1984;(187):223-227. doi:10.1097/00003086-198407000-00035.
18. Gelberman RH, Yamaguchi K, Hollstien SB, et al. Changes in interstitial pressure and cross-sectional area of the cubital tunnel and of the ulnar nerve with flexion of the elbow. An experimental study in human cadavera. *J Bone Joint Surg Am.* 1998;80(4):492-501. doi:10.2106/00004623-199804000-00005.
19. Bartels RH, Verbeek AL. Risk factors for ulnar nerve compression at the elbow: a case control study. *Acta Neurochir (Wien).* 2007;149(7):669-674; discussion 674. doi:10.1007/s00701-007-1166-5.

20. van Rijn RM, Huisstede BM, Koes BW, Burdorf A. Associations between work-related factors and specific disorders at the elbow: a systematic literature review. *Rheumatology (Oxford)*. 2009;48(5):528-536. doi:10.1093/rheumatology/kep013.
21. Soltani AM, Best MJ, Francis CS, Allan BJ, Panthaki ZJ. Trends in the surgical treatment of cubital tunnel syndrome: an analysis of the National Survey of Ambulatory Surgery database. *J Hand Surg Am*. 2013;38(8):1551-1556. doi:10.1016/j.jhsa.2013.04.044.
22. Latinovic R, Gulliford MC, Hughes RA. Incidence of common compressive neuropathies in primary care. *J Neurol Neurosurg Psychiatry*. 2006;77(2):263-265. doi:10.1136/jnnp.2005.066696.
23. McGowan AJ. The results of transposition of the ulnar nerve for traumatic ulnar neuritis. *J Bone Joint Surg Br*. 1950;32-B(3):293-301. doi:10.1302/0301-620X.32B3.293.
24. Staples JR, Calfee R. Cubital tunnel syndrome: current concepts. *J Am Acad Orthop Surg*. 2017;25(10):e215-e224. doi:10.5435/JAAOS-D-15-00261.
25. Gellman H. Compression of the ulnar nerve at the elbow: cubital tunnel syndrome. *Instr Course Lect*. 2008;57:187-197.
26. Buehler MJ, Thayer DT. The elbow flexion test. A clinical test for the cubital tunnel syndrome. *Clin Orthop Relat Res*. 1988;(233):213-216. doi:10.1097/00003086-198808000-00026.
27. Calfee RP, Manske PR, Gelberman RH, Van Steyn MO, Steffen J, Goldfarb CA. Clinical assessment of the ulnar nerve at the elbow: reliability of instability testing and the association of hypermobility with clinical symptoms. *J Bone Joint Surg Am*. 2010;92(17):2801-2808. doi:10.2106/JBJS.J.00097.
28. Beekman R, Van Der Plas JP, Uitdehaag BM, Schellens RL, Visser LH. Clinical, electrodiagnostic, and sonographic studies in ulnar neuropathy at the elbow. *Muscle Nerve*. 2004;30(2):202-208. doi:10.1002/mus.20093.
29. Dellon AL, Hament W, Gittelshon A. Nonoperative management of cubital tunnel syndrome: an 8-year prospective study. *Neurology*. 1993;43(9):1673-1677. doi:10.1212/wnl.43.9.1673.
30. Svernlöv B, Larsson M, Rehn K, Adolfsson L. Conservative treatment of the cubital tunnel syndrome. *J Hand Surg Eur Vol*. 2009;34(2):201-207. doi:10.1177/1753193408098480.
31. Shah CM, Calfee RP, Gelberman RH, Goldfarb CA. Outcomes of rigid night splinting and activity modification in the treatment of cubital tunnel syndrome. *J Hand Surg Am*. 2013;38(6):1125-1130.e1. doi:10.1016/j.jhsa.2013.02.039.
32. Dützmann S, Martin KD, Sobottka S, et al. Open vs retractor-endoscopic in situ decompression of the ulnar nerve in cubital tunnel syndrome: a retrospective cohort study. *Neurosurgery*. 2013;72(4):605-616; discussion 614-616. doi:10.1227/NEU.0b013e3182846dbd.
33. Biggs M, Curtis JA. Randomized, prospective study comparing ulnar neurolysis in situ with submuscular transposition. *Neurosurgery*. 2006;58(2):296-304. doi:10.1227/01.NEU.0000194847.04143.A1.
34. Bartels RH, Verhagen WI, van der Wilt GJ, Meulstee J, van Rossum LG, Grotenhuis JA. Prospective randomized controlled study comparing simple decompression versus anterior subcutaneous transposition for idiopathic neuropathy of the ulnar nerve at the elbow: part 1. *Neurosurgery*. 2005;56(3):522-530. doi:10.1227/01.neu.0000154131.01167.03.
35. King T, Morgan FP. Late results of removing the medial humeral epicondyle for traumatic ulnar neuritis. *J Bone Joint Surg Br*. 1959;41-B(1):51-55. doi:10.1302/0301-620X.41B1.51.
36. Osei DA, Padegimas EM, Calfee RP, Gelberman RH. Outcomes following modified oblique medial epicondylectomy for treatment of cubital tunnel syndrome. *J Hand Surg Am*. 2013;38(2):336-343. doi:10.1016/j.jhsa.2012.11.006.
37. Nabhan A, Ahlhelm F, Kelm J, Reith W, Schwerdtfeger K, Steudel WI. Simple decompression or subcutaneous anterior transposition of the ulnar nerve for cubital tunnel syndrome. *J Hand Surg Br*. 2005;30(5):521-524. doi:10.1016/j.jhsb.2005.05.011.
38. Gervasio O, Gambardella G, Zaccone C, Branca D. Simple decompression versus anterior submuscular transposition of the ulnar nerve in severe cubital tunnel syndrome: a prospective randomized study. *Neurosurgery*. 2005;56(1):108-117; discussion 117. doi:10.1227/01.neu.0000145854.38234.81. [Erratum in *Neurosurgery*. 2005;56(2):409.]
39. Roles NC, Maudsley RH. Radial tunnel syndrome: resistant tennis elbow as a nerve entrapment. *J Bone Joint Surg Br*. 1972;54(3):499-508.
40. Verhaar J, Spaans F. Radial tunnel syndrome. An investigation of compression neuropathy as a possible cause. *J Bone Joint Surg Am*. 1991;73(4):539-544.
41. Lister GD, Belsole RB, Kleinert HE. The radial tunnel syndrome. *J Hand Surg Am*. 1979;4(1):52-59. doi:10.1016/s0363-5023(79)80105-7.
42. Naam NH, Nemani S. Radial tunnel syndrome. *Orthop Clin North Am*. 2012;43(4):529-536. doi:10.1016/j.ocl.2012.07.022.

43. van den Ende KI, Steinmann SP. Radial tunnel syndrome. *J Hand Surg Am.* 2010;35(6):1004-1006. doi:10.1016/j.jhsa.2010.03.020.
44. Jebson PJ, Engber WD. Radial tunnel syndrome: long-term results of surgical decompression. *J Hand Surg Am.* 1997;22(5):889-896. doi:10.1016/S0363-5023(97)80086-X.
45. Lee JT, Azari K, Jones NF. Long term results of radial tunnel release—the effect of co-existing tennis elbow, multiple compression syndromes and workers' compensation. *J Plast Reconstr Aesthetic Surg.* 2008;61(9):1095-1099. doi:10.1016/j.bjps.2007.07.018.
46. Quignon R, Marteau E, Penaud A, Corcia P, Laulan J. Posterior interosseous nerve palsy. A series of 18 cases and literature review [in French]. *Chir Main.* 2012;31(1):18-23. doi:10.1016/j.main.2011.11.004.
47. Umehara F, Yoshino S, Arimura Y, Fukuoka T, Arimura K, Osame M. Posterior interosseous nerve syndrome with hourglass-like fascicular constriction of the nerve. *J Neurol Sci.* 2003;215(1-2):111-113. doi:10.1016/s0022-510x(03)00164-3.
48. Sigamoney KV, Rashid A, Ng CY. Management of atraumatic posterior interosseous nerve palsy. *J Hand Surg Am.* 2017;42(10):826-830. doi:10.1016/j.jhsa.2017.07.026.
49. Hashizume H, Inoue H, Nagashima K, Hamaya K. Posterior interosseous nerve paralysis related to focal radial nerve constriction secondary to vasculitis. *J Hand Surg Br.* 1993;18(6):757-760. doi:10.1016/0266-7681(93)90239-c.
50. Bevelaqua AC, Hayter CL, Feinberg JH, Rodeo SA. Posterior interosseous neuropathy: electrodiagnostic evaluation. *HSS J.* 2012;8(2):184-189. doi:10.1007/s11420-011-9238-8.
51. Wu P, Yang JY, Yu C. Surgical treatment of spontaneous posterior interosseous nerve palsy with hourglass-like constriction. *J Hand Surg Eur Vol.* 2015;40(6):646-647. doi:10.1177/1753193414528154.
52. Ochi K, Horiuchi Y, Tazaki K, et al. Surgical treatment of spontaneous posterior interosseous nerve palsy: a retrospective study of 50 cases. *J Bone Joint Surg Br.* 2011;93(2):217-222. doi:10.1302/0301-620X.93B2.24748.
53. Ferretti A, Cerullo G, Russo G. Suprascapular neuropathy in volleyball players. *J Bone Joint Surg Am.* 1987;69(2):260-263.
54. Martin SD, Warren RF, Martin TL, Kennedy K, O'Brien SJ, Wickiewicz TL. Suprascapular neuropathy. Results of non-operative treatment. *J Bone Joint Surg Am.* 1997;79(8):1159-1165. doi:10.2106/00004623-199708000-00007.
55. Clein LJ. Suprascapular entrapment neuropathy. *J Neurosurg.* 1975;43(3):337-342. doi:10.3171/jns.1975.43.3.0337.
56. Post M, Mayer J. Suprascapular nerve entrapment. Diagnosis and treatment. *Clin Orthop Relat Res.* 1987;(223):126-136.
57. Kraft GH. Axillary, musculocutaneous and suprascapular nerve latency studies. *Arch Phys Med Rehabil.* 1972;53(8):383-387.
58. Antoniadis G, Richter HP, Rath S, Braun V, Moese G. Suprascapular nerve entrapment: experience with 28 cases. *J Neurosurg.* 1996;85(6):1020-1025. doi:10.3171/jns.1996.85.6.1020.
59. Toolanen G, Hildingsson C, Hedlund T, Knibestöl M, Oberg L. Early complications after anterior dislocation of the shoulder in patients over 40 years. An ultrasonographic and electromyographic study. *Acta Orthop Scand.* 1993;64(5):549-552. doi:10.3109/17453679308993690.
60. Flynn LS, Wright TW, King JJ. Quadrilateral space syndrome: a review. *J Shoulder Elbow Surg.* 2018;27(5):950-956. doi:10.1016/j.jse.2017.10.024.
61. Cahill BR, Palmer RE. Quadrilateral space syndrome. *J Hand Surg Am.* 1983;8(1):65-69. doi:10.1016/s0363-5023(83)80056-2.
62. McClelland D, Paxinos A. The anatomy of the quadrilateral space with reference to quadrilateral space syndrome. *J Shoulder Elbow Surg.* 2008;17(1):162-164. doi:10.1016/j.jse.2007.05.013.
63. Brown SA, Doolittle DA, Bohanon CJ, et al. Quadrilateral space syndrome: the Mayo Clinic experience with a new classification system and case series. *Mayo Clin Proc.* 2015;90(3):382-394. doi:10.1016/j.mayocp.2014.12.012.
64. Hoskins WT, Pollard HP, McDonald AJ. Quadrilateral space syndrome: a case study and review of the literature. *Br J Sports Med.* 2005;39(2):e9. doi:10.1136/bjsm.2004.013367.
65. McAdams TR, Dillingham MF. Surgical decompression of the quadrilateral space in overhead athletes. *Am J Sports Med.* 2008;36(3):528-532. doi:10.1177/0363546507309675.
66. Peet RM, Henriksen JD, Anderson TP, Martin GM. Thoracic-outlet syndrome: evaluation of a therapeutic exercise program. *Proc Staff Meet Mayo Clin.* 1956;31(9):281-287.
67. Christo PJ, McGreevy K. Updated perspectives on neurogenic thoracic outlet syndrome. *Curr Pain Headache Rep.* 2011;15(1):14-21. doi:10.1007/s11916-010-0163-1.
68. Brantigan CO, Roos DB. Etiology of neurogenic thoracic outlet syndrome. *Hand Clin.* 2004;20(1):17-22. doi:10.1016/s0749-0712(03)00112-4.

69. Marine L, Valdes F, Mertens R, Kramer A, Bergoeing M, Urbina J. Arterial thoracic outlet syndrome: a 32-year experience. *Ann Vasc Surg.* 2013;27(8):1007-1013. doi:10.1016/j.avsg.2013.06.001.
70. Laulan J, Fouquet B, Rodaix C, Jauffret P, Roquelaure Y, Descatha A. Thoracic outlet syndrome: definition, aetiological factors, diagnosis, management and occupational impact. *J Occup Rehabil.* 2011;21(3):366-373. doi:10.1007/s10926-010-9278-9.
71. Buller LT, Jose J, Baraga M, Lesniak B. Thoracic outlet syndrome: current concepts, imaging features, and therapeutic strategies. *Am J Orthop (Belle Mead NJ).* 2015;44(8):376-382.
72. Novak CB, Collins ED, Mackinnon SE. Outcome following conservative management of thoracic outlet syndrome. *J Hand Surg Am.* 1995;20(4):542-548. doi:10.1016/S0363-5023(05)80264-3.
73. Roos DB. Transaxillary approach for first rib resection to relieve thoracic outlet syndrome. *Ann Surg.* 1966;163(3):354-358. doi:10.1097/00000658-196603000-00005.
74. Terzis JK, Kokkalis ZT. Supraclavicular approach for thoracic outlet syndrome. *Hand (N Y).* 2010;5(3):326-337. doi:10.1007/s11552-009-9253-0.
75. Tender GC, Kline DG. Posterior subscapular approach to the brachial plexus. *Neurosurgery.* 2005;57(4 suppl):377-381. doi:10.1227/01.neu.0000176850.21962.29.

5

Fractures of the Elbow

Nilay A. Patel, MD and John Scolaro, MD, MA

Distal Humerus Fractures

Distal humerus fractures are challenging fractures. Historically, these injuries were managed nonoperatively because of high complication rates following surgical treatment. Advancements in technique and fixation implants dramatically improved outcomes. Currently, open reduction and internal fixation is the standard of care. Anatomic reduction of intra-articular injuries and stable internal fixation allows early range of motion (ROM) and has greatly improved outcomes.

Epidemiology/Mechanism of Injury

- Distal humerus fractures comprise approximately 2% of fractures.[1,2]
- Bimodal age distribution[3,4]
  - 12 to 19 years old
    - Typically, these result from a high-energy mechanism of injury such as motor vehicle collisions, sporting injuries, and falls from height.
  - Ages 80 years and older
    - Typically, these result from a low-energy mechanism of injury such as ground-level fall.
- The most common fracture pattern is extra-articular, followed by bicolumnar or complete articular.

Classification

- AO/Orthopaedic Trauma Association (AO/OTA) classification[5]
  - 13A: extra-articular fracture
    - 13A1: extra-articular, avulsion fracture

Namdari S, Zmistowski B, Omid R, eds.
The Foundations of Shoulder and Elbow Surgery (pp 77-96).

        - 13A2: extra-articular, simple fracture
        - 13A3: extra-articular, wedge or multifragmentary fracture
    - 13B: partial articular
        - 13B1: partial articular, lateral sagittal fracture
        - 13B2: partial articular, medial sagittal fracture
        - 13B3: partial articular, frontal/coronal plane fracture
    - 13C: complete articular
        - 13C1: complete, simple articular, simple metaphyseal fracture
        - 13C2: complete, simple articular, wedge or multifragmentary metaphyseal fracture
        - 13C3: complete, multifragmentary articular, simple, wedge or multifragmentary metaphyseal fracture
- Milch classification (for single-column condyle fractures)[6]
        - Type I: intact lateral trochlear ridge
        - Type II: fractured lateral trochlear ridge
- Jupiter classification (for 2-column distal humerus fractures)[7]
    - High-T
    - Low-T
    - Y
    - H
    - Medial lambda
    - Lateral lambda
    - Multiplane T
- Mehne and Matta classification (based on intraoperative appearance)[8]
    - Intra-articular
    - Extra-articular intracapsular
    - Extracapsular

Diagnosis

- Presentation: elbow pain and swelling
- Physical examination
    - Pain with palpation of elbow
    - Soft-tissue evaluation: ecchymosis; abrasions; open injuries (commonly posterior)
    - Sensory and motor examination (median, radial, and ulnar nerve)
- Imaging
    - Radiographs
        - Anteroposterior (AP) and lateral x-rays of elbow (Figure 5-1A)
        - Humerus, forearm, and wrist radiographs
        - Traction views are often helpful (Figure 5-1B).
    - Computed tomography (CT)
        - May provide further information regarding elements of complex articular fracture patterns: impaction, comminution
        - Three-dimensional reconstructions may be helpful.
        - Helpful in determining decision for open reduction internal fixation (ORIF) vs arthroplasty

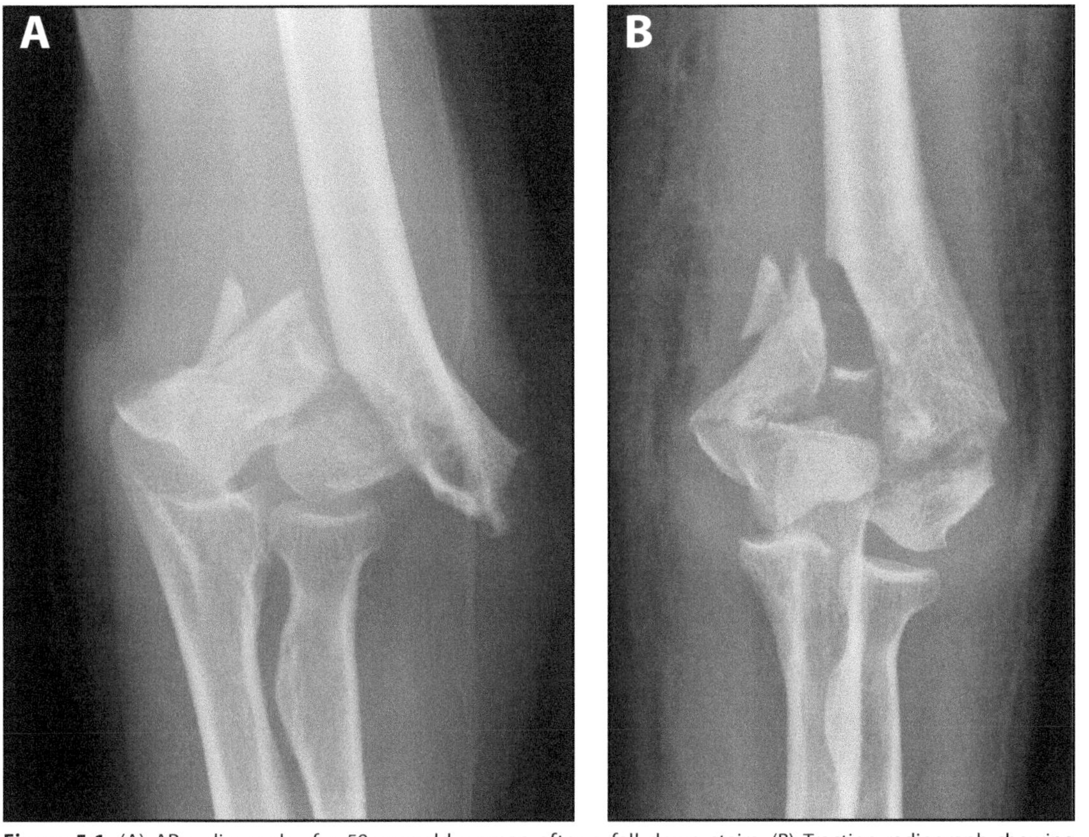

Figure 5-1. (A) AP radiograph of a 59-year-old woman after a fall down stairs. (B) Traction radiograph showing improved identification of the distal humerus fracture fragments.

Applied Anatomy

- The elbow joint is a trocho-ginglymoid joint with rotatory (trochoid) motion through the radiocapitellar joint and proximal radioulnar joint (PRUJ) and hinge-like (ginglymoid) motion through the ulnohumeral joint.
- The distal humeral shaft is triangular in shape and splits into 2 cortical columns; the medial column diverges at approximately 45 degrees from the shaft and the lateral column diverges at approximately 25 degrees from the shaft.
- The medial epicondyle gives rise to the ulnar collateral ligament and the common flexor tendon, which is composed of the following:
    - Pronator teres
    - Flexor carpi radialis
    - Palmaris longus
    - Flexor digitorum superficialis
    - Flexor carpi ulnaris
- The lateral epicondyle gives rise to the lateral (radial) collateral ligament and common extensor tendon, which is composed of the following:
    - Extensor carpi radialis brevis
    - Extensor digitorum communis

    - Extensor digiti minimi
    - Extensor carpi ulnaris
- The distal humerus articular surface is in 4 to 8 degrees of valgus relative to the shaft (trochlea is more distal than the capitellum) and 3 to 8 degrees of internal rotation in the axial plane.
    - The medial portion of the articular surface is named the trochlea. The trochlea articulates with the greater sigmoid notch of ulna.
    - The lateral portion of the articular surface is named the capitellum. The capitellum articulates with the radial head.
- Nervous anatomy
    - Ulnar nerve: travels behind the medial epicondyle to enter the cubital tunnel and then exits between the 2 heads of the flexor carpi ulnaris
    - Radial nerve: enters the spiral groove 20 cm proximal to the medial epicondyle and exits the groove approximately 14 cm proximal to the lateral epicondyle
        - At risk with exposure of proximal extension of distal humerus fractures and application of long posterior/direct lateral plate along the humeral shaft
    - Median nerve: travels with brachial artery between biceps and brachialis and then passes under the bicipital aponeurosis to enter the medial antecubital fossa
        - Relatively protected during fixation of distal humerus fractures by the brachialis muscle
- Vascular anatomy
    - The brachial artery courses with the median nerve. As the brachial artery crosses the cubital fossa, it travels under the brachialis muscle and terminates into the radial and ulnar arteries.

Treatment

- Nonoperative management
    - Technique
        - Cast immobilization: long arm (rarely recommended)
        - Most distal humerus fractures (even nondisplaced) cannot be controlled with cast immobilization and will result in a malunion.
    - Indications
        - Nondisplaced Milch type 1 fractures
        - Older patients with comorbidities precluding operative management[9]
- Operative management
    - Surgical approaches[10] *Recommended reading for understanding the differences in surgical approaches to the distal humerus*
        - Olecranon osteotomy
        - Triceps splitting (Campbell)
        - Triceps sparing
        - Triceps reflecting (Bryan-Morrey)
    - Fixation options
        - Closed reduction and percutaneous pinning
            - Indications
                - Displaced Milch type 1 fractures
        - ORIF
            - Fixation principles[11] *Recommended reading for further understanding of these widely accepted surgical fixation principles*

- Two principles
  - Fixation in the distal fragment must be maximized.
  - All fixation in distal fragments should contribute to stability between the distal fragments and the shaft.
- Eight technical objectives (Figure 5-2)
  1. Every screw in the distal fragments should pass through a plate.
  2. Engage a fragment on the opposite side that is also fixed to a plate.
  3. As many screws as possible should be placed in the distal fragments.
  4. Each screw should be as long as possible.
  5. Each screw should engage as many articular fragments as possible.
  6. The screws in the distal fragments should interdigitate, creating a fixed-angle structure and a biomechanically stable arch.
  7. Plates should be applied so compression is achieved at the supracondylar level for both columns.
  8. The plates must be strong enough and stiff enough to resist breaking or bending before union occurs at the supracondylar level.
- Most biomechanical studies prefer parallel plating vs orthogonal plating.[12-17]
  - Only one randomized clinical study[18]
    - Did not advocate for one technique over the other

- Total elbow arthroplasty
  - Indications[19]
    - Complex/distal fractures in low-functioning older patients with poor bone quality
    - Distal humerus fractures in patients with rheumatoid arthritis
      - Survival rates for elbows with rheumatoid arthritis were 85% at 5 years and 76% at 10 years, and for elbows without rheumatoid arthritis the survival rate was 92% both at 5 and 10 years.[19]
  - Contraindications
    - Active infection
    - Insufficient soft-tissue coverage
  - Five- to 10-pound (2.26 to 4.5 kg) weight-lifting restrictions (5-pounds repetitive lifting and 10-pounds one-time lifting) postoperatively for life
  - Consider a 2-stage reconstruction with use of an interim antibiotic bead-pouch in the setting of an open, nonreconstructable fracture

Olecranon Fractures

Epidemiology/Mechanism of Injury[20]

- Account for approximately 10% of elbow fractures
- Bimodal distribution
  - Young patients likely resulting from high-energy injury
  - Older patients likely resulting from low-energy falls

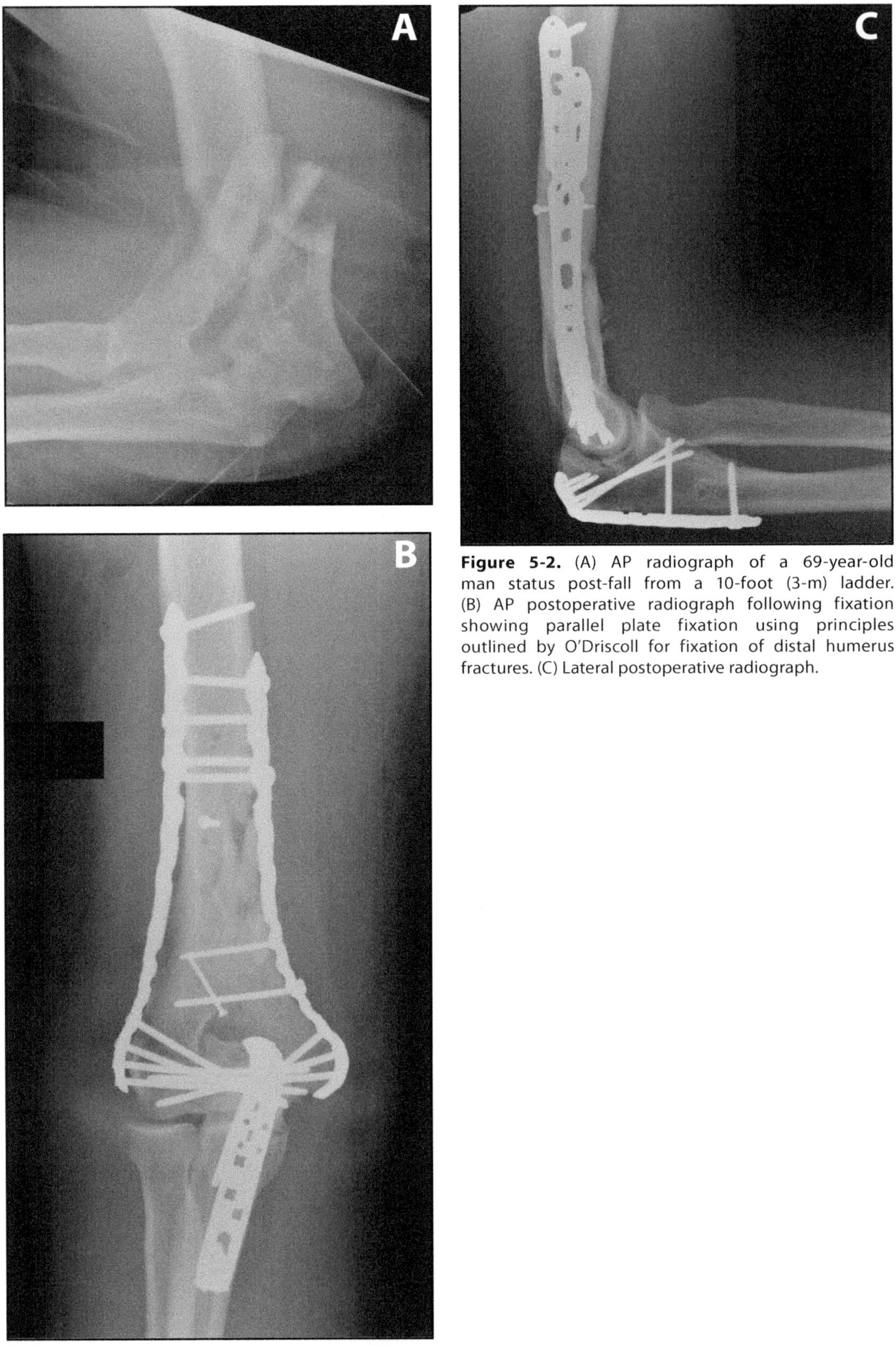

Figure 5-2. (A) AP radiograph of a 69-year-old man status post-fall from a 10-foot (3-m) ladder. (B) AP postoperative radiograph following fixation showing parallel plate fixation using principles outlined by O'Driscoll for fixation of distal humerus fractures. (C) Lateral postoperative radiograph.

Classification

- Mayo classification[21]
  - Type I: undisplaced
  - Type II: displaced, stable
    - A: noncomminuted
    - B: comminuted
  - Type III: unstable
    - A: noncomminuted
    - B: comminuted
- Schatzker-Schmeling classification[22]
  - A: transverse
  - B: transverse-impacted
  - C: oblique
  - D: comminuted
  - E: oblique-distal
  - F: fracture-dislocation
- AO classification: (21-)
  - Type A: extra-articular
  - Type B: intra-articular
  - Type C: intra-articular fractures of both radial head and olecranon

Diagnosis

- Physical examination
  - Comprehensive examination for systemic injuries
  - Examine for open wounds
  - Careful neurovascular exam
  - Evaluate for shoulder, forearm, wrist, and hand injuries.
- Imaging
  - AP and lateral views of elbow (Figure 5-3A)
  - CT scan may be helpful for preoperative planning.

Applied Anatomy

- Proximal ulna has 2 articulations
  - Ulnohumeral joint
  - PRUJ
- Articular surface
  - The greater sigmoid notch is covered in articular cartilage and comprises the ulnohumeral articulation.
    - Bare area at the base of the coronoid process
  - Radial aspect of proximal ulna (lesser sigmoid notch) with articular cartilage that articulates with radial head at the PRUJ
- Olecranon prevents anterior subluxation
  - Excision of more than 87.5% of the olecranon leads to gross instability[23]

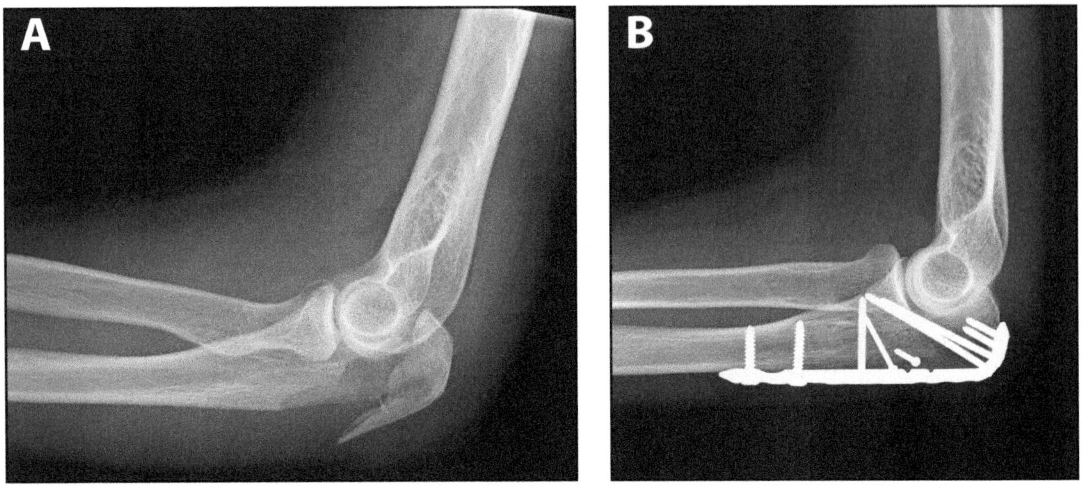

Figure 5-3. (A) Lateral radiograph of a 52-year-old woman status post-fall from bicycle showing a simple oblique olecranon fracture. (B) Lateral postoperative radiograph showing anatomic reduction, lag screw, and neutralization plate fixation of olecranon fracture.

- The triceps tendon broadly inserts onto the proximal ulna. The medial portion of the triceps tendon is more tendinous, whereas the lateral portion of the tendon has a broad fascial expansion.[24]

Treatment

- Nonoperative management
  - Indications
    - Nondisplaced or minimally displaced fracture with maintained reduction with elbow flexion
    - Low-demand older patients with displaced olecranon fractures involving less than 75% of the greater sigmoid notch[25]
  - Technique
    - Elbow splinted for 2 to 3 weeks and then gentle active-assisted flexion. Active extension restricted for first 6 weeks, then active ROM allowed. Resistance exercises started at 3 months.
- Operative management
  - Indications
    - Displaced intra-articular olecranon fracture
  - Operative techniques
    - Olecranon excision and triceps advancement[26]
      - For osteoporotic bone with significant comminution
      - Excised fragment should be less than 75%
      - Heavy, nonabsorbable No. 5 suture placed in triceps tendon and sutured to proximal ulna through 2 mm drill holes. Avoid dorsal placement of knot.
      - Olecranon excision with triceps advancement should rarely be performed.
    - ORIF with tension banding[27]
      - Indicated for simple, transverse, noncomminuted olecranon fractures
    - ORIF with plating (Figure 5-3B)

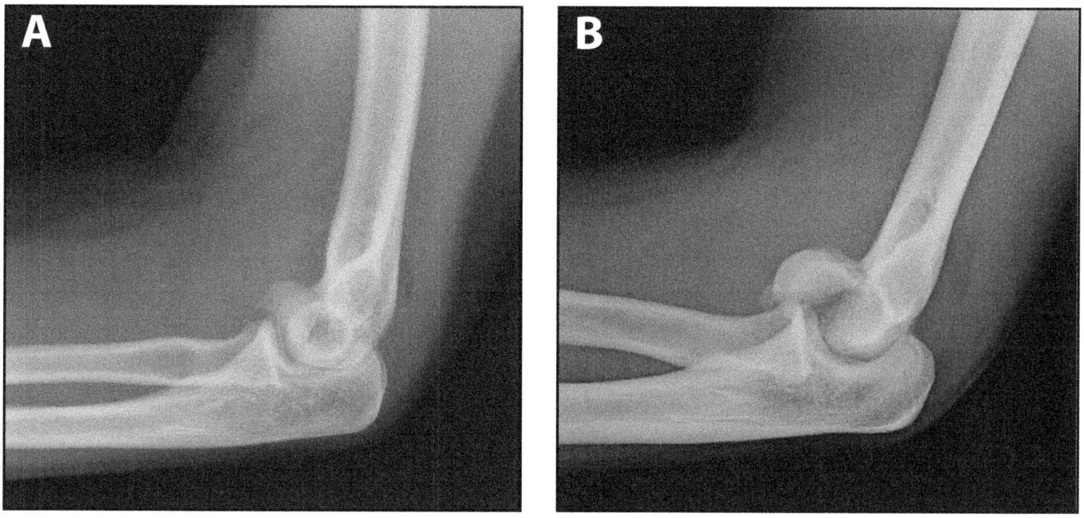

Figure 5-4. Lateral radiograph of Bryan and Morrey (A) type I and (B) type IV capitellum fracture.

- Indicated for olecranon fractures with comminution, elbow instability, and fractures that extend down the ulnar shaft

Capitellum Fractures

Epidemiology/Mechanism of Injury[28]

- Isolated injuries of capitellum are rare (approximately 1% of elbow injuries)
- Patients are generally younger than 12 years old
- More common in girls
- Result of fall on outstretched hand with axial force transmitted to the capitellum by the radial head

Classification

- Bryan and Morrey classification[29]
  - Type I (Hahn-Steinthal): coronal shear fracture resulting in osteochondral fragment (Figure 5-4A)
  - Type II (Kocher-Lorenz): coronal shear fracture with cartilaginous fragment without subchondral bone attached
  - Type III: comminuted capitellar fracture
  - Type IV: coronal shear fracture of the capitellum and trochlea as single fragment (Figure 5-4B)

Diagnosis

- Physical examination
  - May have ecchymosis, swelling, or obvious deformity
  - Evaluate for mechanical block to motion.
  - Perform thorough neurovascular examination.

- Imaging
    - Lateral radiographs of the elbow are usually diagnostic.
    - AP radiograph of elbow may appear normal.
    - CT scan may be performed if helpful for preoperative planning.

Applied Anatomy

- The capitellum is an important static stabilizer involved in longitudinal and valgus stability through the radiocapitellar joint.
- The center of rotation of the capitellum is 12 to 15 mm anterior to the humeral shaft (vulnerable to coronal shearing).

Treatment

- Nonoperative management
    - Indications
        - Nondisplaced type I and II fractures
    - Technique
        - Posterior molded long arm splint immobilization for less than 3 weeks
- Operative management
    - Approaches
        - Lateral column approach (between triceps and brachioradialis)[30]
        - Anterolateral approach (brachialis and brachioradialis proximally and brachioradialis and pronator teres distally)
        - Olecranon osteotomy (preferred for posterior/medial involvement of distal humerus fractures)
    - Treatment options
        - Fragment excision[31]
            - Indicated for displaced type II and III fractures because they are not amenable to fixation
        - ORIF
            - Indicated for displaced type I fractures and type IV fractures
            - Fixation options
                - Headless screws
                - 4 mm partially threaded screws
                - Kirschner wires
                - Absorbable pins
        - Total elbow arthroplasty
            - Indicated for older, low-demand patients with unreconstructable capitellar fractures with medial column instability[32]

Coronoid Fractures

- Coronoid fractures usually occur in association with elbow dislocations.
- They are part of the injury complex known as the "terrible triad."

Epidemiology/Mechanism of Injury

- They occur in approximately 2% to 15% of patients with elbow dislocation.[33]
- Although the specific mechanism of coronoid fracture varies, they are usually associated with elbow dislocations, which tend to occur from high-energy episodes such as falls and motor vehicle accidents.

Classification

- Regan and Morrey[34]
    - Type I: fracture involving the tip of the coronoid
    - Type II: fracture involving more than the tip but less than 50% of the coronoid
    - Type III: fracture involving greater than 50% of the coronoid
- O'Driscoll classification[35]
    - Type I: coronoid tip fracture
        - 1: less than or equal to 2 mm of coronoid bony height
        - 2: greater than or equal to 2 mm of coronoid bony height
    - Type II: anteromedial facet fracture
        - 1: anteromedial rim
        - 2: anteromedial rim + tip
        - 3: anteromedial rim + sublime tubercle ± tip
    - Type III: coronoid base fracture
        - 1: coronoid body and base
        - 2: transolecranon basal coronoid fracture

Diagnosis

- Presentation
    - Swelling, tenderness, and limited elbow ROM
- Physical examination
    - A comprehensive physical examination is warranted because these fractures are associated with high-energy mechanisms.
    - Include a neurologic examination.
    - Assess elbow ROM.
    - Conduct a varus/valgus stability test.
- Imaging
    - AP and lateral radiographs of the elbow should be taken (Figure 5-5)
    - A CT scan may be required to better assess the fracture pattern.

Applied Anatomy

- The coronoid acts as a bony buttress to prevent posterior dislocation of the elbow.
- The anteromedial facet provides restraint to varus instability.
- Three soft-tissue attachments to the coronoid provide stability.
    - Anterior joint capsule of elbow
    - Brachialis muscle

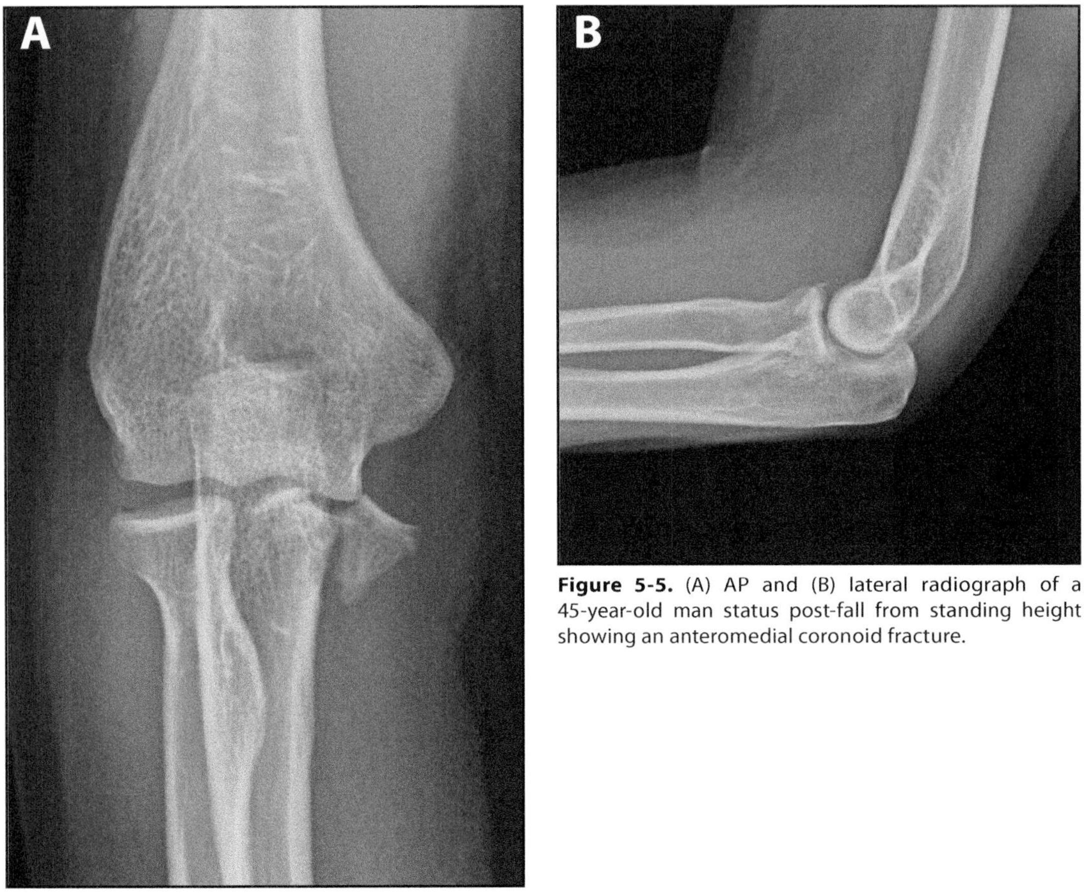

Figure 5-5. (A) AP and (B) lateral radiograph of a 45-year-old man status post-fall from standing height showing an anteromedial coronoid fracture.

- Medial ulnar collateral ligament
    - Attaches to the anteromedial facet of coronoid (sublime tubercle)

Treatment

- Nonoperative management
    - Indications
        - Regan and Morrey types I, II, and III that are nondisplaced and stable
    - Technique
        - A brief period of immobilization followed by early elbow ROM is recommended.
- Operative management[36]
    - Indications
        - Unstable Regan and Morrey type I, II, and III fractures
    - Technique
        - ORIF of coronoid
            - Large coronoid fractures can be rigidly fixed with retrograde cannulated screws or buttress plate fixation.
            - Small or comminuted fractures can be fixed by suturing the bone and anterior capsule to the anterior ulna, using pull-out sutures or suture anchors.

Radial Head Fractures

Epidemiology/Mechanism of Injury[37]

- Most common fractures of the elbow
- Incidence 2.5 to 2.9 per 10,000 people per year
- Most common between 20 and 60 years old
- Mechanisms of radial head injury
  - The valgus load causes impaction of radial head into the capitellum
  - Posterolateral rotary subluxation of the radial head
  - Axial forearm load causes impaction of the radial head into the capitellum

Classification

- Mason classification[38]
  - Type I: fissure or marginal sector fracture without displacement
  - Type II: fissure or marginal sector fracture with displacement
  - Type III: comminuted fracture
  - Type IV: radial head fracture associated with elbow dislocation
- Broberg and Morrey modification[39]
  - Type I: nondisplaced or displaced less than 2 mm that involves less than 30% of articular surface
  - Type II: displaced greater than 2 mm and involves more than 30% of articular surface
  - Type III: comminuted

Diagnosis

- Physical examination
    - Perform a comprehensive examination for systemic injuries.
    - Examine for open wounds.
    - Perform a careful neurovascular exam.
    - Evaluate for mechanical block to motion.
      - Injection of local anesthesia in the elbow joint may assist in evaluation.
    - Evaluate elbow for stability
      - The lateral pivot shift test assesses the lateral ulnar collateral ligament.
      - Valgus stress test to assess the medial collateral ligament
    - Evaluate for shoulder, forearm, wrist, hand injuries.
      - It is important to determine whether there is distal radioulnar joint or interosseous membrane injury.
- Imaging
    - AP and lateral radiographs of the elbow should be taken (Figure 5-6A).
    - A CT scan may be helpful for preoperative planning.

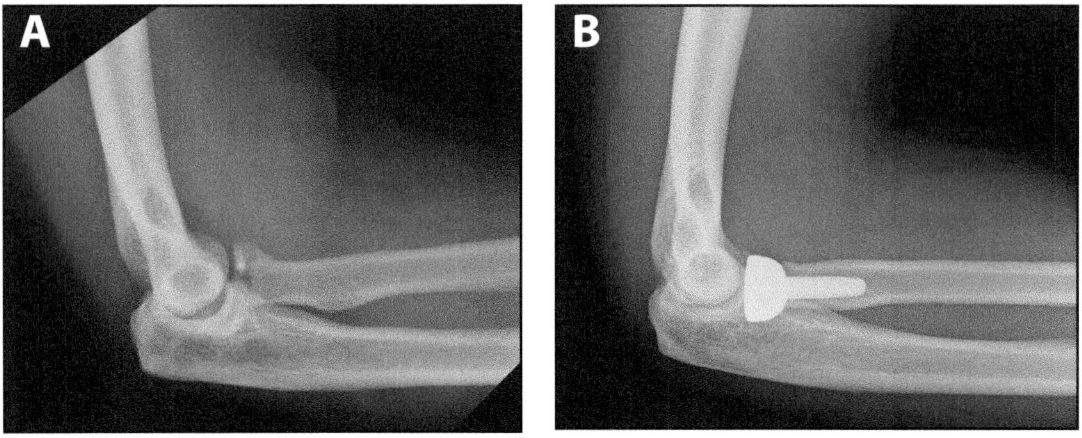

Figure 5-6. (A) Lateral radiograph of a 35-year-old female status post-fall down stairs with a partial articular radial head fracture. (B) Lateral radiograph of a 42-year-old man status post-radial head arthroplasty.

Applied Anatomy

- Radial head
  - The concave dish articulates with the capitellum.
  - The flattened articular margin articulates with the lesser sigmoid notch of ulna.
- The safe zone for placement of a plate on the radial head is a 90- to 110-degree arc from the radial styloid to the Lister tubercle, with the arm in neutral rotation.[40]
- Vascular supply to radial head
    - Branches of radial recurrent artery
    - Branch of ulnar artery

Treatment

- Nonoperative management
  - Indications
    - Nondisplaced or minimally displaced radial head fractures without a block to forearm rotation
  - Technique
    - A short period of immobilization followed by early ROM is recommended.
- Operative management
  - Indications
    - Displaced radial head fractures
    - Radial head fractures with block to motion
  - Approaches
    - Kocher (between extensor carpi ulnaris and anconeus)
    - Kaplan (between extensor digitorum communis and extensor carpi radialis brevis)
  - Treatment options
    - Radial head excision[41]
      - This procedure is rarely indicated but can be used for a displaced fracture that comprises less than 25% of the articular diameter not involved in stability.
      - Elbow stability must be evaluated after excision of the fragment.

- Radial head ORIF with plating[42]
  - This procedure is for displaced, noncomminuted fractures of the radial head with block in forearm rotation.
  - The best candidates are younger patients with good bone quality and 3 or fewer fragments.[43]
- Radial head arthroplasty[44] (Figure 5-6B)
  - This procedure is indicated for comminuted radial head fractures with fewer than 3 articular fragments that are not amenable to fixation or excision.

Monteggia Fractures

- Fracture of the shaft of the ulna associated with an anterior dislocation of the radial head was described by an Italian surgeon, Giovanni Battista Monteggia, in 1814.[45]
- In 1943 Watson-Jones wrote "no fracture presents so many problems; no injury is beset with greater difficulty; no treatment is characterized by more general failure."[46]
- The classification based on the direction of the radial head dislocation was created by José Luis Bado in 1967.[47]

Epidemiology/Mechanism of Injury

- Monteggia fractures account for approximately 1% to 2% of forearm fractures.[48]
- They occur primarily from a fall on an outstretched hand with forced pronation. They may also be associated with high-energy trauma (eg, motor vehicle collisions).

Classification

- Bado classification[47]
  - Type I (60%): fracture of proximal or middle third of ulna with anterior radial head dislocation
  - Type II (15%): fracture of proximal or middle third of ulna with posterior radial head dislocation
  - Type III (20%): fracture of proximal or middle third of ulna with lateral radial head dislocation
  - Type IV (5%): fracture of proximal or middle third of ulna and radius with radial head dislocation in any direction

Diagnosis

- Presentation
  - Pain and swelling of the elbow
- Physical examination
  - A thorough clinical examination is warranted, particularly a complete neurologic exam.
    - The patient may have posterior interosseous neuropathy.
  - Evaluate skin integrity.
- Imaging
  - Plain AP and lateral radiographs of the elbow should be taken (Figure 5-7).
  - Obtain radiographs of the ipsilateral forearm, shoulder, and wrist.

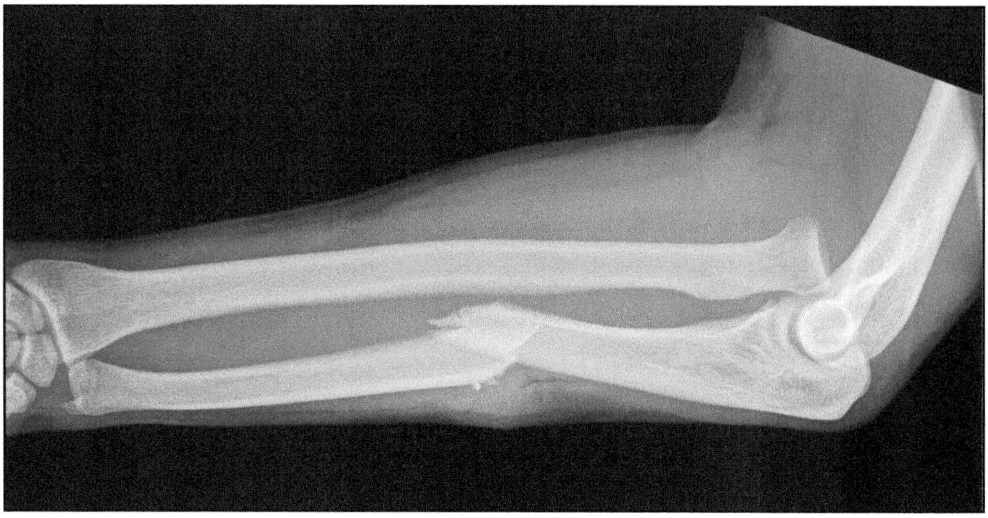

Figure 5-7. Lateral radiograph of a 28-year-old man status post–motor vehicle trauma showing a Monteggia fracture-dislocation; fracture of the middle third of the ulna with radial head dislocation.

- A CT scan of the elbow with 3-dimensional reconstruction may be ordered for preoperative planning.

Applied Anatomy

- The radius and ulna are interconnected at the PRUJ by the annular and quadrate ligaments.
    - The distal radioulnar joint and interosseous membrane remain intact.
        - Anatomic reduction of the ulna generally reduces the radiocapitellar and radioulnar articulations.
- The posterior interosseous nerve travels around the radial neck and splits the supinator as it enters the forearm.

Treatment

- Nonoperative management
    - Closed reduction should be attempted at the initial presentation.
    - Reduction technique
        - Perform supination of the forearm with gentle traction and direct pressure on the radial head.
    - Definitive nonoperative management may be attempted with children if there is anatomic reduction.[49]
- Operative management
    - Indications
        - Open fractures warrant surgery.
        - Most adult fractures are treated operatively.
    - Treatment (Figure 5-8)
        - ORIF of the ulna
            - A 3.5 mm standard or anatomically precontoured proximal ulna plate is recommended.

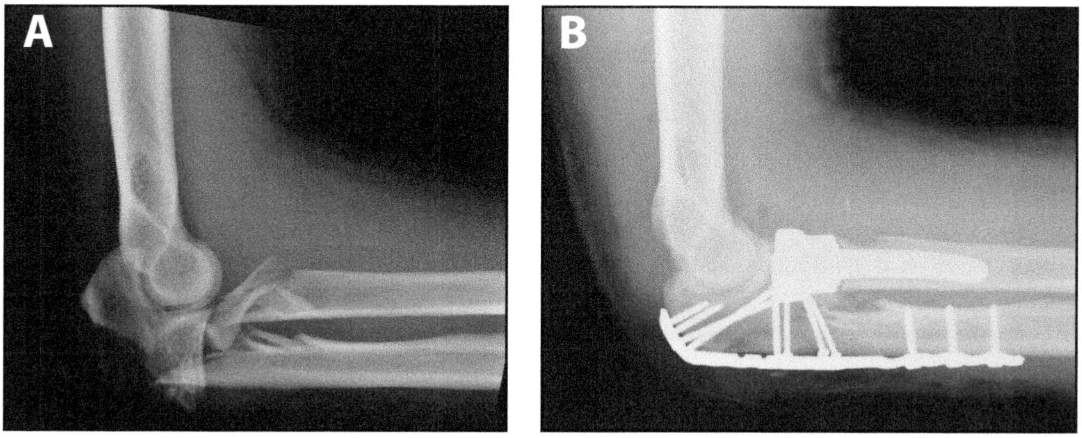

Figure 5-8. (A) Lateral radiograph of a 60-year-old man status post–motor vehicle trauma with a type IV Monteggia fracture-dislocation; fracture of the proximal ulna and radius with dislocation of the radial head. (B) Lateral postoperative radiograph showing plate and screw fixation of the ulna and radial head arthroplasty.

- Anatomic reduction of the ulna generally reduces the radial head.
  - If the radial head does not reduce after reduction of the ulna, ulnar reduction should be reevaluated. If malreduction still persists, interposed capsular tissue may be the cause.
- If the radial head is fractured, use treatment guidelines for radial head fractures.
- Postoperatively, the elbow should be splinted in supination.

Transolecranon Fracture-Dislocation

- Transolecranon fractures were first described by Biga in 1974.[50]
- These are fractures of the olecranon and anterior dislocation of the radiocapitellar joint with intact ligamentous structures, including the PRUJ.
  - Lateral and medial collateral ligaments may also be intact in this injury pattern.
- Transolecranon fractures are often confused with Bado type 1 Monteggia injuries.

Epidemiology/Mechanism of Injury

- These fractures are very rare and often misdiagnosed elbow injuries.
- Usually they are the result of an axial load on the dorsal aspect of the forearm when the elbow is in mid-flexion position.[51]
  - The distal humerus is driven into the greater sigmoid notch.
- Bimodal distribution of injuries
  - Young adults (high-energy mechanism)
  - Older patients (low-energy mechanism such as ground-level fall)

Classification[50]

- Type 1: simple
- Type 2: comminuted

Diagnosis

- Physical examination
  - A thorough neurological exam includes the median, radial, and ulnar nerves.
  - Assess distal pulses and perfusion.
- Imaging
  - AP/lateral plain radiographs of the elbow should be taken.
  - Also obtain ipsilateral plain radiographs of the wrist and forearm to rule out additional injuries.
  - CT of the elbow may be obtained for comminuted fracture-dislocations for surgical planning.

Treatment

- Nonoperative
  - Closed reduction should be attempted at presentation.
    - Closed reduction usually cannot be maintained because this is an inherently unstable injury and usually requires stable, rigid fixation to achieve anatomic reduction.
- Operative
  - ORIF with plating
    - Focus on restoring ulnar length, alignment, rotation, and particularly the greater sigmoid notch.[52]
    - Ring et al reported results of 17 patients who underwent treatment for transolecranon fracture-dislocations.[53]
      - Fifteen out of 17 patients had excellent or good results.

References

1. Rose SH, Melton LJ III, Morrey BF, Ilstrup DM, Riggs BL. Epidemiologic features of humeral fractures. *Clin Orthop Relat Res*. 1982;(168):24-30. doi:10.1097/00003086-198208000-00003.
2. Anglen J. Distal humerus fractures. *J Am Acad Orthop Surg*. 2005;13(5):291-297. doi:10.5435/00124635-200509000-00001.
3. Robinson CM, Hill RMF, Jacobs N, Dall G, Court-Brown CM. Adult distal humeral metaphyseal fractures: epidemiology and results of treatment. *J Orthop Trauma*. 2003;17(1):38-47. doi:10.1097/00005131-200301000-00006.
4. Varecka TF, Myeroff C. Distal humerus fractures in the elderly population. *J Am Acad Orthop Surg*. 2017;25(10):673-683. doi:10.5435/JAAOS-D-15-00683.
5. Meinberg EG, Agel J, Roberts CS, Karam MD, Kellam JF. Fracture and Dislocation Classification Compendium—2018. *J Orthop Trauma*. 2018;32(suppl 1):S1-S170. doi:10.1097/BOT.0000000000001063.
6. Milch H. Fractures and fracture dislocations of the humeral condyles. *J Trauma*. 1964;4:592-607. doi:10.1097/00005373-196409000-00004.
7. Jupiter JB, Mehne DK. Fractures of the distal humerus. *Orthopedics*. 1992;15(7):825-833.
8. Mehne DK, Matta J. Bicolumn fractures of the adult humerus. Paper presented at: 53rd Annual Meeting of the American Academy of Orthopaedic Surgeons; February 20-25, 1986; New Orleans, LA.
9. Batten TJ, Sin-Hidge C, Brinsden MD, Guyver PM. Non-operative management of distal humerus fractures in the elderly: a review of functional outcomes. *Eur J Orthop Surg Traumatol*. 2018;28(1):23-27. doi:10.1007/s00590-017-2006-9.
10. Pollock JW, Athwal GS, Steinmann SP. Surgical exposures for distal humerus fractures: a review. *Clin Anat*. 2008;21(8):757-768. doi:10.1002/ca.20720.
11. O'Driscoll SW. Optimizing stability in distal humeral fracture fixation. *J Shoulder Elbow Surg*. 2005;14(1 suppl S):S186-S194. doi:10.1016/j.jse.2004.09.033.
12. Arnander MW, Reeves A, MacLeod IA, Pinto TM, Khaleel A. A biomechanical comparison of plate configuration in distal humerus fractures. *J Orthop Trauma*. 2008;22(5):332-336. doi:10.1097/BOT.0b013e31816edbce.

13. Penzkofer R, Hungerer S, Wipf F, von Oldenburg G, Augat P. Anatomical plate configuration affects mechanical performance in distal humerus fractures. *Clin Biomech (Bristol, Avon)*. 2010;25(10):972-978. doi:10.1016/j.clinbiomech.2010.07.005.
14. Schemitsch EH, Tencer AF, Henley MB. Biomechanical evaluation of methods of internal fixation of the distal humerus. *J Orthop Trauma*. 1994;8(6):468-475.
15. Schuster I, Korner J, Arzdorf M, Schwieger K, Diederichs G, Linke B. Mechanical comparison in cadaver specimens of three different 90-degree double-plate osteosyntheses for simulated C2-type distal humerus fractures with varying bone densities. *J Orthop Trauma*. 2008;22(2):113-120. doi:10.1097/BOT.0b013e3181632cf8.
16. Stoffel K, Cunneen S, Morgan R, Nicholls R, Stachowiak G. Comparative stability of perpendicular versus parallel double-locking plating systems in osteoporotic comminuted distal humerus fractures. *J Orthop Res*. 2008;26(6):778-784. doi:10.1002/jor.20528.
17. Zalavras CG, Vercillo MT, Jun BJ, Otarodifard K, Itamura JM, Lee TQ. Biomechanical evaluation of parallel versus orthogonal plate fixation of intra-articular distal humerus fractures. *J Shoulder Elbow Surg*. 2011;20(1):12-20. doi:10.1016/j.jse.2010.08.005.
18. Shin SJ, Sohn HS, Do NH. A clinical comparison of two different double plating methods for intraarticular distal humerus fractures. *J Shoulder Elbow Surg*. 2010;19(1):2-9. doi:10.1016/j.jse.2009.05.003.
19. Barco R, Streubel PN, Morrey BF, Sanchez-Sotelo J. Total elbow arthroplasty for distal humeral fractures: a ten-year-minimum follow-up study. *J Bone Joint Surg Am*. 2017;99(18):1524-1531. doi:10.2106/JBJS.16.01222.
20. Rommens PM, Küchle R, Schneider RU, Reuter M. Olecranon fractures in adults: factors influencing outcome. *Injury*. 2004;35(11):1149-1157. doi:10.1016/j.injury.2003.12.002.
21. Morrey BF. Current concepts in the treatment of fractures of the radial head, the olecranon, and the coronoid. *Instr Course Lect*. 1995;44:175-185.
22. Schatzker J. Fractures of the olecranon (12-B1). In: Schatzker J, Tile M, eds. *The Rationale of Operative Fracture Care*. 3rd ed. Berlin, Heidelberg: Springer Berlin Heidelberg; 1987:123-129. doi:https://doi.org/10.1007/3-540-27708-0.
23. Bell TH, Ferreira LM, McDonald CP, Johnson JA, King GJ. Contribution of the olecranon to elbow stability: an in vitro biomechanical study. *J Bone Joint Surg Am*. 2010;92(4):949-957. doi:10.2106/JBJS.H.01873.
24. Keener JD, Chafik D, Kim MH, Galatz LM, Yamaguchi K. Insertional anatomy of the triceps brachii tendon. *J Shoulder Elbow Surg*. 2010;19(3):399-405. doi:10.1016/j.jse.2009.10.008.
25. Duckworth AD, Bugler KE, Clement ND, Court-Brown CM, McQueen MM. Nonoperative management of displaced olecranon fractures in low-demand elderly patients. *J Bone Joint Surg Am*. 2014;96(1):67-72. doi:10.2106/JBJS.L.01137.
26. Iannuzzi N, Dahners L. Excision and advancement in the treatment of comminuted olecranon fractures. *J Orthop Trauma*. 2009;23(3):226-228. doi:10.1097/BOT.0b013e318199e9e1.
27. Claessen FMAP, van den Bekerom MPJ, van Dijk CN, et al. Tension band wiring for simple olecranon fractures: evaluation of surgical technique. *J Orthop Traumatol*. 2017;18(3):275-281. doi:10.1007/s10195-017-0450-2.
28. Carroll MJ, Athwal GS, King GJ, Faber KJ. Capitellar and trochlear fractures. *Hand Clin*. 2015;31(4):615-630. doi:10.1016/j.hcl.2015.07.001.
29. McKee MD, Jupiter JB, Bamberger HB. Coronal shear fractures of the distal end of the humerus. *J Bone Joint Surg Am*. 1996;78(1):49-54. doi:10.2106/00004623-199601000-00007.
30. Mansat P, Morrey BF. The column procedure: a limited lateral approach for extrinsic contracture of the elbow. *J Bone Joint Surg Am*. 1998;80(11):1603-1615. doi:10.2106/00004623-199811000-00006.
31. Garner MR, Schottel PC, Hotchkiss RN, Daluiski A, Lorich DG. Capitellum fracture fragment excision: a case series. *HSS J*. 2015;11(3):204-208. doi:10.1007/s11420-015-9452-x.
32. Frankle MA, Herscovici D Jr, DiPasquale TG, Vasey MB, Sanders RW. A comparison of open reduction and internal fixation and primary total elbow arthroplasty in the treatment of intraarticular distal humerus fractures in women older than age 65. *J Orthop Trauma*. 2003;17(7):473-480. doi:10.1097/00005131-200308000-00001.
33. Morrey B, Sanchez-Sotelo J. *The Elbow and Its Disorders*. 4th ed. Philadelphia, PA: Saunders Elsevier; 2009.
34. Regan W, Morrey B. Fractures of the coronoid process of the ulna. *J Bone Joint Surg Am*. 1989;71(9):1348-1354.
35. O'Driscoll SW, Jupiter JB, Cohen MS, Ring D, McKee MD. Difficult elbow fractures: pearls and pitfalls. *Instr Course Lect*. 2003;52:113-134.
36. Garrigues GE, Wray WH, Lindenhovius AL, Ring DC, Ruch DS. Fixation of the coronoid process in elbow fracture-dislocations. *J Bone Joint Surg Am*. 2011;93(20):1873-1881. doi:10.2106/JBJS.I.01673.
37. Duckworth AD, Clement ND, Jenkins PJ, Aitken SA, Court-Brown CM, McQueen MM. The epidemiology of radial head and neck fractures. *J Hand Surg Am*. 2012;37(1):112-119. doi:10.1016/j.jhsa.2011.09.034.
38. Mason ML. Some observations on fractures of the head of the radius with a review of one hundred cases. *Br J Surg*. 1954;42(172):123-132. doi:10.1002/bjs.18004217203.
39. Broberg MA, Morrey BF. Results of treatment of fracture-dislocations of the elbow. *Clin Orthop Relat Res*. 1987;(216):109-119.
40. Smith GR, Hotchkiss RN. Radial head and neck fractures: anatomic guidelines for proper placement of internal fixation. *J Shoulder Elbow Surg*. 1996;5(2 pt 1):113-117. doi:10.1016/S1058-2746(96)80005-X.

41. Herbertsson P, Josefsson PO, Hasserius R, Besjakov J, Nyqvist F, Karlsson MK. Fractures of the radial head and neck treated with radial head excision. *J Bone Joint Surg Am.* 2004;86(9):1925-1930. doi:10.2106/00004623-200409000-00010.
42. Adams JE, Sems SA, Steinmann SP. Open treatment of radial head fractures. *JBJS Essent Surg Tech.* 2017;7(4):e35. doi:10.2106/JBJS.ST.15.00073.
43. Ring D, Quintero J, Jupiter JB. Open reduction and internal fixation of fractures of the radial head. *J Bone Joint Surg Am.* 2002;84(10):1811-1815. doi:10.2106/00004623-200210000-00011.
44. Heijink A, Kodde IF, Mulder PG, et al. Radial head arthroplasty: a systematic review. *JBJS Rev.* 2016;4(10):e3. doi:10.2106/JBJS.RVW.15.00095.
45. Moteggia GB. Lussazioni delle ossa delle estremita superiori. In: Moteggia GB, ed. *Instituzioni Chirurgiches.* 2nd ed. Vol. 5. Milan, Italy: Maspero; 1814:131-133.
46. Watson-Jones R. *Fractures and Joint Injuries.* 3rd ed. Baltimore, MD: Williams & Wilkins; 1943.
47. Bado JL. The Monteggia lesion. *Clin Orthop Relat Res.* 1967;50:71-86.
48. Bruce HE, Harvey JP, Wilson JC Jr. Monteggia fractures. *J Bone Joint Surg Am.* 1974;56(8):1563-1576.
49. Wilkins KE. Nonoperative management of pediatric upper extremity fractures or 'don't throw away the cast.' *Tech Orthop.* 2005;20(2):115-141. doi:10.1097/01.bto.0000163032.36943.7f.
50. Biga N, Thomine JM. Trans-olecranal dislocations of the elbow [in French]. *Rev Chir Orthop Reparatrice Appar Mot.* 1974;60(7):557-567.
51. Capito NM, Paxton ES, Green A. Transolecranon fracture-dislocations. In: Tashjian RZ, ed. *The Unstable Elbow: An Evidence-Based Approach to Evaluation and Management.* Cham, Switzerland: Springer International Publishing; 2017:99-109. doi:10.1007/978-3-319-46019-2.
52. Scolaro JA, Beingessner D. Treatment of Monteggia and transolecranon fracture-dislocations of the elbow: a critical analysis review. *JBJS Rev.* 2014;2(1). doi:10.2106/JBJS.RVW.M.00049.
53. Ring D, Jupiter JB, Sanders RW, Mast J, Simpson NS. Transolecranon fracture-dislocation of the elbow. *J Orthop Trauma.* 1997;11(8):545-550. doi:10.1097/00005131-199711000-00001.

6

Elbow Arthritis

Jared R. Thomas, MD and Matthew L. Ramsey, MD

Pathophysiology

- Normal elbow function requires a pain-free, stable articulation capable of completing a functional arc of motion. Compromise of one or more of these properties leads to functional impairment of the elbow. Patients with arthritic elbows describe difficulty or even inability to use the affected limb because of lack of motion and pain.
- As with arthritis of other joints, the primary pathology involves progressive loss and degeneration of articular cartilage followed by osteophyte formation and eventually joint erosion. This results in progressive loss of range of motion, crepitus, and worsening pain.
    - Clinically significant arthritis is less common in the elbow than in other large joints such as the hip, knee, or shoulder.
        - Elbow arthritis is grouped into 3 major types:
            - Primary osteoarthritis (OA)
            - Post-traumatic arthritis
            - Rheumatoid arthritis (RA; inflammatory)

Presentation, Demographics, and Diagnosis

- Primary OA
    - Primary OA of the elbow is uncommon, typically representing fewer than 2% of elbow arthritides.[1,2] This number may be underestimated because it can often be misattributed to post-traumatic arthropathy.
    - The primary pathology of elbow OA involves loss of articular cartilage with osteophyte formation on the olecranon and coronoid as well as in their respective fossae.

Namdari S, Zmistowski B, Omid R, eds.
The Foundations of Shoulder and Elbow Surgery (pp 97-114).

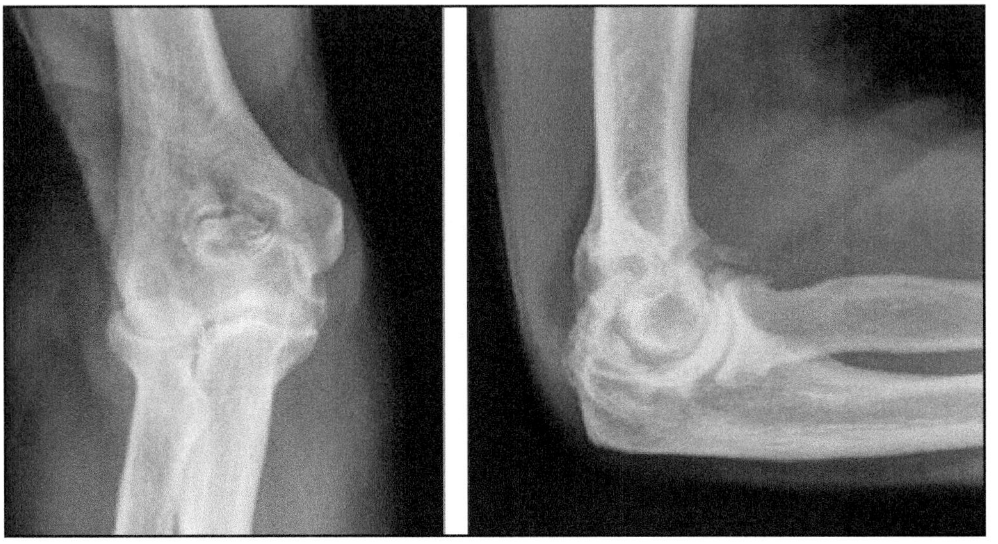

Figure 6-1. Anteroposterior and lateral x-ray of an arthritic elbow. (Reprinted with permission from Matthew L. Ramsey, MD.)

- Secondary resultant changes involve osteophyte formation at the radial head margin and the eventual formation of intra-articular loose bodies.
- Although rare, primary OA of the elbow follows a consistent presentation:
  - The typical patient is a middle-aged (around 50 years old), male, and a heavy laborer.[3,4] The condition is rarely seen in women.
  - Exposure to occupations that involve repetitive use of the upper extremities, heavy lifting, and vibration is commonly reported.[5]
- The dominant extremity is involved in 80% to 90% of patients, with bilateral involvement in 25% to 60% of patients.[6,3]
- Osteoarthritic patients will often have a loss of elbow motion, and most patients complain of pain at the extremes of motion.
  - Terminal extension pain is believed to occur when osteophytes on the olecranon and within the olecranon fossa impinge on each other or interposed soft tissue, whereas terminal flexion pain can be due to similar osteophyte impingement involving the coronoid and the coronoid fossa.
    - Pain with terminal flexion is less frequent than extension pain in primary OA of the elbow.
  - It is common for patients to present with a substantial flexion contracture, often with greater than a 30-degree extension deficit.
  - Forearm pronation and supination is commonly preserved or minimally effected.
  - Ulnar nerve irritation can be observed and has been reported in roughly 10% of patients with OA of the elbow and is thought to be due to local encroachment secondary to excessive humeral osteophyte formation.[7,8]
  - Routine labs including white blood cell count and inflammatory markers are normal.
  - X-rays are diagnostic, and the main characteristic of primary OA is marginal osteophyte formation (Figure 6-1).
    - Routine anteroposterior and true lateral x-rays should be obtained on all patients.
    - Lateral x-rays commonly reveal the following:

Table 6-1

Osteoarthritis and Post-Traumatic Arthritis Classification Systems for the Elbow

BROBERG AND MORREY	HASTINGS AND RETTIG
Grade 1: mild joint space narrowing with minimal osteophyte formation	Class I: degeneration in the margins of the ulnotrochlear joint with the presence of coronoid and olecranon spurring; absence of degenerative changes within the radiocapitellar joint
Grade 2: moderate joint space narrowing with moderate osteophyte formation	Class II: class I with mild joint space narrowing within the radiocapitellar joint, without subluxation of the radial head
Grade 3: severe degenerative change with gross destruction of the joint	Class III: class II with radiocapitellar subluxation

- Anterior osteophytes of the coronoid and distal humerus
- Posterior osteophytes of the olecranon process[9] and distal humerus

▫ Anteroposterior x-rays commonly reveal the following:
- Ossification and osteophyte formation of the olecranon and coronoid fossa

▫ Broberg and Morrey and Hastings and Rettig radiographic classification systems have shown good intraobserver and interobserver reliability (Table 6-1) for both OA and post-traumatic arthritis.[10]

▫ More recently, a computed tomography scan has been recommended after an increased appreciation of the 3-dimensional nature of the disease process.
- Computed tomography scan as well as 3-dimensional reconstructions (Figure 6-2) are helpful when planning surgical resection of impinging osteophytes.[11] *Recommended reading for important change in best practices*

- Inflammatory arthritis
  - The most common and well-described inflammatory arthritis of the elbow is RA, which is considered to be the most common cause of elbow arthritis.
  - Unlike primary OA, RA frequently affects the elbow and can be bilateral.
  - The underlying etiology of RA is that of a synovitis that leads to progressive destruction of the elbow joint.
    - RA primarily involves the ulnohumeral joint early in the disease process, with the remaining segments of the elbow joint becoming involved as the disease progresses.
  - Most patients with RA of the elbow have painful loss of motion and function.
    - Patients will often demonstrate a mild but persistent flexion contracture due to effusion and synovitis, which causes patients to adopt an obligate flexed position to minimize painful joint capsule distention.[12]
    - Neuropathy may be present because inflamed synovium can invade the soft tissues and directly or indirectly lead to compression of the radial and ulnar nerves.
    - With disease progression, ligamentous destruction can also occur, leading to instability.
    - X-rays are diagnostic and several radiographic staging systems have been described:

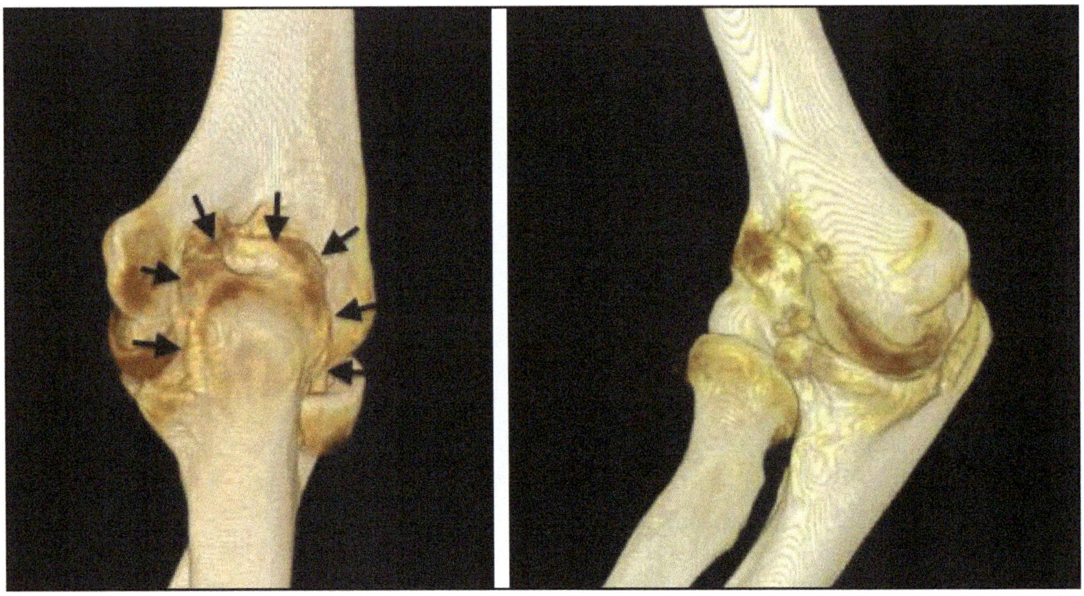

Figure 6-2. Preoperative computed tomography scan 3-dimensional reconstruction showing osteophytes for planned resection. (Reprinted with permission from Matthew L. Ramsey, MD.)

Table 6-2

Mayo Classification of Radiographic Grading of Rheumatoid Arthritis of the Elbow

GRADE	DESCRIPTION
I	Synovitis, but no radiographic changes other than osteoporosis
II	Synovitis persists with narrowing of the joint and intact architecture
III	Variable synovitis with architectural changes of the joint
IV	Gross destruction of the joint
V	Ankylosis of elbow

    - The most commonly used staging systems are the Mayo Classification of Radiographic Grading of Rheumatoid Arthritis of the Elbow (Table 6-2), the Larsen Grading System for Rheumatoid Arthritis (Table 6-3), and the Sharp Classification (Table 6-4).
        - A recent study showed good intraobserver and interobserver reliability with both the Larsen and Sharp classifications.[13]
  - Modern treatment by rheumatologists with disease-modifying anti-rheumatologic drugs (DMARDs) has become the mainstay of treatment and reduced the number of patients requiring surgical intervention.[14]
- Post-traumatic arthritis
  - Unlike the aforementioned types of elbow arthritis, post-traumatic arthritis of the elbow can affect patients of any age or sex.

Table 6-3	
Larsen Grading System for Rheumatoid Arthritis	
GRADE	**DESCRIPTION**
1	Soft-tissue changes with near normal x-rays
2	Periarticular erosions and mild cartilage loss, evidence of soft-tissue swelling, and osteopenia
3	Marked joint space narrowing
4	Advanced erosion with penetration of the subchondral plate
5	Advanced joint damage and loss of articular contour

Table 6-4	
Sharp Classification	
JOINT SPACE NARROWING	**EROSION**
Normal = 0	Normal = 0
Focal joint narrowing = 1	Discrete erosions = 1
Narrowing < 50% of joint = 2	Larger erosion (by surface area) = 2 to 3
Narrowing > 50% of joint = 3	Erosions passing midline = 4
Ankylosis = 4	Complete collapse = 5
Total score = Joint space narrowing score + erosion score. Higher score indicates greater severity.	

- It is most commonly encountered as the sequela of comminuted, intra-articular fractures of the elbow but may also be seen after an elbow dislocation.
- Residual ligamentous insufficiency and resultant instability may also lead to articular wear and progressive arthritis in the post-traumatic elbow.
- Despite the occasional presence of instability, stiffness is often the main complaint in patients with post-traumatic arthritis of the elbow, followed by pain.
- Whereas treatment for OA and RA is more standardized, treatment for post-traumatic arthrosis is individualized depending on the functional demands, age, occupation, and degree of injury.

Treatment

Nonoperative Management

- The goal of nonoperative management of elbow arthritis is to preserve range of motion and function while alleviating stiffness and minimize pain and inflammation.
- Several modalities exist to treat the painful and stiff arthritic elbow:

- Symptoms may be controlled by activity modification, medications, and intra-articular corticosteroid injections.
- Range of motion may improve with physical therapy and dynamic or static splinting.
- Physical therapy
  - Physical therapy is aimed at improving motion and decreasing pain and inflammation in the arthritic elbow.
  - Caution should be used because aggressive physical therapy of an arthritic, stiff elbow can worsen inflammation, increase pain, and even lead to soft-tissue injury.
  - Helpful approaches include active assist range of motion, as well as gentle passive stretch, coupled with modalities to reduce pain such as heat, cold treatments, or iontophoresis or phonophoresis.
- Splinting
  - A popular nonoperative method of treating elbow stiffness is static or dynamic splinting.
  - Splinting is typically continued for 6 to 12 months as long as progress is observed.
  - Similar to physical therapy, exercise caution with dynamic splinting to prevent worsening inflammation, soft-tissue injury, and increased pain.
  - A recent systematic review of post-traumatic elbow stiffness showed range of motion improvement of 36 degrees and 37 degrees respectively for static and dynamic splinting.[15]
- Medical/symptomatic management
  - As with arthritis in other joints, nonsteroidal anti-inflammatory drugs are commonly used to control pain.
    - Long-term use may increase risks of gastrointestinal complications.
  - Agents such as antimalarial drugs, gold salts, and immunosuppressives such as corticosteroids are more aggressive options that have proven beneficial, especially in the treatment of RA.
    - These medications fall into the category of the aforementioned DMARDs and should be managed by a rheumatologist.
  - Injections
    - Corticosteroid injections can prove useful in alleviating symptoms of acute arthritic flairs; however, effects typically diminish over time.
    - Viscosupplementation has not been effective for use in the arthritic elbow and is not currently approved by the Food and Drug Administration for the treatment of elbow arthritis.[16]

Operative Management

- Indications for surgery
  - Surgical management of elbow arthritis is considered in patients with painful, limited range of motion not responsive to nonoperative management.
  - Treatment options are based on the underlying pathology and the extent of the disease process.
  - Periarticular- and synovial-based symptoms are treated with surgery directed at managing the disease process to limit symptoms and preserve the articular cartilage.
  - Articular-based symptoms are managed surgically by addressing the joint surface.
- Patients who fail nonoperative are candidates for surgical intervention.

- Young patients (less than 60 years old for OA and less than 40 years old for RA), high-demand, or patients with early-stage arthritis should be managed with procedures other than total elbow arthroplasty (TEA) in most cases.
- Currently, there are 3 main surgical alternatives to TEA:
  - Open debridement/synovectomy
  - Arthroscopic debridement/synovectomy
  - Interposition arthroplasty
- Other options for treating painful arthritic elbows include resection arthroplasty and arthrodesis; however, both are rarely indicated and are now primarily considered to be salvage procedures.
- The ulnar nerve requires evaluation in all patients with elbow stiffness. Patients with less than 90 degrees of flexion preoperatively should have an ulnar nerve decompression or transposition as part of the surgical procedure.

- Open debridement
  - Open debridement is performed with the aim of removing loose bodies and osteophytes from the humerus and ulna (and occasionally the radius) to improve the impingement-free arc of the elbow.
    - This procedure is contraindicated in patients with symptomatic cartilage destruction with significant loss of motion and pain throughout the mid-arc of motion. Other important contraindications include the following:
      - Instability, especially in patients with advanced RA.
    - A number of procedures have been described, the most common currently being used are discussed in the following bullet points.
  - Outerbridge-Kashiwagi procedure (O-K) and ulnohumeral arthroplasty
    - O-K and ulnohumeral arthroplasty are indicated in the patient with painful osteophyte impingement and subsequent loss of motion.
    - Originally described by Outerbridge and then reported in 1978 by Kashiwagi, the O-K procedure allows for debridement of osteophytes on the olecranon, olecranon fossa, and coronoid.
    - Modified by Morrey to include osteophyte removal from the ulnar and humeral articular margins (altering the joint, hence making it an arthroplasty) as well as the use of a trephine, the procedure was termed ulnohumeral arthroplasty.
    - The technique of ulnohumeral arthroplasty can be combined with a lateral column or medial over-the-top approach.
  - Ulnohumeral arthroplasty (modified O-K) technique
    - The modified O-K technique includes posterior exposure of the elbow via a triceps-splitting or medial triceps-reflecting approach.
    - The tip of the olecranon and surrounding osteophytes are removed.
      - A trephine is used to widen and deepen the olecranon fossa, eventually penetrating through the anterior cortex of the distal humerus.
      - One must be cognizant of the contour of trochlea and direct the trephine proximally to compensate for the anterior flare of the distal humerus.
        - Errant trephine placement can result in increased risks:
          - Fracture if the trajectory is too medial or lateral, compromising either osseous column
          - Articular damage if trajectory is too distal, resulting in violation of the trochlea or capitellar cartilage

    - Working through the trephined hole in the distal humerus, transhumeral debridement of the coronoid fossa, coronoid osteophytes, and supracapitellar recess is performed.
    - Anterior capsular contracture is difficult to address through this exposure.
    - The ulnar nerve can be decompressed and/or transposed through the same surgical approach when compressive neuropathy is present.
    - Most reports indicate substantial improvement in pain relief and improvement in painless range of motion (especially terminal extension pain) in the short- and mid-term.[17]
        - However, long-term studies have found the initial success wanes for some patients over time.[18]
        - Minami and colleagues reported 90% patients had marked pain relief in the early postoperative period after treatment with the O-K procedure.[7] However, only 55% of patients had enduring improvement at 10-year follow-up.
- Column procedure
    - The column procedure is most useful for anterior and posterior capsulectomy in patients with extrinsic contractures.
        - It may also be used for intrinsic sources of stiffness such as debridement of osteophytes, removal of loose bodies, and recontouring of the distal humerus and proximal olecranon.
    - Principles are to remove bony impingement, improve range of motion, and reshape articular segments if necessary.
    - Technique
        - A lateral incision is made directly over the lateral column of the distal humerus and extended distally along a standard Kocher approach.
        - The anterior interval uses release of the extensor carpi radialis longus from the lateral column with distal extension into the common extensor tendons.
        - The posterior interval uses an extended Kocher approach on the lateral elbow.
        - Take care to preserve the lateral ulnar collateral ligament.
        - Anterior and posterior capsules are removed, as are osteophytes.
    - This procedure allows for debridement of the anterior ulnohumeral, posterior ulnohumeral, and radiocapitellar joint spaces.
        - Capsular contracture may be addressed by capsulectomy.
            - Take care to protect the radial and median nerve during anterior capsulectomy and the ulnar nerve during posterior capsulectomy.
    - The radial head is often not involved (especially in primary OA), and resection is rarely indicated or advised.
    - Predictable improvements in range of motion and pain relief from bony impingement are expected.
        - Oka reported an average of 24 degrees of improvement in motion and good pain relief in 50 laborers and athletes treated with open debridement. Long-term follow-up was limited; however, 90% had minimal pain, preserved motion, and all resumed their prior occupation or sport.[19]
        - Tsuge and Mizuseki similarly reported 34 degrees of improvement in motion and good pain relief in patients followed for 64 months.[20]
    - A medial approach can also be helpful.
        - It allows access to the ulnar nerve.

        - In cases in which elbow flexion remains limited after capsulectomy, the medial approach allows for release of the posterior band of the medial collateral ligament, which has been shown to markedly improve elbow flexion in this setting.[21,22]
        - In addition to medial access, an "over-the-top" approach described by Hotchkiss and Kasparyan[23] allows for access to anterior and posterior structures.
            - The obvious drawback to using a medial-only approach is the inability to address laterally based pathology, especially osteophytes in the lateral gutter and along the posterior aspect of the capitellum.
- Arthroscopic debridement
- Historically, indications for arthroscopic debridement consisted primarily of loose body removal and modest debridement.
- More recently, improved techniques have led to expanded indications for the use of arthroscopy to treat a variety of elbow pathologies.
- Indications for arthroscopic debridement are similar to that of open debridement.
- It is contraindicated in some patients:
    - Those with prior elbow surgery or trauma resulting in distorted anatomy (especially neurovascular anatomy)
    - Those with previous ulnar nerve transposition, which may be overcome by open exposure of the nerve prior to establishing medial portals
    - Those with inadequate joint space to allow cannula entry and/or joint distention
- Technique
    - Patient positioning is per surgeon preference.
        - Lateral decubitus with arm over padded bolster
        - Prone, or supine with the arm suspended or supported
    - A tourniquet is recommended.
    - Prior to establishing portals, the joint is insufflated via posterolateral "soft spot" with 10 to 25 cm^3 of normal saline, depending on the underlying pathology.
    - The arthroscope is then introduced via proximal anteromedial portal for anterior joint inspection.
    - Proximal anterolateral or anterolateral portals are established under direct visualization as working portals.
        - Accessory medial and lateral portals may be necessary for additional access or retractor placement.
    - Next, the posterior joint is visualized after establishing a midline posterior portal 3 cm proximal to the olecranon fossae.
        - A posterolateral working portal is also established.
    - Debridement, removal of loose bodies, reshaping of distal humerus, synovectomy, and capsulotomy all can be performed.
- Overall results of arthroscopic debridement are similar to open procedures for pain relief, range of motion, and patient satisfaction.[24-26]
    - Arthroscopy, however, provides the possible benefit of decreased perioperative pain and earlier onset of motion/therapy.
        - Savoie and colleagues reported an average increase of 81 degrees of motion and a significant decrease in pain in 24 patients.[27]
        - A prospective study comparing the O-K procedure with an arthroscopic variant found no difference in patient satisfaction between procedures. However, the authors

noted more complete debridement/release in the open O-K procedure, and as a result, significantly more flexion was seen in these patients postoperatively.[28]

- Synovectomy
    - Synovectomy is primarily indicated in patients with early-stage RA who present with painful synovitis that has been refractory to nonoperative measures.
    - The primary goal is to relieve pain.
    - Improved medical management of RA has lessened the role of surgical synovectomy.
    - It may be performed in open fashion or arthroscopically.
    - Technique
        - Open synovectomy is typically performed via a Kocher approach. Historically, exposure involved resection of radial head to allow access to medial synovium.
        - The anterior and posterior synovium is then removed.
        - Recent literature has found that radial head resection alters elbow kinematics and may lead to more rapid onset of ulnohumeral instability and degeneration.[29]
    - Arthroscopic synovectomy offers comparable results to open synovectomy, with the benefit of potentially faster rehabilitation and excellent exposure without radial head excision.
        - Excellent pain relief and subjective patient reported outcomes have been reported in greater than 75% and 93%, respectively, especially in patients with early-stage radiographic changes. These effects diminished with long-term follow-up.[30,31]
        - Several complications have been reported during arthroscopic synovectomy with the most dreaded being nerve palsy. Kelly and colleagues found that the *most significant risk factor* for development of postoperative nerve palsy after elbow arthroscopy was in patients with RA of the elbow with contracture.[32] *Recommended reading for clinical relevance for surgeons new to elbow arthroscopy in this setting*

- Interposition arthroplasty
    - Interposition arthroplasty is performed in patients with painful arthritic elbows who are in too high demand (laborers) or too young for TEA who have failed nonoperative treatment.
        - Patients will often have prior open or arthroscopic debridement prior to considering interposition arthroplasty.
    - Contraindications
        - Inadequate bone stock
        - Gross elbow instability
        - Postseptic arthritis with residual infection
        - Patients unwilling or unable to follow postoperative guidelines, including care of external fixator
        - The need for operative elbow for weight bearing or ambulation assistance is considered a relative contraindication.
    - Technique
        - Several graft options have been described.
            - Achilles tendon allograft
                - The Achilles tendon allograft offers the advantage of no donor site morbidity and can be fashioned to reconstruct collateral ligaments as needed.
            - Autogenous dermal (cutis) or fascia lata graft
            - Commercially available dermal allograft tissue

- Local autograft from interposition of the anconeus into the radiocapitellar and/or proximal radioulnar joints has been described as a separate procedure with good results.[33]
- Exposure is obtained through a posterior skin incision followed by an extensile Kocher approach or through a triceps reflecting approach such as the Bryan-Morrey or triceps-reflecting anconeus pedicle approach.
- The ulnar nerve is isolated and protected.
- The distal humerus articular surface is exposed and prepared by reshaping the distal humerus into a smooth, single articular surface that conforms to the olecranon.
- The graft of choice is then placed over the distal humerus and secured with sutures.
  - Excess tissue tails can then be fashioned to reconstruct the collateral ligaments.
- The radial head is usually left intact.
- A distraction, hinged external fixator is then applied.
- Prior to fascial and skin closure, the triceps (if reflected) is repaired through bone tunnels in the proximal ulna.

- Postoperatively range of motion is started immediately, and may be assisted with a continuous passive motion machine.
  - External fixation is left in place for approximately 4 weeks, and then removed in the operating room to allow for assessment of elbow stability and motion under anesthesia.
  - Rehabilitation is continued with concentration on obtaining and maintaining functional range of motion.
- Results
  - Studies report 70% satisfaction rate among patients with respect to pain relief, and 80% of patients regain functional range of motion.[34,35]
  - Cheng and Morrey found 67% of patients treated for RA had satisfactory relief of pain, and 75% of patients treated for OA were satisfied at 5-year follow-up.[36]
  - Ljung and associates found similar results but found that the long-term results (greater than 10 years) were inferior to TEA in patients with RA, especially in those with concomitant instability.[37]
- Complications in the literature have been reported to occur in up to 25% of patients[38]:
    - Superficial pin tract infection
    - Deep infection
    - Progressive instability
    - Ulnar nerve irritation
    - Heterotopic bone formation
    - Resorptive bone loss that occurs most commonly about the distal humeral condyles; this may complicate future arthroplasty
    - Most commonly reported complication is recurrence of pain.
- Interposition arthroplasty is widely regarded as a technically demanding procedure with a substantial learning curve.
  - The salvage procedure for failed interposition arthroplasty is a TEA.

Table 6-5

Commonly Used Elbow Prostheses Organized by Design

LINKED	UNLINKED	CONVERTIBLE (LINKED AND UNLINKED)
Coonrad-Morrey	Capitellocondylar	Latitude
Nexel	Kudo	
Discovery	Souter-Strathclyde	
GSB-III		

Total Elbow Arthroplasty

Design and History

- The goal of total elbow replacement surgery is to obtain a stable joint with a painless functional arc of at least 30 to 130 degrees. Modern total elbow implant designs are either linked or unlinked.
  - Unlinked
    - Previously referred to as unconstrained, this type of prosthesis resurfaces the distal humeral and proximal ulnar surfaces with no hinge attachment.
    - Stability of the implant requires integrity of the medial and lateral collateral ligaments.
      - Stability is afforded by the geometry of the implant and the surrounding soft tissues (the collateral ligaments and muscles crossing the elbow joint).
      - This type of implant is a less theoretic risk for component loosening.
      - The trade-off for a decreased loosening rate is a higher risk of instability.
    - Currently used unlinked prostheses are shown in Table 6-5.
  - Linked
    - Linked designs evolved initially from constrained implants and now are "semi-constrained." These prostheses are coupled between the humeral and ulnar component but allow for multidirectional play to avoid the loosening problems in early constrained designs.
    - Linked designs allowing conversion from an unlinked to linked prosthesis are also used and may hold particular value in the revision setting.
  - Cement fixation with an appropriate mantle to adequately fix the implant is required.
    - First-generation cement techniques are still used at times because of the limitations of implant plug design and inherent difficulty with pressurization of the humeral and ulnar canals.
    - However, at least one study exists that demonstrates improved fixation with the use of advanced cementing techniques with the use of cement restrictor and pressurization.[39]
  - Prosthetic elbow replacement was first described in 1947 when the distal portion of the humerus was replaced with an acrylic hemiarthroplasty.
  - The first TEA was performed by Dee in 1972 with a cemented constrained prosthesis he designed.
  - Early constrained prosthetic designs, like the one designed by Dee, failed early because of aseptic loosening (likely from rotational and varus/valgus stresses).

    - This resulted in excessive load at the bone-cement-prosthesis interface, resulting in early failure.
    - These early failures, along with an increased appreciation of the biomechanics of the native elbow, led to the design of unlinked as well as less-constrained, linked prostheses.[40]
  - Another important design innovation that has been found to resist the posterosuperior moment across the elbow, thus decreasing strain at the cement mantle, is an anterior flange on the prosthesis.[41]
    - This flange further allows for improvement in rotational stability of the implant.[42]
    - A wedge of bone or cement is placed between the anterior surface of the humerus and the flange. Finite elemental analysis shows that stress and strain in the distal humerus and distal cement mantle can be reduced 10% to 30% when using a bone graft compared with no bone graft between the anterior flange and the bone cortex.[42]
- Ultimately, implant choice is determined based on underlying etiology, patient bony and soft-tissue deformity, and surgeon preference.
- Anatomic considerations are of the utmost important when selecting an implant.
  - Distal humeral anatomy will at times dictate choice of implant.
    - Special note should be made of the integrity of the humeral condyles and collateral ligaments.
      - Lack of ligamentous integrity requires reconstruction or use of a linked device.
      - Loss of intact distal humeral condyles necessitates a linked prosthesis.
        - Certain linked designs can be implanted with up to 8 cm of distal humeral loss before custom designs are needed.[43]

Indications

- The primary indication for TEA is debilitating pain, with additional consideration given to the goal of improving of motion, function, and joint stability.
  - Indications for TEA have broadened more recently and in appropriately selected patients can include the following:
    - RA
    - Post-traumatic conditions
      - Post-traumatic arthritis
      - Malunion/nonunion
      - Dysfunctional instability
      - Chronic dislocation
    - Acute distal humerus fractures
      - Good long-term outcomes have been shown in acute fractures with severe comminution in low-demand, older patients.[44]
      - Nonunion
    - Primary OA
- Contraindications for TEA include the presence of persistent infection and the inability to actively flex the elbow joint.
- Relative contraindications included high-demand patients, patients who are unable to comply with postoperative restrictions, and very young patients.

Surgical Approaches

- Most arthroplasty procedures require wide exposure of the articular surface of the elbow.
- The majority of approaches use a posterior skin incision over the elbow that extends slightly medial or lateral to the tip of the olecranon.
- Approaches most pertinent to elbow arthroplasty include the Bryan-Morrey, triceps preserving, and triceps-splitting approaches.
    - Regardless of approach used, certain key steps are critical to a successful outcome.
        - Preservation of triceps function by meticulous preservation of its attachments and/or reconstruction during closure is paramount.
        - Collateral ligament integrity is critical to successful outcome when using unlinked implants.
        - Routine transposition of the ulnar nerve is often recommended.
- Technical considerations of unlinked design TEA implantation
    - A tourniquet is used on the upper arm.
    - A variety of approaches are available.
        - Dislocation of the joint necessitates release of one of the collateral ligaments, often the lateral ulnar collateral ligament.
    - Humeral preparation is performed first.
        - The central portion of trochlea is removed with a sagittal saw, allowing access to the humeral canal.
        - Reaming is then performed with maintenance of integrity of medial and lateral columns of the distal humerus.
        - Depending on implant, various amounts of the distal humeral articular surface are then resected with the help of cutting blocks or jigs.
        - Trial implantation is performed with special attention given to placement in the appropriate axis of rotation.
            - The anterior humeral cortex is used as reference to ensure the implant is placed in the appropriate flexion axis.
            - The humeral condyles are referenced to recreate anatomic rotation.
    - Ulnar preparation is then performed.
        - A burr or awl used to gain entry into ulnar canal
        - The tip of the olecranon is often resected for easier canal entry.
        - The canal is then broached, and trial implantation is performed.
            - The posterior aspect of the proximal ulnar cortex is used to orient the ulnar implant perpendicular to the flexion axis.
    - Some unlinked designs resurface the radial head to match corresponding capitellar resurfacing, whereas others maintain the native radial head.
    - Trial reduction assesses stability and soft-tissue tension.
        - Pistoning indicates a flexion axis mismatch.
        - Stability of the elbow must be assessed throughout arc of motion.
            - Alignment and contact of the humerus and ulna through arc of motion should be observed.
    - After trialing, final components are cemented into place.
    - Reconstruction of the collateral ligament and triceps is performed during closure.

- Wound closure over a drain is recommended.
- Technical considerations of linked TEA implantation
  - As with unlinked TEA, a tourniquet should be used.
  - A variety of surgical approaches are available.
    - The opportunity to leave the triceps mechanism intact exists in some cases of acute fracture or nonunion.
  - Ulnar nerve is transposed followed by resection of the collateral ligaments.
  - Humeral and ulnar preparation is performed first as described in the unlinked TEA technical considerations.
    - Though the inherent stability of the implant makes the precision of bone resection somewhat less critical, most systems still employ cutting blocks and jigs to direct bone cuts.
  - Trial reduction
    - Assess soft-tissue balance, rotational orientation, and stability of the implant.
  - Cement final components, then the humerus followed by the ulna.
  - Repair the triceps through bone tunnels.
  - Wound closure over a drain is again recommended.

Complications

- Complications after TEA are common.
  - Gschwend et al reviewed 828 TEA performed from 1986 to 1992 and found a 43% complication rate.[45]
  - A more recent systematic review included nearly 3000 total elbow arthroplasties and found an overall complication rate of $24.3 \pm 5.8\%$. The main complications reported in descending order of frequency were the following[46]:
    - Aseptic loosening (higher in linked designs)
    - Instability (higher in unlinked designs)
    - Deep infection
    - Intraoperative fracture
    - Prosthesis fracture
    - Ulnar nerve complications
    - Other complications include the following:
      - Delayed healing
      - Postoperative periprosthetic fracture
      - Triceps insufficiency or rupture
      - Bushing wear
      - Heterotopic ossification
- After primary TEA an infection rate of between 2% and 8% has been reported,[46-50] which is notably higher than other major joint arthroplasty. The most frequent organisms isolated are *Staphylococcus epidermidis* or *Staphylococcus aureus*,[51] with *Staphylococcus epidermidis* thought to be the more virulent organism in this setting.[52]
- These patients often require a staged revision using antibiotics, although a patient with an early *S. aureus* infection can sometimes be treated with aggressive irrigation and debridement.[53]

Conclusion

- The treatment of elbow arthritis has seen significant advancement both in diagnosis and treatment in recent times.
- An increased understanding of the anatomy and biomechanics of the elbow joint have allowed for refined surgical management both with arthroplasty and nonarthroplasty options, whereas the use of DMARDs has led to improved medical management of inflammatory arthritis.
- Clinicians charged with treating the arthritic elbow find themselves with numerous options that have been proven to reduce pain and restore function.

References

1. Delal S, Bull M, Stanley D. Radiographic changes at the elbow in primary osteoarthritis: A comparison with normal aging of the elbow joint. *J Shoulder Elbow Surg.* 2007;16(3):358-361. doi:10.1016/j.jse.2006.08.005.
2. Collins DH. Incidence of cartilage changes and osteoarthritis in joints at different ages. In: Collins DH. *The Pathology of Articular and Spinal Diseases.* London, England: Edward Arnold & Co; 1949:354-356.
3. Morrey BF. Primary arthritis of the elbow. Treated by ulnohumeral arthroplasty. *J Bone Joint Surg Br.* 1992;74(3):409-413.
4. Wysocki RW, Cohen MS. Primary osteoarthritis and posttraumatic arthritis of the elbow. *Hand Clin.* 2011;27(2):131-137. doi:10.1016/j.hcl.2011.02.001.
5. Spahn G, Lipfert JU, Maurer C, et al. Risk factors for cartilage damage and osteoarthritis of the elbow joint: case-control study and systematic literature review. *Arch Orthop Trauma Surg.* 2017;137(4):557-566. doi:10.1007/s00402-017-2654-6.
6. Doherty M, Preston B. Primary osteoarthritis of the elbow. *Ann Rheum Dis.* 1989;48(9):743-747. doi:10.1136/ard.48.9.743.
7. MinamiM,KatoS,KashiwagiD.Outerbridge-Kashiwagi'smethodforarthroplastyofosteoarthritisoftheelbow—44elbows followed for 8-16 years. *J Orthop Sci.* 1996;1(1):11-15. doi:10.1007/BF01234111.
8. Kawanishi Y, Miyake J, Omori S, Murase T, Shimada K. The association between cubital tunnel morphology and ulnar neuropathy in patients with elbow osteoarthritis. *J Shoulder Elbow Surg.* 2014;23(7):938-945. doi:10.1016/j.jse.2014.01.047.
9. Minami NM. Roentgenological studies of osteoarthritis of the elbow joint [in Japanese]. *Nippon Seikeigeka Gakkai Zasshi. [Jpn Orthop Assoc.]* 1977;51:1223-1236.
10. Amini MH, Sykes JB, Olson ST, et al. Reliability testing of two classification systems for osteoarthritis and post-traumatic arthritis of the elbow. *J Shoulder Elbow Surg.* 2015;24(3):353-357. doi:10.1016/j.jse.2014.10.015.
11. Miyake J, Shimada K, Oka K, et al. Arthroscopic debridement in the treatment of patients with osteoarthritis of the elbow, based on computer simulation. *Bone Joint J.* 2014;96-B(2):237-241. doi:10.1302/0301-620X.96B2.30714.
12. O'Driscoll SW, Morrey BF, An KN. Intraarticular pressure and capacity of the elbow. *Arthroscopy.* 1990;6(2):100-103. doi:10.1016/0749-8063(90)90007-z.
13. Jew NB, Hollins AM, Mauck BM, et al. Reliability testing of the Larsen and Sharp classifications for rheumatoid arthritis of the elbow. *J Shoulder Elbow Surg.* 2017;26(1):140-143. doi:10.1016/j.jse.2016.07.074.
14. da Silva E, Doran MF, Crowson CS, O'Fallon WM, Matteson EL. Declining use of orthopedic surgery in patients with rheumatoid arthritis? Results of a long-term, population-based assessment. *Arthritis Rheum.* 2003;49(2):216-220. doi:10.1002/art.10998.
15. Veltman ES, Doornberg JN, Eygendaal D, van den Bekerom MP. Static progressive versus dynamic splinting for posttraumatic elbow stiffness: a systematic review of 232 patients. *Arch Orthop Trauma Surg.* 2015;135(5):613-617. doi:10.1007/s00402-015-2199-5.
16. van Brakel RW, Eygendaal D. Intra-articular injection of hyaluronic acid is not effective for the treatment of post-traumatic osteoarthritis of the elbow. *Arthroscopy.* 2006;22(11):1199-1203. doi:10.1016/j.arthro.2006.07.023.
17. Raval P, Ellanti P, Harrington P. Ulnohumeral debridement arthroplasty: a retrospective study and midterm outcome results. *Eur J Orthop Surg Traumatol.* 2015;25(5):847-850. doi:10.1007/s00590-015-1593-6.
18. Antuña SA, Morrey BF, Adams RA, O'Driscoll SW. Ulnohumeral arthroplasty for primary degenerative arthritis of the elbow: long-term outcome and complications. *J Bone Joint Surg Am.* 2002;84(12):2168-2173. doi:10.2106/00004623-200212000-00007.
19. Oka Y. Debridement arthroplasty for osteoarthrosis of the elbow: 50 patients followed mean 5 years. *Acta Orthop Scand.* 2000;71(2):185-190. doi:10.1080/000164700317413175.
20. Tsuge K, Mizuseki T. Debridement arthroplasty for advanced primary osteoarthritis of the elbow. Results of a new technique used for 29 elbows. *J Bone Joint Surg Br.* 1994;76(4):641-646. doi:10.1302/0301-620x.76b4.8027156.

21. Itoh Y, Saegusa K, Ishiguro T, Horiuchi Y, Sasaki T, Uchinishi K. Operation for the stiff elbow. *Int Orthop.* 1989;13(4):263-268. doi:10.1007/bf00268509.
22. Wada T, Ishii S, Usui M, Miyano S. The medial approach for operative release of post-traumatic contracture of the elbow. *J Bone Joint Surg Br.* 2000;82(1):68-73. doi:10.1302/0301-620x.82b1.9782.
23. Hotchkiss RN, Kasparyan GN. The medial "over the top" approach to the elbow. *Tech Orthop.* 2000;15(2):105-112. doi:10.1097/00013611-200015020-00003.
24. Sochacki KR, Jack RA 2nd, Hirase T, et al. Arthroscopic debridement for primary degenerative osteoarthritis of the elbow leads to significant improvement in range of motion and clinical outcomes: a systematic review. *Arthroscopy.* 2017;33(12):2255-2262. doi:10.1016/j.arthro.2017.08.247.
25. Lim TK, Koh KH, Lee HI, Shim JW, Park MJ. Arthroscopic débridement for primary osteoarthritis of the elbow: analysis of preoperative factors affecting outcome. *J Shoulder Elbow Surg.* 2014;23(9):1381-7. doi: 10.1016/j.jse.2014.01.009.
26. Merolla G, Buononato C, Chillemi C, Paladini P, Porcellini G. Arthroscopic joint debridement and capsular release in primary and post-traumatic elbow osteoarthritis: a retrospective blinded cohort study with minimum 24-month follow-up. *Musculoskelet Surg.* 2015;99(suppl 1):S83-S90. doi: 10.1007/s12306-015-0365-0.
27. Savoie FH III, Nunley PD, Field LD. Arthroscopic management of the arthritic elbow: indications, technique, and results. *J Shoulder Elbow Surg.* 1999;8(3):214-219. doi:10.1016/S1058-2746(99)90131-3.
28. Cohen AP, Redden JF, Stanley D. Treatment of osteoarthritis of the elbow: a comparison of open and arthroscopic debridement. *Arthroscopy.* 2000;16(7):701-706. doi:10.1053/jars.2000.8952.
29. Schiffern A, Bettwieser SP, Porucznik CA, Crim JR, Tashjian RZ. Proximal radial drift following radial head resection. *J Shoulder Elbow Surg.* 2011;20(3):426-433. doi:10.1016/j.jse.2010.11.008.
30. Horiuchi K, Momohara S, Tomatsu T, Inoue K, Toyama Y. Arthroscopic synovectomy of the elbow in rheumatoid arthritis. *J Bone Joint Surg Am.* 2002;84(3):342-347. doi:10.2106/00004623-200203000-00002.
31. Lee BP, Morrey BF. Arthroscopic synovectomy of the elbow for rheumatoid arthritis. A prospective study. *J Bone Joint Surg Br.* 1997;79(5):770-772. doi:10.1302/0301-620x.79b5.7466.
32. Kelly EW, Morrey BF, O'Driscoll SW. Complications of elbow arthroscopy. *J Bone Joint Surg Am.* 2001;83(1):25-34. doi:10.2106/00004623-200101000-00004.
33. Baghdadi YM, Morrey BF, Sanchez-Sotelo J. Anconeus interposition arthroplasty: mid- to long-term results. *Clin Orthop Relat Res.* 2014;472(7):2151-2161. doi:10.1007/s11999-014-3629-3.
34. Chen DD, Forsh DA, Hausman MR. Elbow interposition arthroplasty. *Hand Clin.* 2011;27(2):187-197. doi:10.1016/j.hcl.2011.01.002.
35. Larson AN, Morrey BF. Interposition arthroplasty with an Achilles tendon allograft as a salvage procedure for the elbow. *J Bone Joint Surg Am.* 2008;90(12):2714-2723. doi:10.2106/JBJS.G.00768.
36. Cheng SL, Morrey BF. Treatment of the mobile, painful arthritic elbow by distraction interposition arthroplasty. *J Bone Joint Surg Br.* 2000;82(2):233-238. doi:10.1302/0301-620x.82b2 .9507.
37. Ljung P, Jonsson K, Larsson K, Rydholm U. Interposition arthroplasty of the elbow with rheumatoid arthritis. *J Shoulder Elbow Surg.* 1996;5(2 pt 1):81-85.
38. Nolla J, Ring D, Lozano-Calderon S, Jupiter JB. Interposition arthroplasty of the elbow with hinged external fixation for post-traumatic arthritis. *J Shoulder Elbow Surg.* 2008;17(3):459-464. doi:10.1016/j.jse.2007.11.008.
39. Faber KJ, Cordy ME, Milne AD, Chess DG, King GJ, Johnson JA. Advanced cement technique improves fixation in elbow arthroplasty. *Clin Orthop Relat Res.* 1997;(334):150-156.
40. O'Driscoll SW, An KN, Korinek S, Morrey BF. Kinematics of semi-constrained total elbow arthroplasty. *J Bone Joint Surg Br.* 1992;74(2):297-299. doi:10.1302/0301-620X.74B2.1544973.
41. Quenneville CE, Austman RL, King GJ, Johnson JA, Dunning CE. Role of an anterior flange on cortical strains through the distal humerus after total elbow arthroplasty with a latitude implant. *J Hand Surg Am.* 2008;33(6):927-931. doi:10.1016/j.jhsa.2008.02.020.
42. Herren DB, Ploeg H, Hertig D, Klabunde R. Modeling and finite element analysis of a new revision implant for the elbow. *Clin Orthop Relat Res.* 2004;(420):292-297. doi:10.1097/00003086-200403000-00041.
43. Kamineni S, Morrey BF. Distal humeral fractures treated with noncustom total elbow replacement. *J Bone Joint Surg Am.* 2004;86(5):940-947. doi:10.2106/00004623-200405000-00009.
44. Barco R, Streubel PN, Morrey BF, Sanchez-Sotelo J. Total elbow arthroplasty for distal humeral fractures: a ten-year-minimum follow-up study. *J Bone Joint Surg Am.* 2017;99(18):1524-1531. doi:10.2106/JBJS.16.01222.
45. Gschwend N, Simmen BR, Matejovsky Z. Late complications in elbow arthroplasty. *J Shoulder Elbow Surg.* 1996;5(2 pt 1):86-96. doi:10.1016/S1058-2746(96)80002-4.
46. Voloshin I, Schippert DW, Kakar S, Kaye EK, Morrey BF. Complications of total elbow replacement: a systematic review. *J Shoulder Elbow Surg.* 2011;20(1):158-168. doi:10.1016/j.jse.2010.08.026.
47. Sanchez-Sotelo J, Baghdadi YM, Morrey BF. Primary linked semiconstrained total elbow arthroplasty for rheumatoid arthritis: a single-institution experience with 461 elbows over three decades. *J Bone Joint Surg Am.* 2016;98(20):1741-1748. doi:10.2106/JBJS.15.00649.
48. Morrey BF, Bryan RS. Infection after total elbow arthroplasty. *J Bone Joint Surg Am.* 1983;65(3):330-338. doi:10.2106/00004623-199804000-00004.
49. Ewald FC, Simmons ED Jr, Sullivan JA, et al. Capitellocondylar total elbow replacement in rheumatoid arthritis. Long-term results. *J Bone Joint Surg Am.* 1993;75(4):498-507. doi:10.2106/00004623-199304000-00004.

50. Aldridge JM III, Lightdale NR, Mallon WJ, Coonrad RW: Total elbow arthroplasty with the Coonrad/Coonrad-Morrey prosthesis. A 10- to 31-year survival analysis. *J Bone Joint Surg Br.* 2006;88(4):509-514. doi:10.1302/0301-620X.88B4.17095.
51. Cheung EV, Adams RA, Morrey BF. Reimplantation of a total elbow prosthesis following resection arthroplasty for infection. *J Bone Joint Surg Am.* 2008;90(3):589-594. doi:10.2106/JBJS.F.00829.
52. Yamaguchi K, Adams RA, Morrey BF. Infection after total elbow arthroplasty. *J Bone Joint Surg Am.* 1998;80(4):481-491. doi:10.2106/00004623-199804000-00004.
53. Streubel PN, Simone JP, Morrey BF, Sanchez-Sotelo J, Morrey ME. Infection in total elbow arthroplasty with stable components: outcomes of a staged surgical protocol with retention of the components. *Bone Joint J.* 2016;98-B(7):976-983. doi:10.1302/0301-620X.98B7.36397.

7

Humeral Shaft Fractures

E. Scott Paxton, MD and Kalpit N. Shah, MD

Demographics

- Demographics of patients who suffer humeral shaft fractures demonstrate a bimodal distribution[1]:
  - Younger men typically tend to sustain these fractures secondary to high-energy injuries.
  - Older women suffer humeral shaft fractures after low-energy falls in the setting of osteopenia or osteoporosis.

Anatomy

- The average length of the humeral shaft has been reported to be 30.4 cm, with an average transverse diameter of 1.8 cm and a cortical thickness of 4.4 mm.[2,3]
- The proximal and middle third of the humeral shaft are cylindrical in shape.
- The distal third of the humeral shaft flattens into the more triangular-shaped supracondylar area.
- The spiral groove for the radial nerve is located on the dorsal aspect of the humeral shaft.[4]
  - It has been noted to be about 20 cm proximal to the medial epicondyle and 14 cm proximal to the lateral epicondyle.

Namdari S, Zmistowski B, Omid R, eds.
The Foundations of Shoulder and Elbow Surgery (pp 115-127).

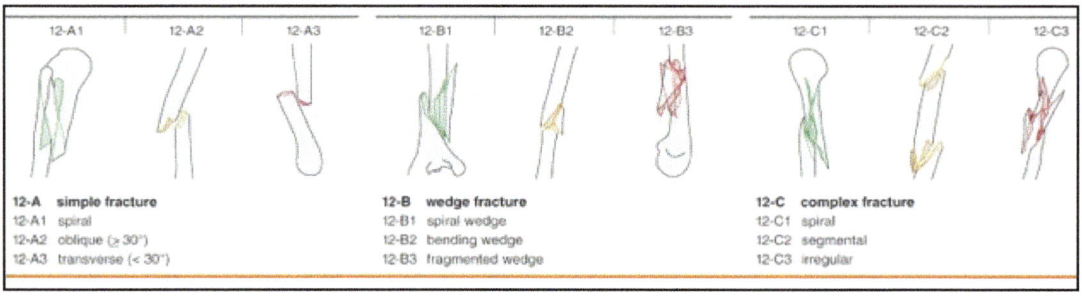

Figure 7-1. AO classification for humeral shaft fracture. (Source: AO Surgery Reference, www.aosurgery.org. Copyright by AO Foundation, Switzerland.)

Biomechanics

- Rotational forces are the most common cause for these fractures.
- Displacement of the fractured segments of the humeral shaft depends on the level of the fracture.
  - If the fracture is proximal to the deltoid insertion, the following occur:
    - The proximal fragment externally rotates and abducts.
    - The distal fragment translates medially and flexes anteriorly.
  - If the fracture is distal to the deltoid insertion, the proximal segment abducts.
  - Both of these mechanisms combined with the patient's body habitus typically result in a varus deformity.

Examination

- Neurovascular examination is critical in patients with humeral shaft fractures.
- Radial nerve injuries are common.[5]
  - Motor function is best tested by examining the extensor carpi radialis longus, extensor digitorum comminus, and the extensor pollicis longus (extension of the wrist, thumb, and fingers at the metacarpophalangeal joints, respectively).
  - Sensory function is best tested by assessing sensation over the dorsum of the hand in the first web space.

Imaging

- Standard anteroposterior and lateral radiographs of the humerus are often sufficient and are the imaging modality of choice.
- The shoulder and the elbow should also be imaged to rule out injury to the adjacent joints.
- Classification system
  - Arbeitsgemeinschaft für Osteosynthesefragen, better known as the AO Classification, can be used to describe the pattern (Figure 7-1)
  - As in other fractures, characteristics of fracture orientation, comminution, displacement, and distraction at the fracture site are important in assessing these injuries.
  - Spiral fractures of the distal one-third humeral shaft are called Holstein-Lewis fractures.[6]

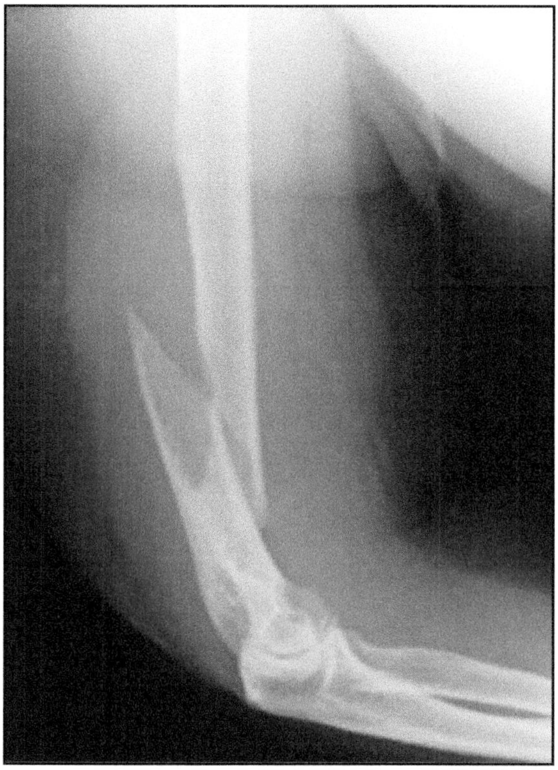

Figure 7-2. Anteroposterior radiograph of a right humerus showing a distal one-third humeral shaft fracture with a spiral pattern, often referred to as a Holstein-Lewis fracture.

- These fractures are associated with neuropraxia of the radial nerve (22%) because the fracture typically occurs through an area where the radial nerve has limited mobility (Figure 7-2).
    - This is the area between the area of direct contact of the nerve with the posterior humeral shaft and the lateral intramuscular septum (which the nerve transverses to pass from the posterior compartment of the arm to the anterior compartment).[6]

Treatment

- Emergent or urgent surgical management is reserved for the following:
    - Open fractures, with the aim of decreasing the infection rate by timely debridement
    - Concomitant vascular injury, which requires emergent exploration and repair by a vascular surgeon. The humeral shaft fracture should be addressed at the same time to provide skeletal stability.
- Initial management
    - Humeral shaft fractures are immobilized initially using a coaptation splint or a hanging arm cast (Figure 7-3). Although some may prefer to treat the fracture with a fracture brace initially.
    - Previously published acceptable radiographic parameters on postreduction and immobilization radiographs include the following (although the basis for these is unclear)[7]:
        - 20-degree anterior angulation
        - 30-degree varus angulation

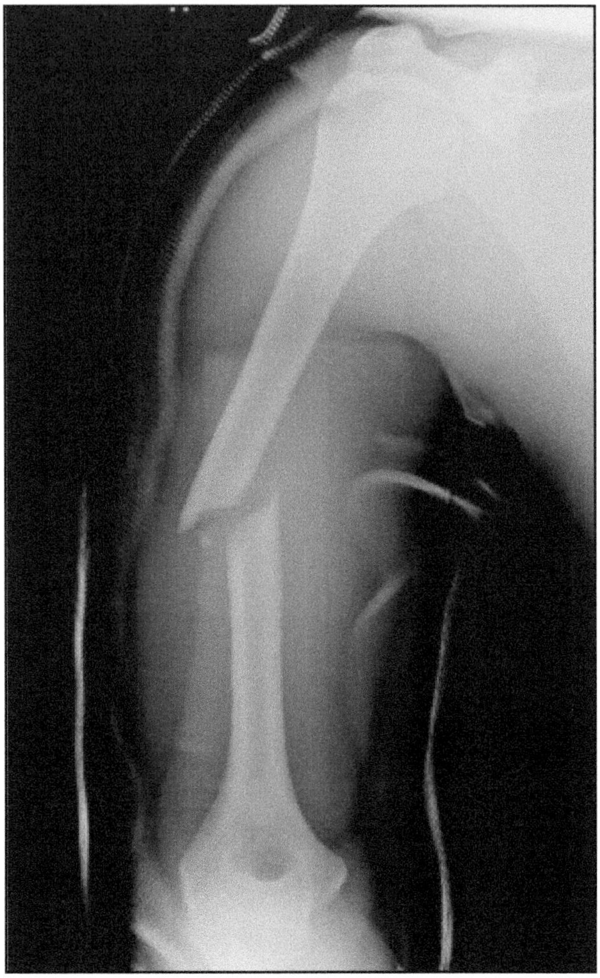

Figure 7-3. Anteroposterior radiograph of a right midshaft humeral fracture with a short spiral pattern with fracture distraction and varus deformity immobilized in a coaptation splint.

        - 15-degree malrotation
        - 3-cm shortening
- Nonoperative
    - Patients are often initially placed in a coaptation splint or a hanging arm cast.
        - Patients are typically transitioned to a functional brace after 7 to 10 days from the injury once the majority of initial swelling has subsided (Figure 7-4).
    - Sarmiento et al[8] reported their experience with 620 patients treated with a functional arm brace.
        - Less than 2% of the 465 patients with closed humeral shaft fractures were found to have a nonunion with the use of a functional arm brace.[8] *Recommended reading for historical importance*
        - At final follow-up, 98% of the patients had limitations in their shoulder motion of 25 degrees or less.
        - However, these results have not been reproducible universally for nonoperative treatment of humeral shaft fractures.[9-11]
    - Quicker return to function has been advocated after operative management but no difference in outcomes at 1 year.[9]

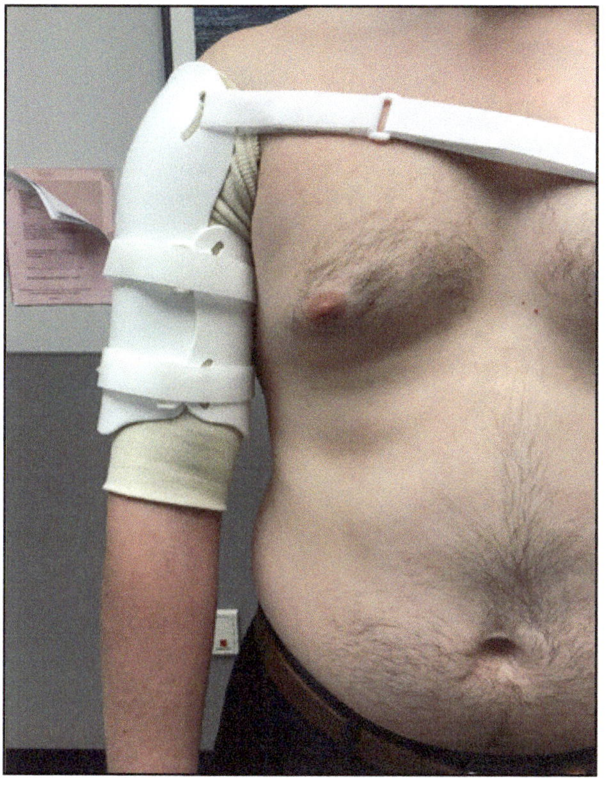

Figure 7-4. Patient in a well-fitted functional fracture brace that is often used for closed management of humeral shaft fractures.

- Complications
  - Coaptation splints can be associated with axillary skin irritation and even full-thickness skin loss secondary to abrasion. It is imperative that the superior aspect of the brace be well padded.
  - Hanging arm casts can overdistract the fracture.
  - Delayed union is often common with functional bracing.
- Operative
  - Operative management is recommended in the following settings:
    - Open fracture: Surgery may facilitate a thorough debridement to minimize the risk of soft-tissue infection and osteomyelitis.
    - Skin injury or soft-tissue considerations may preclude treatment in a functional arm brace.
    - Vascular injury: Surgery may allow for exploration, repair, and skeletal stabilization.
    - Highly functional patients with suboptimal alignment may benefit from surgery.
    - Multiple-injured patients with the presence of bilateral fractures, "floating" shoulder or elbow, an expected long recovery in the supine position (typically patients in the intensive care unit), patients with multiple-injured extremities to allow for weight bearing through the humerus, and large body habitus that prevents adequate reduction all may be candidates for surgery.
    - Some have advocated for early exploration and fixation in the setting of a radial nerve palsy with irreducible fractures or unacceptable reduction, associated vascular injuries, or radial nerve palsy after manipulation or intractable neurogenic pain.[12,13]

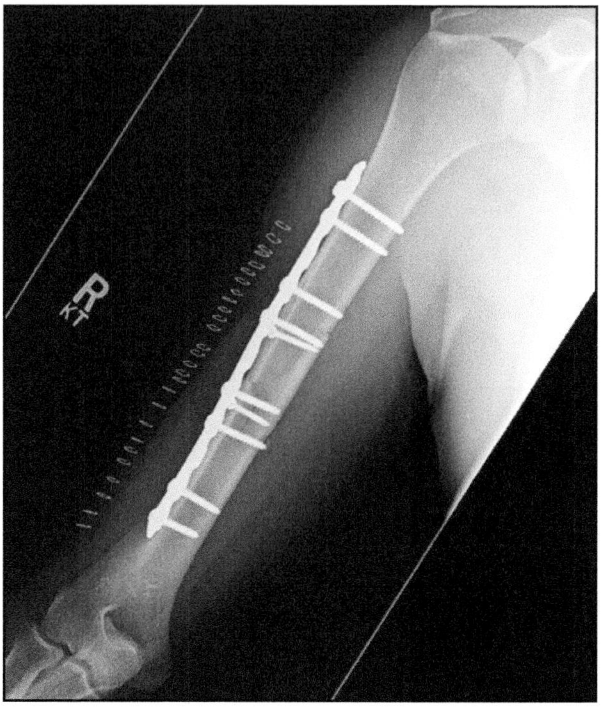

Figure 7-5. Anteroposterior radiograph of a right humeral shaft fracture with a butterfly fragment that was treated with a compression plate construct using multiple 3.5-mm lag screws and a 4.5-mm limited contact dynamic compression plate with at least 4 cortical screws on each side of the fracture.

- A recent randomized, controlled trial evaluated the use of a minimally invasive osteosynthesis with a bridge plate to a functional brace for humeral shaft fractures.[14]
  - The bridge plate group had a significantly more favorable nonunion rate (0% vs 15%).
  - The authors report that the bridge plate group's Disabilities of the Arm, Shoulder, and Hand (DASH) score was statistically superior to that of the functional brace group only at 6 months.
  - No difference between the groups was detected with regard to the 36-Item Short Form Health Survey score, pain level, or Constant-Murley score.
- Plate osteosynthesis (Figure 7-5)
  - Typically, a 4.5 mm direct contact plate is used for most humeral shaft fracture because it imparts significantly more stiffness to the construct than a 3.5 mm direct contact plate.[15]
  - It is recommended that at least 4 bicortical, nonlocking screws or 2 bicortical, locking screws be applied to each side of the fracture during compression plating and bridge plating, respectively.[15-17]
  - Fracture of the distal third of the humerus can be treated with a "90 to 90" degree dual-plating construct, typically with a malleable lateral plate used for reduction and a stronger posterolateral plate.[18]
  - Compression plates are typically used for simple fractures, whereas comminuted fractures are often treated with a bridge construct. Unstable fractures or those in osteopenic patients may be treated with a locked or hybrid plate fixation, although in patients with normal bone, nonlocking screws and conventional locking screws have shown similar biomechanical properties in cortical bone.[16]
  - Surgical approach
    - Anterior approach
      - This approach can be used for proximal and middle third humeral shaft fractures.

- Incision starts at the deltopectoral groove and runs distally along the lateral aspect of the long biceps tendon and its muscle belly distally.
- After retracting the muscle belly of the biceps medially to protect the neurovascular structures on the medial aspect of the arm, the brachialis is split roughly one-third of the muscle width away from the lateral aspect to gain access to the humeral shaft.
  - The lateral portion of the brachialis is innervated by the radial nerve and the medial portion by the musculocutaneous nerve, allowing for split in the muscle with low risk of denervation.
- The lateral antebrachial cutaneous nerve (continuation of the musculocutaneous nerve) is medial to the humerus between the brachialis and biceps muscles.
- The radial nerve is between the brachialis and brachioradialis muscle laterally and should be protected.

- Posterolateral approach (Figure 7-6)
  - This exposure can be used for middle and distal third humeral shaft fractures.[19] *Recommended reading for understanding of humeral shaft approaches*
  - The incision is centered over the posterior aspect of the humerus and taken distally to the olecranon.
  - After dividing the subcutaneous tissues, the interval between the triceps muscle and the lateral intermuscular septum is taken down the humerus.
  - Take care when elevating the deeper, medial head of the triceps off the humerus as the radial nerve courses medial to lateral at its cranial border.
  - The radial nerve usually runs with the profunda brachii artery and can be found roughly 20 cm proximal to the medial epicondyle and 14 cm proximal to the lateral epicondyle along the posterior aspect of the humerus.[19]
  - At the lateral aspect of the humerus, the radial nerve usually has 3 branches: one to the medial head of the triceps, another that continues as the lateral brachial cutaneous nerve, and the third, which is the continuation of the radial nerve proper into the distal arm and forearm.
  - The radial nerve traverses through the lateral intermuscular septum 11 cm proximal to the lateral epicondyle.[20]
- Anterolateral minimally invasive approach
  - This approach is used to create a bridging construct with minimal soft-tissue dissection with hopes of better cosmesis and earlier rehabilitation.[21]
  - Proximally, a small deltopectoral approach is taken between the deltoid and the pectoralis major or a lateral deltoid split approach is employed.
  - Distally, the interval between the brachialis and the brachioradialis muscle is taken.
  - As discussed previously, the radial nerve courses between those two muscles. Take care to identify the nerve to avoid iatrogenic injury.

- Intramedullary nail
  - This is an alternative to minimally invasive plate osteosynthesis.
  - Anterograde nailing[22] (Figure 7-7)
    - These are inserted using a small anterolateral incision, using a deltoid split approach anterolateral to the acromion.
    - Straight nails are inserted at the apex of the humerus (Figure 7-8).
    - Proximally curved nails are inserted by the bone-cartilage interface of the humeral head and historically have gone through the rotator cuff insertion, which should be

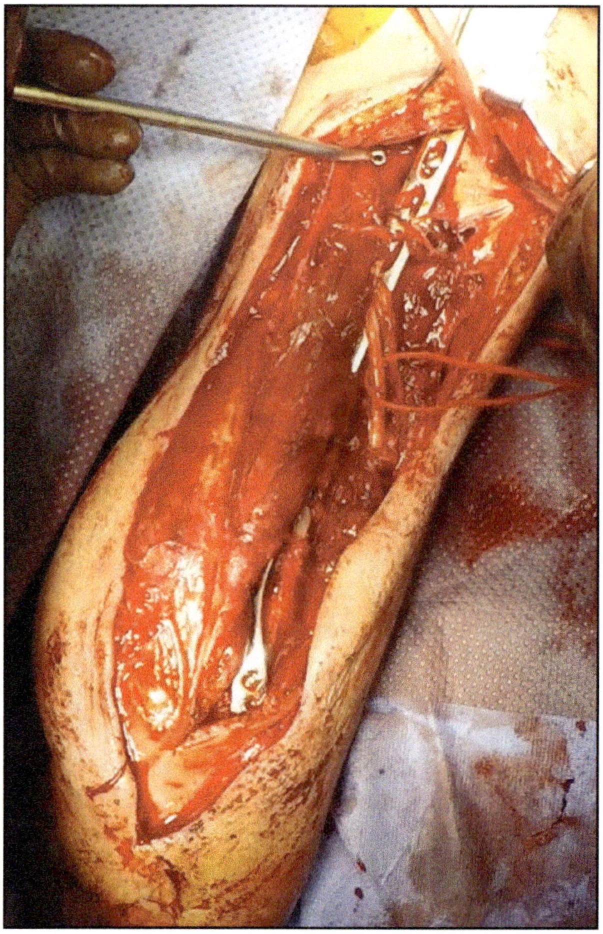

Figure 7-6. Surgical image of a patient undergoing open reduction internal fixation with a plate and screw construct via the posterolateral approach. The radial nerve and the profunda brachii artery were tagged with a vessel loop as they course around the humeral shaft, over the top of the plate.

avoided and can lead to the rotator cuff complaints seen with this modality. The authors prefer straight nails.

- The axillary nerve is 6 cm distal to the anterolateral acromion and must be protected when placing the proximal interlocking screws.
- The median nerve, ulnar nerve, and the brachial artery are at risk when inserting the distal interlocking screws, which are typically placed in an anterior-to-posterior direction.

- Retrograde nailing
  - An incision just proximal to the olecranon is made over the distal humerus.
  - The triceps tendon is split and the humeral intramedullary cavity is entered just proximal to the olecranon fossa.
  - Given the relatively thin profile of the supracondylar area, the most common complication of this method is a fracture in that area.
- Plate osteosynthesis vs nailing
  - A Cochrane Review evaluated 5 randomized, controlled trials that compared compression plating to locked intramedullary nailing.[23]
    - There was no difference in the union rate, operating time, blood loss during surgery, iatrogenic radial nerve injury, return to preinjury occupation, or American Shoulder and Elbow Surgeons scores between the 2 groups.

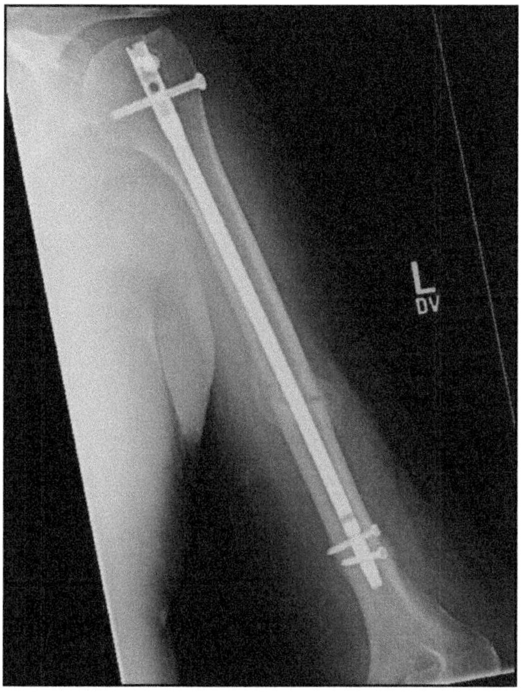

Figure 7-7. Anteroposterior radiograph of a left humeral shaft fracture treated with a straight intramedullary nail showing good callous formation at the fracture site.

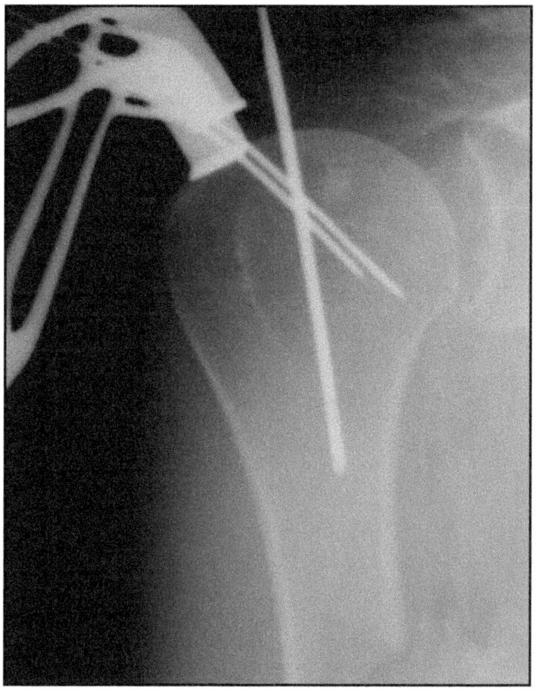

Figure 7-8. Intraoperative fluoroscopic image demonstrating the entry point at the apex of the humeral head for an antegrade intramedullary humeral nail; this is medial to the rotator cuff attachment.

- There was an increase in shoulder impingement and removal of hardware in the intramedullary nailing group compared with the plating group.
- Another meta-analysis included 10 studies comparing compression plating to intramedullary nailing for humeral shaft fractures.[24]
  - In the 439 patients included in this analysis, nailing was associated with a risk of shoulder impingement pain and decreased motion in comparison with plating.
  - The authors did not find a significant difference in postoperative infection, nonunion, delayed union, radial nerve palsy, iatrogenic fracture comminution, or implant failure between groups.
- External fixation
  - External fixation is often used in emergent situations for which definitive fixation is prohibitive or when there is compromise of the soft-tissue envelope.
  - Proximally, 2 pins must be placed though an anterolateral trajectory, which is the safest approach.
  - Distally, pins can be placed dorsally or transcondylarly to avoid damage to the neurovascular structures traversing in that area.
- Rehabilitation
  - For patients treated in a functional fracture brace, motion of the shoulder and elbow should be encouraged after the first week.

        - The patient should be instructed on appropriate use of the functional brace and the importance of compliance to take advantage of the incompressible fluid effect of the soft tissues.
        - Pendulum motion can be initiated after the first week.
        - Active-assisted mobilization should begin after the second week if pain is manageable.
        - Brace is usually left in place for 8 to 12 weeks until there is clinical and radiographic evidence of fracture healing.
        - Strengthening exercises may be initiated at that point.
    - Patients treated with plate osteosynthesis or intramedullary nailing may start working on passive and active-assisted range of motion immediately.
        - If necessary, polytrauma patients treated surgically may start weight bearing as soon as possible.[25]
        - Strengthening may be initiated once there is radiographic and clinic evidence of fracture healing.

Complications

- Radial nerve palsy
    - Shao and colleagues reported an incidence of 11.8%, for primary radial nerve palsy noted initially in the setting of humeral shaft fractures.
        - The authors described transverse and spiral fracture patterns and those in the middle and middle-distal humeral shaft as significant associated with radial nerve palsy.
    - It has been estimated that roughly 73% to 92% of patients will regain radial nerve function after 4 months of conservative management of a humeral shaft fracture with concomitant, primary radial nerve palsy.[12]
        - As such, it is recommend that patients who typically would have been managed without surgical intervention should be observed in the setting of a radial nerve palsy.[4,12]
        - Brachioradialis muscle is the usually the first to recover, and the extensor indicis propius is the last muscle to recover.
    - In patients without any signs of recovery, clinical diagnosis can be confirmed with electromyography only after 3 to 5 weeks because some time is needed for pathologic motor potentials to develop after the initial injury.[26]
    - Exploration after 3 months of no functional recovery of the radial nerve is recommended.
        - Most patients do not gain significant radial nerve function despite nerve repair in the setting of injury to the nerve. Hence, tendon transfers may be recommended to improve the functional capacity of the upper extremity.[12,27]
    - Early exploration of the radial nerve in the setting of a radial nerve palsy is recommended for open fractures, those that are irreducible fractures or found to have unacceptable radiographic parameters, associated vascular injuries, radial nerve palsy that develops after manipulative reduction, or patients with intractable neurogenic pain.[12]
- Nonunion
    - A nonunion rate of 10% to 20% can be expected with nonoperative management of humeral shaft fractures.[9,11,28]

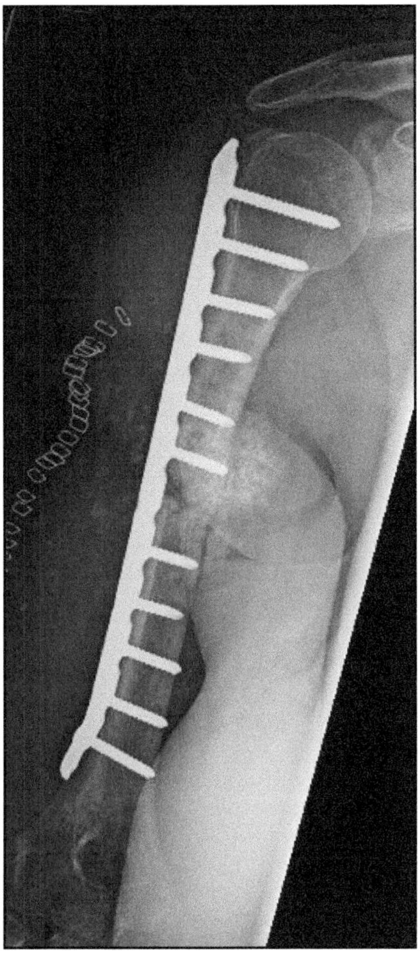

Figure 7-9. Postoperative anteroposterior radiograph of a right humeral shaft nonunion treated with open reduction internal fixation with a 4.5-mm limited contact dynamic compression plate and bone grafting.

    - Some authors have suggested that transverse fracture patterns may be associated with nonunion because that pattern has a lesser contact area between the fractured bone ends.[5,8]
- After operative fixation, the nonunion rate has been reported to be between 0% and 10%.[9,28-30]
    - No difference in fracture union has been found between plating and intramedullary nailing.[23,30,31]
- The most common reason for a nonunion of the humeral shaft has been theorized to be diminished vascularity secondary to damage to the main nutrient artery to the humeral shaft, which is usually found in the middle to distal third of the humeral shaft.[32]
- Plate osteosynthesis with bone graft is recommended for treatment of nonunions[31] (Figure 7-9).

Outcomes

- Shields et al found no statistically significant difference between operative (55 patients) and nonoperative patients (32 patients) in terms of functional outcome scores.[33]
- Matsunaga and colleagues conducted the first randomized trial between operative (minimally invasive plate osteosynthesis) and nonoperative management (functional brace).[14]
  - They reported a 15% nonunion rate in the functional brace group vs a 0% nonunion rate in the bridge plate group.
    - The 7 patients who had a nonunion following functional brace application were treated with a compression plate to promote union, all of which were successful.
  - The authors did find a 6-point difference favoring operative management in the DASH questionnaire at the 6-month follow-up only; however, it has been well established that the minimal clinically important difference in the DASH questionnaire is roughly 10 points. There were no differences in the other outcomes measures or complications between the 2 groups.
- Benegas et al randomly assigned patients undergoing operative fixation for their humeral shaft fractures to either antegrade nailing or minimally invasive plate osteosynthesis.[30]
  - They found no differences in the patient outcomes as measured by the University of California, Los Angeles scale, elbow function, or shoulder stiffness.

References

1. Tytherleigh-Strong G, Walls N, McQueen MM. The epidemiology of humeral shaft fractures. *J Bone Joint Surg Br.* 1998;8080(2):249-253. doi:10.1302/0301-620X.80B2.8113.
2. Singh A, Nagar M, Kumar A. An anthropometric study of the humerus in adults. *Res Rev J Med Health Sci.* 2012;3(3):77-82. http://www.rroij.com/peer-reviewed/an-anthropometric-study-of-the-humerus-in-adults-34958.html. Accessed February 17, 2018.
3. Tingart MJ, Apreleva M, von Stechow D, Zurakowski D, Warner JJ. The cortical thickness of the proximal humeral diaphysis predicts bone mineral density of the proximal humerus. *J Bone Joint Surg Br.* 2003;85(4):611-617. doi:10.1302/0301-620X.85B4.12843.
4. Acklin YP, Sommer C. Fracture of the humeral shaft. In: Browner B, Jupiter J, Krettek C, Anderson P, eds. *Skeletal Trauma: Basic Science, Management and Reconstruction.* 5th ed. Philadelphia, PA: Saunders Elsevier; 2014:1389-1405.
5. Ekholm R, Adami J, Tidermark J, Hansson K, Törnkvist H, Ponzer S. Fractures of the shaft of the humerus. An epidemiological study of 401 fractures. *J Bone Joint Surg Br.* 2006;88(11):1469-1473. doi:10.1302/0301-620X.88B11.17634.
6. Ekholm R, Ponzer S, Törnkvist H, Adami J, Tidermark J. The Holstein-Lewis humeral shaft fracture: aspects of radial nerve injury, primary treatment, and outcome. *J Orthop Trauma.* 2008;22(10):693-697. doi:10.1097/BOT.0b013e31818915bf.
7. Klenerman L. Fractures of the shaft of the humerus. *J Bone Joint Surg Br.* 1966;48(1):105-111. doi:10.1302/0301-620X.48B1.105.
8. Sarmiento A, Zagorski JB, Zych GA, Latta LL, Capps CA. Functional bracing for the treatment of fractures of the humeral diaphysis. *J Bone Joint Surg Am.* 2000;82(4):478-486. doi:10.2106/00004623-200004000-00003.
9. van Middendorp JJ, Kazacsay F, Lichtenhahn P, Renner N, Babst R, Melcher G. Outcomes following operative and non-operative management of humeral midshaft fractures: a prospective, observational cohort study of 47 patients. *Eur J Trauma Emerg Surg.* 2011;37(3):287-296. doi:10.1007/s00068-011-0099-0.
10. Ekholm R, Tidermark J, Törnkvist H, Adami J, Ponzer S. Outcome after closed functional treatment of humeral shaft fractures. *J Orthop Trauma.* 2006;20(9):591-596. doi:10.1097/01.bot.0000246466.01287.04.
11. Ali E, Griffiths D, Obi N, Tytherleigh-Strong G, Van Rensburg L. Nonoperative treatment of humeral shaft fractures revisited. *J Shoulder Elbow Surg.* 2014;24(2):1-5. doi:10.1016/j.jse.2014.05.009.
12. Korompilias AV, Lykissas MG, Kostas-Agnantis IP, Vekris MD, Soucacos PN, Beris AE. Approach to radial nerve palsy caused by humerus shaft fracture: is primary exploration necessary? *Injury.* 2013;44(3):323-326. doi:10.1016/j.injury.2013.01.004.

13. Chang G. Radial nerve palsy after humeral shaft fractures: the case for early exploration and a new classification to guide treatment and prognosis. *Hand Clin.* 2018;34(1):105-112. doi:10.1016/J.HCL.2017.09.011.
14. Matsunaga FT, Tamaoki MJS, Matsumoto MH, Netto NA, Faloppa F, Belloti JC. Minimally invasive osteosynthesis with a bridge plate versus a functional brace for humeral shaft fractures: a randomized controlled trial. *J Bone Joint Surg Am.* 2017;99(7):583-592. doi:10.2106/JBJS.16.00628.
15. Catanzarite J, Alan R, Baig R, Forno P, Benson L. Biomechanical testing of unstable humeral shaft fracture plating. *J Surg Orthop Adv.* 2009;18(4):175-181.
16. Spiguel AR, Steffner RJ. Humeral shaft fractures. *Curr Rev Musculoskelet Med.* 2012;5(3):177-183. doi:10.1007/s12178-012-9125-z.
17. Hak DJ, Althausen P, Hazelwood SJ. Locked plate fixation of osteoporotic humeral shaft fractures: are two locking screws per segment enough? *J Orthop Trauma.* 2010;24(4):207-211. doi:10.1097/BOT.0b013e3181bdd1da.
18. Prasarn ML, Ahn J, Paul O, et al. Dual plating for fractures of the distal third of the humeral shaft. *J Orthop Trauma.* 2011;25(1):57-63. doi:10.1097/BOT.0b013e3181df96a7.
19. Gerwin M, Hotchkiss R, Weiland AJ. Alternative operative exposures of the posterior aspect of the humeral diaphysis with reference to the radial nerve. *J Bone Joint Surg Am.* 1996;78(11):1690-1695. doi:10.1017/CBO9781107415324.004.
20. Artico M, Telera S, Tiengo C, et al. Surgical anatomy of the radial nerve at the elbow. *Surg Radiol Anat.* 2009;31(2):101-106. doi:10.1007/s00276-008-0412-8.
21. Kobayashi M, Watanabe Y, Matsushita T. Early full range of shoulder and elbow motion is possible after minimally invasive plate osteosynthesis for humeral shaft fractures. *J Orthop Trauma.* 2010;24(4):212-216. doi:10.1097/BOT.0b013e3181c2fe49.
22. Sobel AD, Shah KN, Paxton ES. Fixation of a proximal humerus fracture with an intramedullary nail. *J Orthop Trauma.* 2017;31(suppl 3):S47-S49. doi:10.1097/BOT.0000000000000909.
23. Kurup H, Hossain M, Andrew JG. Dynamic compression plating versus locked intramedullary nailing for humeral shaft fractures in adults. *Cochrane Database Syst Rev.* 2011;(6):CD005959. doi:10.1002/14651858.CD005959.pub2.
24. Ouyang H, Xiong J, Xiang P, Cui Z, Chen L, Yu B. Plate versus intramedullary nail fixation in the treatment of humeral shaft fractures: an updated meta-analysis. *J Shoulder Elbow Surg.* 2013;22(3):387-395. doi:10.1016/j.jse.2012.06.007.
25. Tingstad EM, Wolinsky PR, Shyr Y, Johnson KD. Effect of immediate weightbearing on plated fractures of the humeral shaft. *J Trauma.* 2000;49(2):278-280. doi:10.1097/00005373-200008000-00014.
26. Thomsen NO, Dahlin LB. Injury to the radial nerve caused by fracture of the humeral shaft: timing and neurobiological aspects related to treatment and diagnosis. *Scand J Plast Reconstr Surg Hand Surg.* 2007;41(4):153-157. doi:10.1080/02844310701445586.
27. Ring D, Chin K, Jupiter JB. Radial nerve palsy associated with high-energy humeral shaft fractures. *J Hand Surg Am.* 2004;29(1):144-147. doi:10.1016/j.jhsa.2003.09.013.
28. Denard A Jr, Richards JE, Obremskey WT, Tucker MC, Floyd M, Herzog GA. Outcome of nonoperative vs operative treatment of humeral shaft fractures: a retrospective study of 213 patients. *Orthopedics.* 2010;33(8). doi:10.3928/01477447-20100625-16.
29. McCormack RG, Brien D, Buckley RE, McKee MD, Powell J, Schemitsch EH. Fixation of fractures of the shaft of the humerus by dynamic compression plate or intramedullary nail. A prospective, randomised trial. *J Bone Joint Surg Br.* 2000;82(3):336-339. doi:10.1302/0301-620x.82b3.9675.
30. Benegas E, Ferreira Neto AA, Gracitelli ME, et al. Shoulder function after surgical treatment of displaced fractures of the humeral shaft: a randomized trial comparing antegrade intramedullary nailing with minimally invasive plate osteosynthesis. *J Shoulder Elbow Surg.* 2014;23(6):767-774. doi:10.1016/j.jse.2014.02.010.
31. Martínez ÁA, Cuenca J, Herrera A. Treatment of humeral shaft nonunions: nailing versus plating. *Arch Orthop Trauma Surg.* 2004;124(2):92-95. doi:10.1007/s00402-003-0608-7.
32. Xue Z, Ding H, Hu C, Xu H, An Z. An anatomical study of the nutrient foramina of the human humeral diaphysis. *Med Sci Monit.* 2016;22:1637-1645. doi:10.12659/MSM.898361.
33. Shields E, Sundem L, Childs S, et al. Factors predicting patient-reported functional outcome scores after humeral shaft fractures. *Injury.* 2015;46(4):693-698. doi:10.1016/j.injury.2015.01.027.

SECTION II

Shoulder

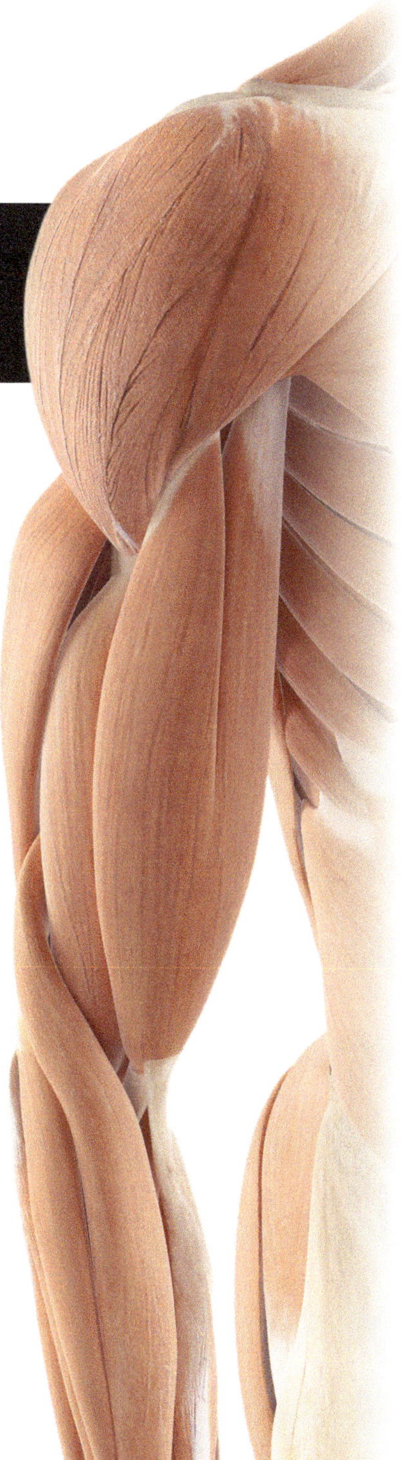

8

Anatomy and Physical Examination

Benjamin Hendy, MD and J. Gabriel Horneff III, MD

Osteology

- Clavicle
  - The clavicle is the first bone to ossify and last to fuse. Acromial edge fuses at 19 to 20 years old, and sternal edge fuses at 25 years old.
  - Muscle origins
    - Deltoid
    - Sternocleidomastoid
    - Pectoralis major
    - Sternohyoid
  - Muscle insertions
    - Trapezius
    - Subclavius
  - Neurovascular structures
    - Subclavian artery and vein
    - Brachial plexus
- The scapula is tilted anteriorly 30 degrees relative to chest and upward 3 degrees and forward flexed 20 degrees.
  - Coracoid process
    - The coracoid process ossifies from the middle portion.
      - The coracoid process ossifies at 15 to 18 months old.
      - The coracoid process fuses at 15 years old.
    - Anatomic landmark or "lighthouse" to shoulder surgery[1,2]

Namdari S, Zmistowski B, Omid R, eds.
The Foundations of Shoulder and Elbow Surgery (pp 131-173).

        - Muscle origins
            - Conjoined tendon: short head of biceps and coracobrachialis tendons on the tip of coracoid process
        - Soft-tissue attachments
            - Lateral side: coracoacromial (CA), coracohumeral (CHL) ligament
            - Medial side: pectoralis minor
            - Tip: conjoined tendon
            - Base: coracoclavicular (CC) ligaments (conoid inserts at the medial base)
    - Glenoid
        - The glenoid has a 5-degree upward tilt and 2-degree to 7-degree retroversion.[3,4]
    - Spine of scapula
        - Muscle origins
            - Posterior deltoid
        - Muscle insertions
            - Trapezius
        - The spine of scapula divides the supraspinatus and infraspinatus fossa.
    - Acromion
        - Three ossification centers unite to form the acromion.
            - Meta-acromion: base
            - Mesoacromion: middle
            - Preacromion: anterior tip
            - The os acromiale is an unfused secondary ossification of the acromion and is most commonly seen at the junction of the mesoacromion and meta-acromion. It has a 3% incidence with 60% bilaterally.
        - Bigliani et al defined 3 types of acromion morphologie[5]:
            - Type 1: relatively flat
            - Type 2: gentle curve
            - Type 3: hooked
                - Type 3 is associated with rotator cuff pathology (correlation but no causation with degenerative cuff tears).
                - The suprascapular notch is another type 3 morphology.
        - The superior transverse ligament can ossify and cause compression of the suprascapular nerve; it is associated with supraspinatus and infraspinatus atrophy.
    - Spinoglenoid notch
        - The spinoglenoid notch joins the supraspinous and infraspinatus fossa.
- Proximal humerus
    - Muscle insertions (Figure 8-1)
        - Pectoralis major: lateral lip of intertubercular groove
        - Latissimus dorsi: floor of intertubercular groove
        - Teres major: medial lip of intertubercular groove
        - Deltoid: lateral aspect of the humerus distal to the insertion of the pectoralis and latissimus dorsi
        - Coracobrachialis: medial aspect of the humerus corresponding to the level of the deltoid
    - The proximal humeral physis provides approximately 80% of the growth of the humerus.
    - Humeral head retroversion is 20 degrees to 40 degrees in reference to the transepicondylar axis.

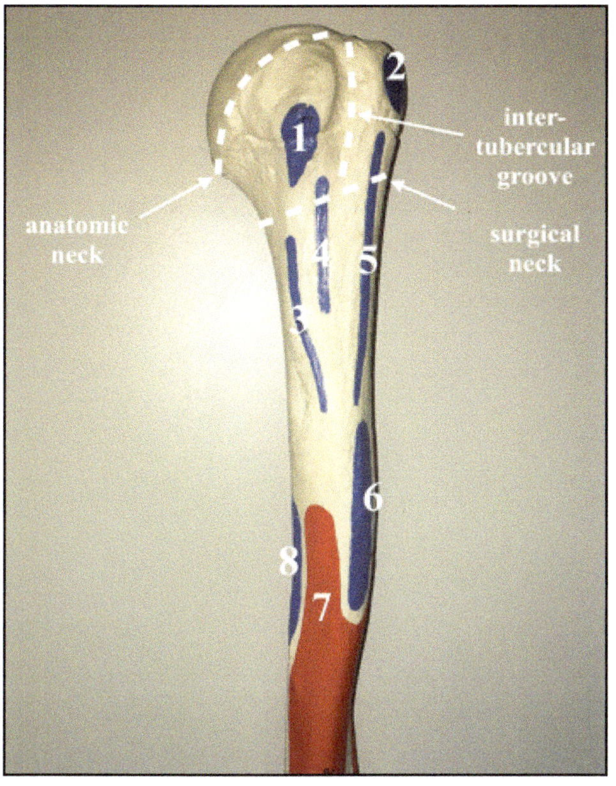

Figure 8-1. Proximal humerus muscle insertions and origins. (1) Subscapularis insertion on lesser tuberosity. (2) Posterosuperior rotator cuff insertion on greater tuberosity. (3) Teres major insertion medial lip of intertubercular groove. (4) Latissimus dorsi insertion on floor of intertubercular groove. (5) Pectoralis major insertion on lateral lip on intertubercular groove. (6) Deltoid insertion on deltoid tuberosity. (8) Brachialis origin on midshaft to distal shaft of humerus. (9) Coracobrachialis insertion on medial shaft of humerus.

- The head-shaft angle averages 135 degrees.
- The surgical neck is a weakened area of bone that marks transition to the humeral shaft, just distal to the tuberosities (Figure 8-2).
  - The *surgical neck* is so termed because of the frequency of fractures at this level.
- The anatomic neck is the space between humeral head articular cartilage and ligamentous and tendon attachment.
- Greater tuberosity is the insertion site of the supraspinatus, infraspinatus, and teres minor from anterior to posterior.
- Lesser tuberosity is the insertion site of the subscapularis tendon.
- The intertubercular (bicipital) groove internally rotates as it courses distally 10 degrees to 15 degrees (between the groove at the anatomic neck and the surgical neck).
  - The intertubercular groove serves as a landmark for orientation during surgical reduction of proximal humerus fractures.
- Proximal humerus fracture “parts”
  - Codman[6] described 4 parts that were later used in the classification system of proximal humerus fractures by Neer.[7]
  - To qualify as a “part,” each fragment requires either 45-degree angulation or 1 cm displacement.
    - Articular fragment (humeral head)
    - Greater tuberosity
    - Lesser tuberosity
    - Humeral shaft

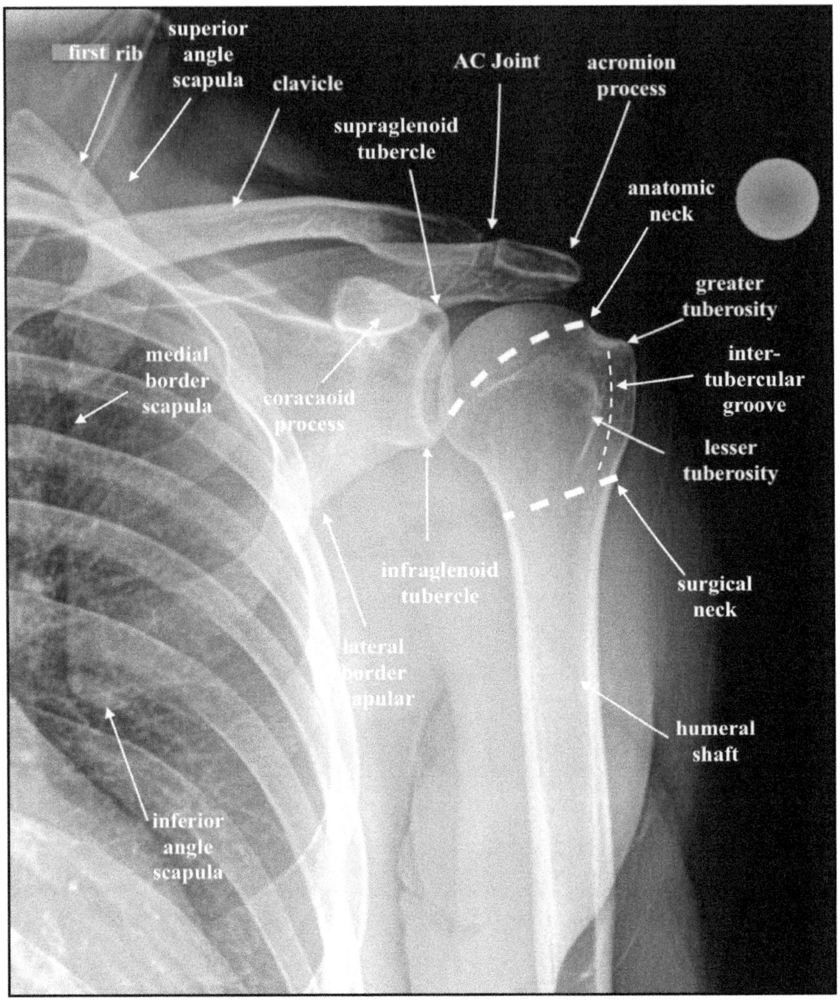

Figure 8-2. Anterior-to-posterior shoulder radiograph with anatomic landmarks labeled.

Joints and Ligaments

- Glenohumeral (GH) joint
  - The GH joint is inherently unstable to allow a large range of motion (ROM).
  - Stability is provided by static and dynamic stabilizers.
    - Dynamic stabilizers
      - Rotator cuff via joint concavity compression, periscapular muscles
    - Static stabilizers
      - Glenoid labrum, articular version, articular conformity, negative intra-articular pressure, capsule/GH ligaments/rotator interval (RI)
  - Glenoid labrum
    - The glenoid labrum is a fibrous ring that is an anchor attachment point for capsuloligamentous structures.
    - It deepens the glenoid cavity and reduces excess GH translation.
    - Excision of the labrum decreases the depth of the GH socket by 50% and reduces resistance to instability by 20%.[8,9]

- GH capsule
  - The surface area of the joint capsule is twice that of the humeral head, and the average fluid volume that the capsule can hold is 10 to 20 mL.
  - Normally the joint contains less than 1 mL of fluid, and the pressure in the joint is below atmospheric (negative intra-articular pressure provides stability).
    - An increase in the intra-articular pressure (eg, effusion or hematoma) can disrupt this stability.
  - The arm position in space can tension various portions of the capsule, which resists humeral translation.
    - Adduction: Superior capsule is taut and inferior capsular is lax.
    - Abduction: Inferior capsule is taut and superior capsule is lax.
    - External rotation (ER): Anterior capsule is taut.
    - Internal rotation (IR): Posterior capsule is taut.
  - Pathologic tightness of the capsule can cause humeral head translation in the opposite direction (ie, tight anterior capsule causes the head to subluxate posteriorly and eccentrically wear the posterior aspect of the glenoid).
- GH ligaments
  - The inferior glenohumeral ligamentous (IGHL) complex is the primary stabilizer for anterior stability in 90-degree abduction.
    - As the arm is abducted and in ER, the anterior band tightens and resists anterior translation.
    - With IR of the abducted arm, the posterior band becomes taut, and posterior translation is resisted. The IGHL complex is the most important restraint to ER in either neutral or abduction.
  - The middle GH ligament is the primary stabilizer to anterior translation and ER with arm in midranges (45 to 60 degrees).
    - Limits ER of the adducted arm.
    - Limits inferior translation of the adducted and ER arm.
    - Limits anterior and posterior translation of midrange (45 to 60 degrees) abduction and ER.
  - The superior glenohumeral ligament (SGHL) is the primary stabilizer to inferior translation with arm at the side.
  - The CHL is similar in function to the SGHL but also the primary restraint to posterior subluxation with the arm in forward flexion (FF) and IR.
    - CHL is a significant restraint to ER, especially in the neutral adducted position.
    - SGHL and CHL are reinforcing structures of the RI and limit the following:
      - Inferior translation and ER when arm is adducted
      - Posterior translation when arm is FF, adducted, and IR
- RI
  - The RI is the space between the anterior edge of the supraspinatus and superior edge of the subscapularis.
  - The RI contains the following:
    - Joint capsule
    - SGHL (deep)
    - CHL (superficial)

      - Long head of the biceps tendon (LHBT) traverses the space intra-articularly from the supraglenoid tubercle, exiting the intertubercular groove distally.
    - The dimensions of the RI change with rotation, becoming smaller with IR. It is recommended that RI closure be performed in ER because imbricating the RI with the arm in IR may lead to overtightening, with loss of ER.
    - Release of the RI causes increased FF and ER.
    - A sulcus sign with an adducted ER arm suggests RI insufficiency.
    - Imbrication of the RI causes decreased inferior and posterior translation of the humeral head.
      - RI imbrication should be considered in the surgical treatment of patients with multidirectional instability.
      - In general, 1 cm of capsular plication results in an approximately 20-degree loss of rotation.
  - CA ligament
    - The CA helps contain the humeral head from excessive superior translation.
    - It restrains anterior and inferior translation through interaction with the CHL via the falx (a thickening of the clavipectoral fascia connecting the conjoined tendon, the CA ligament, and the CHL).
      - Be cautious when releasing the CA ligament in patients with subacromial symptoms when there is concomitant rotator cuff pathology and proximal humeral migration.
    - The medial aspect of the CA ligament contains the acromial branch of the thoracoacromial artery.
    - The CA ligament is separated from the overlying deltoid by a layer of adipose tissue, and this can be used as a reliable landmark for avoiding iatrogenic injury to the CA ligament with a surgical approach.
- Acromioclavicular (AC) joint
  - CC ligaments are primarily responsible for vertical stability of the AC joint.
    - The AC joint is composed of trapezoid and conoid ligaments.
      - The trapezoid is lateral to the conoid ligament.
        - The average trapezoid ligament beginning distance from lateral end of the clavicle is 1.0 cm and ends 2.6 cm medial.[10]
        - The average conoid ligament beginning distance from lateral end of the clavicle is 2.6 cm and ends 4.7 cm medial.[10]
      - The trapezoid is the stronger of the 2 ligaments.
  - The AC ligaments are primarily responsible for anteroposterior (AP) plane stability of the AC joint.
    - Superior
      - The superior ligament is the most important for stabilization in the AP plane.
    - Posterior
      - The posterior ligament is the second most important for AP stabilization.
    - Anterior
    - Inferior
    - These insert about 7 to 10 mm from the joint and can become damaged during aggressive distal clavicle resection, leading to AC joint instability.

- Sternoclavicular joint
  - The sternoclavicular joint is a synovial joint with a fibrocartilaginous articular disc, or meniscus.
  - The major constraint to sternoclavicular motion is the costoclavicular ligament, which resists upward as well as posterior displacement.
  - If the CC ligaments are competent, there is sufficient stability of the proximal clavicle to allow resection of the medial clavicle in cases of arthrosis. However, if the CC ligaments are disrupted (AC dislocation), then excision of the medial clavicle will lead to clavicular instability.
- Scapulothoracic joint
  - The medial border of the scapula articulates with the posterior aspect of the second to seventh ribs.
  - Two major scapulothoracic bursa are sometimes causes of pain and snapping scapula syndrome.
  - The ratio of GH to scapulothoracic motion during abduction of the arm is 2:1, and the ratio can become altered in cases of shoulder pathology.

Muscles

- The shoulder girdle and rotator cuff muscles are detailed in Tables 8-1 and 8-2, respectively.

Nerves

- The brachial plexus is described in Table 8-3 and shown in Figure 8-3.

Arteries

- Arteries of the shoulder are detailed in Table 8-4.

Anatomic Spaces

- Anatomic spaces around the shoulder are detailed in Table 8-5 and shown in Figure 8-4.

Surgical Anatomy

- Open approaches
  - Deltopectoral approach
    - Internervous plane
      - The deltoid muscle is supplied by the axillary nerve.
      - The pectoralis major is supplied by the medial and lateral pectoral nerves.

Table 8-1

Shoulder Girdle Muscles

MUSCLE	ORIGIN	INSERTION	NERVE	FUNCTION	COMMENT
Trapezius	Spinous process C7 to T12 vertebrae	Clavicle, acromion, scapular spine	Spinal accessory (cranial nerve XI)	Elevate, rotate and retract scapula	Lateral scapular winging result of weakness
Rhomboid minor	Spinous process C7 to T1	Medial border of scapula at the spine	Dorsal scapular	Retract and elevate scapula	
Rhomboid major	Spinous process T2 to T5	Medial border scapula	Dorsal scapular	Retract and elevate scapula	
Levator scapula	Transverse process C1 to C4	Superior angle of scapula	Dorsal scapular	Elevate scapula	
Serratus anterior	Anterolateral ribs 1 to 8	Anteromedial boarder of scapula	Long thoracic	Protracts scapula	Medial scapular winging result of weakness
Pectoralis minor	Ribs 3 to 5, anterior	Medial coracoid process	Medial pectoral	Protraction and downward rotation of scapula	
Deltoid *Anterior*	Lateral clavicle	Deltoid tuberosity of humerus	Axillary	Abduct arm, GH joint stability	
Middle	Acromion				
Posterior	Spine of scapular				
Pectoralis major *Upper third*	Medial clavicle	Lateral lip of bicipital groove	Medial and lateral pectoral	Adducts arm, IR, flexion	
Middle third	Manubrium and sternum				
Lower third	Distal sternum				

(continued)

Table 8-1 (continued)

Shoulder Girdle Muscles

MUSCLE	ORIGIN	INSERTION	NERVE	FUNCTION	COMMENT
Latissimus dorsi	Spinous process T7 to T12, iliac crest, sacrum	Medial crest and floor of bicipital groove	Thoraco-dorsal	Adduct, IR, extend humerus	
Teres major	Inferior angle of scapula, lateral border	Medial lip of bicipital groove	Lower subscapular	IR, adduct, extend humerus	
Coraco-brachialis	Tip of coracoid as conjoined tendon	Anteromedial midportion of humerus	Musculo-cutaneous	Flexion and adduction humerus	
Biceps brachii			Musculo-cutaneous	Supination and flexion of elbow	
Long head	Supraglenoid tubercle	Radial tuberosity			
Short head	Coracoid tip as conjoined tendon				
Triceps brachii			Radial	Extension of elbow	
Long head	Infraglenoid tubercle	Olecranon			
Lateral head	Posterior humerus (proximal)				
Medial head	Posterior humerus (distal)				

Table 8-2

Rotator Cuff Muscles

MUSCLE	ORIGIN	INSERTION	NERVE	FUNCTION	COMMENT
Supraspinatus	Supraspinous fossa	Anterior greater tuberosity	Suprascapular	Shoulder elevation	
Infraspinatus	Infraspinous fossa	Middle greater tuberosity	Suprascapular	ER, depresses humeral head, stabilizes GH joint	
Teres minor	Inferolateral border of scapula	Posterior greater tuberosity	Axillary, posterior branch	ER, stabilizes GH joint	
Subscapularis[a]	Subscapularis fossa	Lesser tuberosity	Upper and lower subscapular	IR	

[a]The subscapularis fibers act as a sling around the LHBT, so if the LHBT is not in the intertubercular groove you must consider a subscapularis tear.

- Incision
  - The incision should start between the clavicle and coracoid, along the lateral edge of the coracoid to deltoid insertion (straight incision when the arm in abducted 30 to 40 degrees, not curved) and be about 10 to 15 cm long.
- Surgical dissection
  - Incise the skin and subcutaneous fat.
  - Locate the cephalic vein firmly embedded in deltoid in the deltopectoral interval (Figure 8-5).
    - Usually retract it laterally because there are more venules to the deltoid than the pectoralis.
    - An alternative is retraction medially to relieve tension on the vein.
  - Free the deltoid from the pectoralis, starting from the clavicle extending to the humeral shaft insertion.
  - Superficial dissection: Identify acromion, CA ligament, coracoid process, and conjoined tendon attaching to the lateral coracoid process (Figure 8-6).
  - The lateral edge of the conjoined tendon is identified.
    - Usually it is in a muscular portion laterally.
  - The conjoint tendon represents the origin of the short head of biceps and coracobrachialis muscle (musculocutaneous nerve).
- Deep dissection: Identify the proximal end of the humerus, rotator cuff, and LHBT sheath.
- The LHBT is an excellent landmark to identify the interval between the lesser and greater tuberosity.
- It is essential to identify and protect the musculocutaneous and axillary nerves:

Table 8-3

Cranial Nerve Contribution to Shoulder and Brachial Plexus by Subdivision

CRANIAL NERVE				
NAMED NERVE	**NERVE ROOT CONTRIBUTIONS**	**MOTOR INNERVATION**	**SENSORY DISTRIBUTION**	**NOTES**
Spinal accessory	Cranial nerve XI	Trapezius, sternocleidomastoid	None	Paralysis results in lateral scapular winging
BRACHIAL PLEXUS				
Subdivided into roots, trunks, divisions, cords, and branches				
ROOTS				
C5 to C8 and T1 ventral rami				
NAMED NERVE	**NERVE ROOT CONTRIBUTIONS**	**MOTOR INNERVATION**	**SENSORY DISTRIBUTION**	**NOTES**
Dorsal scapular	C5	Levator scapula, rhomboid minor/major	None	Comes off C5 nerve root
Long thoracic	C5, C6, C7	Serratus anterior	None	Paralysis results in medial scapular winging
TRUNKS				
Roots combine to form 3 trunks: superior (C5, C6), middle (C7), and inferior (C8, T1) Trunks emerge between anterior and middle scalene muscles above first rib				

(continued)

Table 8-3 (continued)

Cranial Nerve Contribution to Shoulder and Brachial Plexus by Subdivision

NAMED NERVE	NERVE ROOT CONTRIBUTIONS	MOTOR INNERVATION	SENSORY DISTRIBUTION	NOTES
Suprascapular	C5, C6 form superior trunk	Supraspinatus, Infraspinatus	GH joint capsule	Passes under transverse scapular ligament in suprascapular notch
Nerve to subclavius	C5, C6	Subclavius	None	
DIVISIONS				
Each trunk gives one anterior and one posterior division (3 anterior, 3 posterior) No named nerves branch off divisions				
CORDS				
Named in anatomic relationship to axillary artery: posterior, lateral, and medial cords				
NAMED NERVE	**NERVE ROOT CONTRIBUTIONS**	**MOTOR INNERVATION**	**SENSORY DISTRIBUTION**	**NOTES**
Upper subscapular	Posterior cord C5, C6	Subscapularis	None	
Thoracodorsal	Posterior cord C6, C7, C8	Latissimus dorsi	None	Runs with thoracodorsal artery
Lower subscapular	Posterior cord C5, C6	Subscapularis and teres major	None	
Lateral pectoral	Lateral cord C5, C6, C7	Pectoralis major	None	Communicates with medial pectoral nerve
Medial pectoral	Medial cord C8, T1	Pectoralis minor and major	None	Pierces through pectoralis minor

(continued)

Table 8-3 (continued)

Cranial Nerve Contribution to Shoulder and Brachial Plexus by Subdivision

NAMED NERVE	NERVE ROOT CONTRIBUTIONS	MOTOR INNERVATION	SENSORY DISTRIBUTION	NOTES
Medial cutaneous nerve of arm	Medial cord T1	None	Medial arm	
Medial cutaneous nerve of forearm	Medial cord C8, T1	None	Medial forearm	
TERMINAL BRANCHES				
NAMED NERVE	**NERVE ROOT CONTRIBUTIONS**	**MOTOR INNERVATION**	**SENSORY DISTRIBUTION**	**NOTES**
Musculocutaneous	Lateral cord C5, C6, C7	Biceps brachii, coracobrachialis, brachialis (medial portion)	Lateral forearm as the lateral antebrachial cutaneous nerve	Enters coracobrachialis muscle about 5.6 cm from tip of the coracoid[11]
Axillary	Posterior cord C5, C6	Deltoid, teres minor	Superior lateral arm	Travels under GH joint capsule with posterior circumflex artery through quadrangular space
Radial	Posterior cord C5, C6, C7, T1	Triceps brachii, brachialis (lateral portion), anconeus, BR, ECRL, ECRB. Becomes PIN in forearm and supplies ED, EDM, ECU, APL, EPB, EPL, and EI.	Posterior arm via posterior cutaneous nerve of arm and lateral arm via inferior lateral cutaneous nerve or arm. SRN innervated back of hand, including first web space.	Runs with deep artery of the arm in triangular interval to radial groove on posterior humerus. Radial nerve branches into SRN and PIN at level of radiohumeral joint line.

(continued)

Table 8-3 (continued)

Cranial Nerve Contribution to Shoulder and Brachial Plexus by Subdivision

NAMED NERVE	NERVE ROOT CONTRIBUTIONS	MOTOR INNERVATION	SENSORY DISTRIBUTION	NOTES
Median	Lateral and medial cords C5, C6, C7, T1	Forearm: PT, FCR, PL, FDS, FDP (radial half), FPL (AIN), PQ (AIN) Fingers: first to second lumbricals Thenar: OP, APB, FPB	Digital cutaneous branches: supply radial 3 half digits (palmar) Palm, PCB: supplies lateral palm Recurrent branch: supplies thenar mass	Runs in medial arm, anterior compartment. Terminal branches include AIN, PCB, recurrent branch, and digital cutaneous branches.
TERMINAL BRANCHES				
NAMED NERVE	**NERVE ROOT CONTRIBUTIONS**	**MOTOR INNERVATION**	**SENSORY DISTRIBUTION**	**NOTES**
Ulnar	Medial cord C7, C8, T1	Forearm: FCU, FDP (ulnar half) Thenar: AP, deep head of FPB Fingers: IO (dorsal and palmar), third to fourth lumbricals Hypothenar: ADM, PDM, FDM	Supplies small finger and ulnar half of ring finger and corresponding part of palm Palm: DCB supplies dorsal medial hand and dorsum of short finger and ring finger PCB supplies	Runs from anterior to posterior in medial compartment of arm. Terminal branches include AIN, DCB, and PCB.

Abbreviations: ADM, abductor digiti minimi; AIN, anterior interosseous nerve; AP, adductor pollicis; APB, abductor pollicis brevis; APL, abductor pollicis longus; BR, brachioradialis; DCB, dorsal cutaneous branch; ECRB, extensor carpi radialis brevis; ECRL, extensor carpi radialis longus; ECU, extensor carpi ulnaris; ED, extensor digitorum; EDM, extensor digiti minimi; EI, extensor indicis; EPB, extensor pollicis brevis; EPL, extensor pollicis longus; FCR, flexor carpi radialis; FCU, flexor carpi ulnaris; FDM, flexor digiti minimi; FDP, flexor digitorum profundus; FDS, flexor digitorum superficialis; FPB, flexor pollicis brevis; FPL, flexor pollicis longus; IO, interossei; ODM, opponens digiti minimi; OP, opponens pollicis; PCB, palmar cutaneous branch; PIN, posterior interosseous nerve; PL, palmaris longus; PT, pronator teres; SRN, superficial radial nerve.

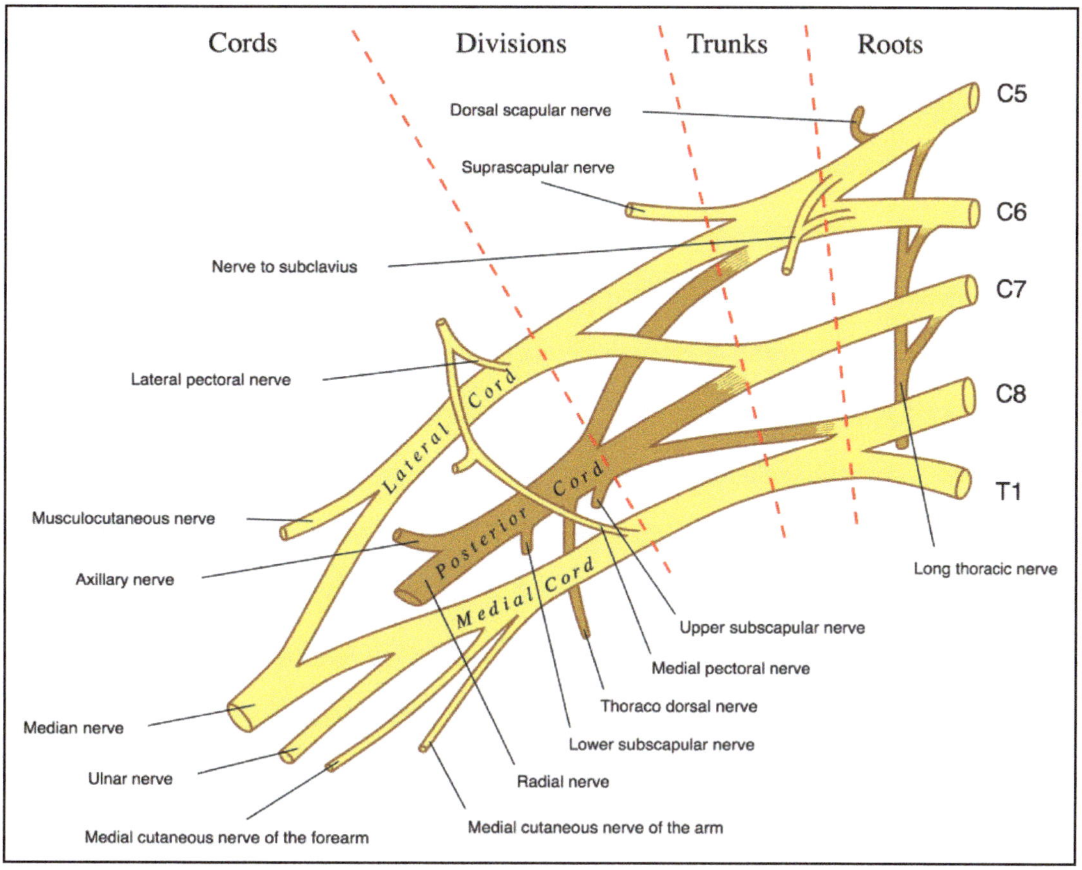

Figure 8-3. The brachial plexus. (Reprinted with permission from https://commons.wikimedia.org/wiki/File:Brachial_plexus_2.svg.)

- The musculocutaneous nerve averages 4 cm distal to the tip of the coracoid and is palpated as it comes into the posteromedial aspect of the conjoined tendon (but can enter as high as 1.5 to 2 cm from the tip). Place index finger under the conjoined tendon hooked anteriorly to palpate it.
- The axillary nerve is located by passing the volar surface of the index finger (hooked anteriorly) down along the anterior surface of the subscapularis.

- The anterior humeral circumflex artery runs horizontal and anterior to the subscapularis tendon (Figure 8-7).
  - The artery and its 2 accompanying veins are termed the *3 sisters*.
- The subscapularis tendon can be managed several ways to gain access to the GH joint.
  - Peel off the lesser tuberosity insertion.
  - Perform a lesser tuberosity osteotomy.
  - Perform a tenotomy 1 to 2 cm medial to the lateral insertion of the subscapularis on the lesser tuberosity.
  - Split in line with muscle fibers.

Table 8-4

Arteries of the Shoulder

SUBCLAVIAN ARTERY		
Branches off the aorta on the left and brachiocephalic artery on the right. Travels above the first rib between anterior and middle scalene muscles with the brachial plexus. Divided into 3 parts based on location of anterior scalene muscle: medial; posterior; and lateral.		
	NAMED ARTERY BRANCHES	**SUPPLY, NOTES**
First part	Vertebral	Spinal cord, brainstem, brain
	Internal thoracic	Anterior chest wall
	Thyrocervical	Two branches
	Suprascapular	Travels above transverse scapular ligament to rotator cuff muscles
	Transverse cervical	Neck
Second part	Costocervical trunk	
Third part	Dorsal scapular	Levator scapula, rhomboids, trapezius
AXILLARY ARTERY		
Continuation of subclavian artery after the first rib. Becomes the brachial artery at the inferior border of the teres major muscle. Divided into 3 parts based on location to pectoralis minor muscle. Number of branches corresponds to part number (eg, first part: one branch). First part proximal: 1 branch; second part behind: 2 branches; third part distal: 3 branches.		
	NAMED ARTERY BRANCHES	**SUPPLY, NOTES**
First part	Superior thoracic	Serratus anterior and pectoralis muscles
Second part	Thoracoacromial	Four branches
	Clavicular	At risk with clavicle fractures and surgery
	Acromial	Runs near the CA ligament, at risk during subacromial decompression
	Deltoid	Runs near deltopectoral interval
	Pectoral	Runs with lateral pectoral nerve
	Lateral thoracic	Runs with long thoracic nerve to serratus anterior

(continued)

Table 8-4 (continued)

Arteries of the Shoulder

	NAMED ARTERY BRANCHES	SUPPLY, NOTES
Third part	Subscapular	Two branches
	Thoracodorsal	Runs with thoracodorsal nerve
	Circumflex scapular	Runs in triangular space
	Anterior humeral circumflex[a]	Important surgical landmark marking transition of the upper tendinous subscapularis tendon from lower muscular insertion
	Posterior circumflex humeral[a]	

[a]Original studies postulated the predominant supply to the humeral head was via the anterolateral branch of the anterior humeral circumflex artery.[11,12] However, more recent studies show the predominant supply to the humeral head is provided by the posterior humeral circumflex artery.[13]

Table 8-5

Anatomic Spaces

SPACE	BORDERS	STRUCTURES
Triangular space	Teres minor Teres major Triceps (long head)	Circumflex scapular artery
Quadrangular space[a]	Teres minor Teres major Triceps (long head) Triceps (lateral head)	Axillary nerve Posterior circumflex artery
Triangular interval	Teres major Triceps (long head) Triceps (lateral head)	Radial nerve Deep artery of arm

[a]The quadrangular space borders differ when looking from them anteriorly rather than posteriorly. Anteriorly, the superior border is the subscapularis (not the teres minor), and posteriorly the border is teres minor.

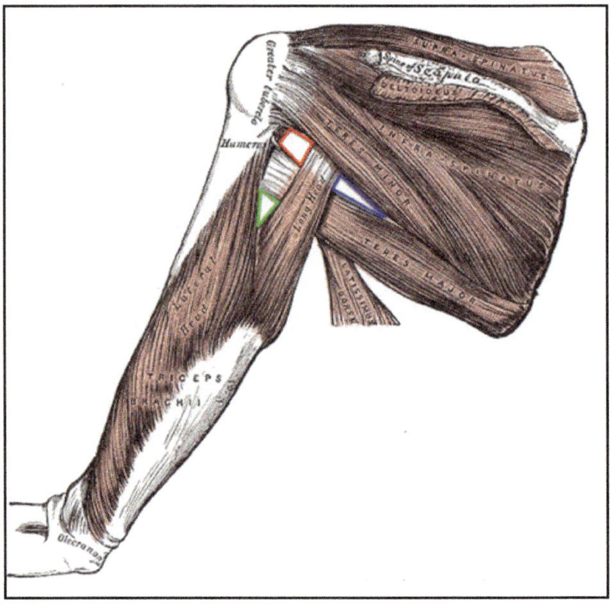

Figure 8-4. Anatomic spaces of the shoulder. Quadrangular space border highlighted in red. Triangular space border highlighted in blue. Triangular interval border highlighted in green. (Reprinted with permission from https://commons.wikimedia.org/wiki/File:Arm_shoulder_gray.png.)

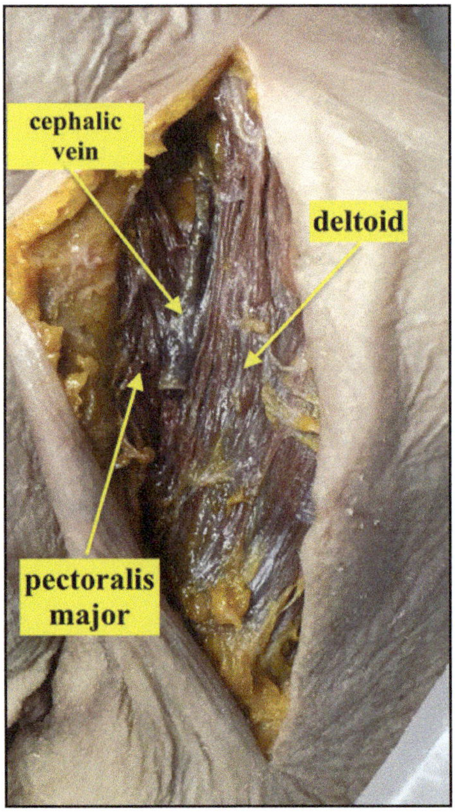

Figure 8-5. A deltopectoral incision with cephalic vein, deltoid, and pectoralis major identified.

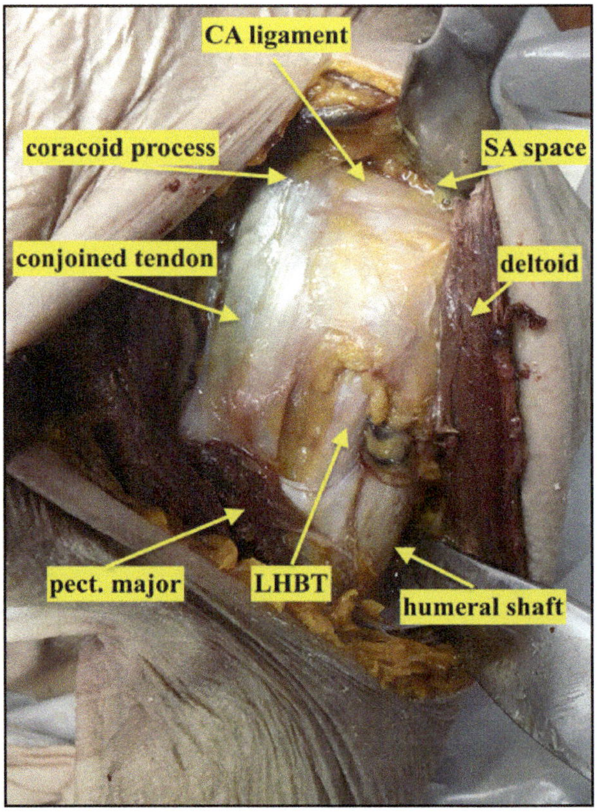

Figure 8-6. Superficial exposure of the deltopectoral approach with conjoined tendon, CA ligament, LHBT, humeral shaft, pectoralis major, and deltoid identified. Abbreviation: SA, subacromial.

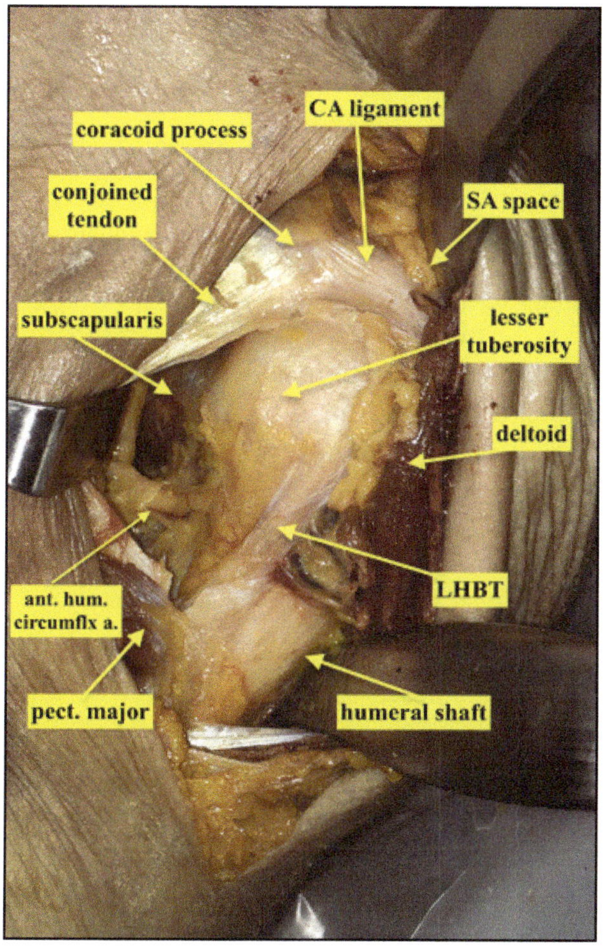

Figure 8-7. Deeper exposure with conjoined tendon retracted medially reveals subscapularis muscle attaching to lesser tuberosity and anterior humeral circumflex artery. Abbreviation: SA, subacromial.

- Superolateral approach
  - Internervous plane
    - There is no internervous plane: Dissection is through the deltoid muscle proximal to innervation. Typically performed in the split between the raphe of the anterior and middle deltoid fibers.
  - Incision
    - Skin incision is performed from the tip of the acromion at the posterior edge of the clavicle.
  - Dissection
    - Superficial dissection: Avoid dissection beyond 5 cm from the lateral acromial edge because the axillary nerve passes laterally around the humeral head in this region. Often a stay suture in the inferior apex of the incision can prevent propagation.
    - Deep dissection: Subacromial or subdeltoid bursa can be excised to gain access to the rotator cuff and greater tuberosity.
    - In cases of proximal humeral fracture fixation with a locking plate, a distal window is commonly created and the plate is slid underneath the neurovascular bundle.

- Posterior approach
  - Internervous plane
    - The infraspinatus is innervated by the suprascapular nerve and the teres minor is innervated by the axillary nerve.
  - Incision
    - A vertical or horizontal incision can be used based on pathology and surgeon preference.
    - A horizontal incision is made along the scapular spine to the posterolateral corner of the acromion.
    - A vertical incision made in line with the GH joint "soft spot."
  - Surgical dissection
    - Superficial dissection: The origin of the deltoid is identified on the scapular spine.
      - There are several ways to manage the deltoid:
        - Detach the deltoid off the scapular spine.
        - Split the deltoid in line with muscle fibers.
        - Retract the deltoid superiorly.
      - Identify the infraspinatus and teres minor muscles.
      - The axillary nerve enters the quadrangular space inferior to the teres minor.
        - The posterior humeral circumflex artery travels with the axillary nerve.
    - Deep dissection: Develop the plane and retract the infraspinatus muscle superior and teres minor muscle inferior.
      - The posterior GH capsule should be visualized.
- Arthroscopic portals
  - Outline anatomy
    - Coracoid
    - Acromion
      - Posterolateral corner of the acromion (easiest to find)
      - Anterolateral corner of the acromion
    - Confluence of the distal clavicle and scapular spine
      - At the supraclavicular fossa
      - Posterior aspect of the AC joint
      - Just lateral to "Nevaiser" supraclavicular portal
    - Recall the axillary nerve is 5.5 cm distal to the lateral edge of the acromion (but can be as close as 3.1 cm).[14]
  - The posterior portal is the primary entry portal for the shoulder.
      - It allows examination of most of the joint and assists in the placement of subsequent portals.
      - Place 2 cm inferior and 2 cm medial to the posterolateral tip of the acromion angled toward the coracoid process.
        - Some place it 1.5 cm inferior and 1 cm medial; it may be placed more laterally for rotator cuff repairs.
      - Both locations attempt to pass through the posterior soft spot between the infraspinatus and teres minor muscles.
      - By placing the portal 1 to 2 cm medial to the posterolateral acromion, the portal can be made approximately parallel to the glenoid articular surface, making for easier passage of the arthroscopic instrumentation to the anterior part of the joint.

- The anterior portal is essential to allow observation of the posterior capsule and the rotator cuff and for an anterior view of the GH ligaments and the subscapularis tendon.
  - This portal is placed slightly lateral to a point halfway between the anterolateral tip of the acromion and the coracoid process.
  - It is 1 to 2 cm inferomedial to the anterolateral acromion and lateral to the coracoid.
  - The cannula passes through the anterior soft spot, which corresponds to an interarticular triangle bounded by the interarticular portion of the biceps tendon superiorly, the superior intra-articular portion of the subscapularis tendon inferiorly, and the anterior edge of the glenoid at the base (placed within the RI).
  - It is established with a spinal needle (outside in) or with a Wissinger rod (inside out).
- The anterolateral (or lateral) portal is the primary working portal for the subacromial space.
  - It is located 1 cm posterior and 2 to 3 cm distal to the anterolateral border of the acromion.
  - Accessory portals can be made anteriorly or posteriorly as necessary.
  - Outside-in portal placement is frequently used in current arthroscopic techniques because it is useful in identifying the ideal placement of the arthroscopic portals.
- The posteroinferior portal is for in-flow cannula during arthroscopy in the beach chair position.
  - It is located 2 cm above the posterior axillary fold and enters the joint in the axillary recess.
  - As long as the portal is directed caudally, the axillary nerve and posterior humeral circumflex artery are safe.
  - The axillary nerve and posterior circumflex humeral artery enter the axilla through the quadrangular space, and they should be approximately 3 cm from the posterior portal.
- The anteroinferior (5 o'clock) portal is described by Davidson and Tibone[15] as an accessory portal for stabilization procedures that improves access to the inferior aspect of the GH joint, the IGHL (for Bankart repair), and the anteroinferior aspects of the glenoid rim and scapular neck.
  - The portal is placed just lateral and usually slightly superior to the coracoid.
  - It is created under direct visualization from inside out by passing a blunt Wissinger rod through the anterior capsule directed to the leading edge of the anteroinferior IGHL with the arm adducted.
  - This portal passes lateral to the conjoint tendon and through the lower subscapularis muscle.
  - Risks
    - It is within 14 mm of the axillary nerve
    - It is within 12 mm of the musculocutaneous nerve
    - Abduction decreases both distances so it is vital to create this portal with the arm adducted.
  - In a cadaver study, all test portals were safe for the neurovascular structures; however, using the anterior or 5 o'clock portal could jeopardize the cephalic vein.
  - Safety of the 5 o'clock portal was reported by Mehta,[16] who found no clinically detectable neurovascular injuries associated with the use of the 5 o'clock portal after 48 consecutive Bankart repairs.
- The posteroinferior (7 o'clock) portal is described by Davidson and Rivenburgh[17] as an accessory portal to access the inferior GH joint for loose body removal, posteroinferior labral fixation, capsular shrinkage, and capsulotomy.

        - The inside-to-outside 7 o'clock portal is created by using a switching stick passed through the 2 o'clock portal and directed posteroinferiorly.
        - The switching stick is then brought through a small skin incision and left in place.
        - Risks
            - It is within 39 mm of the axillary nerve and posterior circumflex artery
            - It is within 29 mm of the suprascapular nerve
            - Differential flexion/extension or abduction-adduction had no effect on the distances between the portal and the neurovascular structures.
    - The superior (Neviaser) portal is the most useful as an in-flow site but may also allow limited viewing of the posterior glenoid labrum, posterior humeral head, and posterior aspect of the rotator cuff.
        - The portal penetrates the trapezius muscle and then passes through the supraspinatus muscle belly (the tendon is safe with this portal).
        - Entry is in the soft spot between the most lateral aspect of the triangle formed between the clavicle and acromion and angled posteriorly.
- Arthroscopic anatomy
    - LHBT
        - The LHBT originates from the posterosuperior labrum and supraglenoid tubercle (recall the long head of the triceps originates from the infraglenoid tubercle).
        - The tendon is widest at its origin and has a variable origin:
            - Habermeyer showed the LHBT.[18]
                - Fifty percent originated completely from the labrum.
                - Twenty percent originated completely from the supraglenoid tubercle.
                - Thirty percent originated from both.
            - Vangsness showed the LHBT.[19]
                - Forty to 60% arose from both the labrum and supraglenoid tubercle.
                - Forty to 60% arose from the labrum alone.
                - Type 1 (22%): entirely posterior
                - Type 2 (33%): mostly posterior with some anterior
                - Type 3 (37%): equal anterior and posterior
                - Type 4 (8%): mostly anterior some posterior
        - Regardless of the exact labral origin, when the articular cartilage of the superior glenoid rim is extended, it always blends superiorly with the biceps tendon origin.
        - The LHBT arches over the humeral head to exit the joint encased in a synovial sheath beneath the transverse humeral ligament.
        - The synovial sheath ends in a blind pouch at the intertubercular groove. The LHBT is therefore intra-articular and extrasynovial.
        - Pathologic changes are commonly seen within the groove so it is essential to draw this portion of the tendon into the joint during arthroscopy (pull with probe or alternatively place an Allis clamp into the joint and clasp around the tendon and rotate to pull the tendon into the joint).
- RI
    - A recent study divided the RI into 2 portions[19]:
        - The medial portion is composed of 2 layers:
            - Superficial CHL
            - Deeper SGHL

- The lateral portion is composed of 4 layers:
  1. Layer 1, the most superficial layer, is made up of superficial fibers of the CHL that extend lateral to the insertion of the subscapularis and supraspinatus.
  2. Layer 2 is composed of tendon fibers of the subscapularis and supraspinatus.
  3. Layer 3 is made up of deep fibers of the CHL.
  4. Layer 4 is the deepest layer and consists of the SGHL and capsule.
- Externally, the CHL is seen to originate as a band 1 to 2 cm wide from the proximal third of the dorsolateral aspect of the coracoid process, which travels anterior and superficial to the biceps tendon to insert onto the tuberosities.
- Tetro and colleagues found that the fibers of the CHL are extra-articular medially but laterally become interlaced and indistinguishable from those of the capsule and SGHL.[21] Therefore, to perform an arthroscopic RI release, the fibers of the CA ligament must be visualized from within the GH joint.
  - The measured distance from the RI to the CA ligament is 3.5 mm.
- The SGHL, the medial head of the CHL, and the insertion of the subscapularis tendon become confluent and support the biceps tendon as the medial sheath at the proximal aspect of the intertubercular groove.
- The subscapularis tendon inserts onto the lesser tuberosity just inferior to the articular cartilage and medial to the SGHL/CHL complex.
- The lateral head of the CHL crosses the bicipital groove to insert with the fibers of the supraspinatus onto the greater tuberosity.

- Glenoid labrum
  - Although somewhat variable, the labrum is peripherally continuous with the joint capsule and the periosteum of the scapular neck.
  - Centrally, the labrum is in continuity with the hyaline cartilage on the surface of the glenoid fossa.
  - The most common type of detachment of the labrum is the central detachment type, seen in 60% of patients.
    - In this variant, the labrum is secured peripherally to the joint capsule but centrally at its free margin; a probe can be placed between its edge and the superior glenoid rim.
  - The key to distinguishing this normal variant from a true superior labrum anterior and posterior (SLAP) lesion is to recognize the presence of normal hyaline articular cartilage extending over the glenoid's superior rim and smooth transition to the labral undersurface.
  - The labrum may appear to be loose and in fact is often quite mobile, but this is entirely normal and should not be confused with a SLAP lesion.
  - The "peel-back" injury described by Burkhart can be seen only with dynamic assessment of the joint.
    - The labrum peels back medially along the glenoid when the arm is placed in the throwing position (abduction and ER).
  - The anterosuperior labrum is commonly variable, so be aware of anatomic variants (see following section) in this region. Pathology in this region is rare.
  - The most significant variation of capsular attachments to the labrum was shown in a study of 52 fetal shoulders. Seventy-seven percent of labrums had direct capsular attachment, and 23% had capsular attachment to the scapular neck with a freestanding labrum, creating an anterior pouch.[22]

- GH ligaments
  - When viewed externally, the GH capsule is featureless, but when viewed arthroscopically, the deep capsule has discrete thickenings (GH ligaments) that are defined by their humeral insertions as superior (SGHL), middle (MGHL), or inferior (IGHL).
  - The superior GH ligament is almost always present (94% to 100%) but varies in thickness.
    - The SGHL arises near the supraglenoid tubercle and inserts just superior to the lesser tuberosity in close association with the CHL, forming an anterior band around the biceps tendon, which is the main restraint to medial biceps subluxation (primary restraint to inferior translation in adduction; also resists posterior and inferior humeral head displacement).
    - Variations of the SGHL have to do with its origin:
      - It may originate from the superior glenoid tubercle, anterior to the LHBT.
      - It may originate solely from the glenoid labrum at the 1 o'clock position, possibly sharing a common origin with the MGHL.
  - The middle glenohumeral ligament is not seen as consistently (85%) as is the SGHL, though it is significantly larger and more variable in size (thin wisp of tissue or as thick as the biceps tendon).
    - The MGHL arises from the glenoid labrum immediately below the origin of the SGHL or from the adjacent glenoid neck and inserts just medial to the lesser tuberosity, crossing over and occasionally blending into the subscapularis tendon.
    - It functions as the main restraint to anterior translation in the midrange of shoulder function (especially if the IGHL has been damaged). It has the greatest number of normal variants (9% of the population has a cordlike MGHL).
    - The Buford complex is seen in 1.5% of patients and consists of a cordlike MGHL with deficient anterosuperior labrum.
  - The inferior glenohumeral ligament is a complex consisting of an anterior band, a posterior band, and intervening axillary pouch.
    - It originates from the glenoid, the labrum, or the neck of the glenoid just adjacent to the labrum:
      - The anterior band of the IGHL originates between 2 and 4 o'clock.
      - The posterior band of the IGHL originates between 7 and 9 o'clock.
      - As a complex, the IGHL originates between 3 and 8 o'clock in more than 90% of shoulders.
    - A distinct IGHL ligament is found in 72% of patients, a thickening of the capsule is found in 21% of patients, and no ligament or thickening is found in 7%.
    - The IGHL inserts in 1 of 2 configurations:
      - Onto the anatomic neck of the humerus as a collar just inferior to the articular margin
      - Onto the anatomic neck of the humerus as a "V" with the axillary pouch inserting distal to the articular cartilage
    - The IGHL is best demonstrated with the arm in abduction; the posterior band becomes more prominent with IR and the anterior band becomes more prominent with ER.
    - The humeral avulsion of GH ligaments lesion is seen in up to 9.3% of patients and is best seen from an anterior portal or with the use of a 70-degree scope from the traditional posterior portal.[23]
    - The classic pattern of distinct ligament of the SGHL, MGHL, and IGHL with synovial reflections between them is seen in 66% of patients.

    - Seven percent of patients have a pattern of "confluence" in which the MGHL and IGHL are confluent as one ligament without an intervening recess.
    - Eight percent have no discernible ligaments.
- Rotator cuff
- Footprint anatomy[24] *Recommended reading for pertinent anatomic review*
  - The supraspinatus is triangular in shape, with an average maximum medial to lateral length of 6.9 mm and an average maximum AP width of 12.6 mm.
  - The infraspinatus is trapezoidal in shape, with an average maximum medial to lateral length of 10.2 mm and an average maximum AP width of 32.7 mm.
  - The teres minor is triangular in shape, with an average maximum medial to lateral length of 29 mm and an average maximum width of 21 mm.
  - The subscapularis is a comma-shaped insertion, with an average maximum medial to lateral length of 40 mm and an average maximum width of 20 mm.
- Subscapularis
  - The superior two-thirds of the subscapularis muscle inserts as a tendon onto the lesser tuberosity, and the inferior one-third has a direct muscular attachment along the surgical neck.
  - The distal 1.5 cm of the subscapularis is tendinous.
  - The most superior tendon fibers interdigitate at their insertion with the supraspinatus because these muscles send fibers to both the lesser and greater tuberosity.
  - The subscapularis bursa is a structure between the glenoid and the tendon and is lined with synovial membrane. It is best seen from an anterior portal and can be the site of loose bodies.
- Supraspinatus
  - The supraspinatus consists of a large anterior fusiform muscle belly and smaller unipennate posterior muscle belly.
  - The anterior muscle has a thicker tendon and contributes to the majority of contractile force, which is a reason it may be the most important part to repair.
  - The posterior tendon fibers of the supraspinatus merge with the tendon of the infraspinatus about 15 mm from their insertion and are indistinguishable at the junction.
- Infraspinatus
  - The infraspinatus is bipennate.
- Teres minor
  - The teres minor is fusiform and, like the subscapularis, its tendinous insertion is supplemented by a direct muscular attachment onto the surgical neck.
- Rotator cable
  - Proximal to the terminal rotator cuff insertion is a thickened, capsular structure known as the rotator cable.
  - The intact rotator cuff demonstrates an arching, cable-like thickening surrounding a thinner crescent of tissue that inserts into the greater tuberosity of the humerus; this is known as the cable-crescent complex.[25]
  - This cable-like structure represents a thickening of the CHL and consistently is located at the margin of the avascular zone. The rotator cable extends from its anterior attachment just posterior to the biceps tendon to its posterior attachment near the inferior border of the infraspinatus tendon.
  - This rotator cable may function in a way that is analogous to a load-bearing suspension bridge.

        - By this model, stress is transferred from the cuff muscles to the rotator cable as a distributed load, thereby stress-shielding the thinner, avascular crescent tissue, particularly in older individuals.
        - The synovial vasculature of the undersurface of the rotator cuff stops at the rotator cable. The thinner rotator crescent is avascular.
        - A rotator cuff tear similarly can be modeled after a suspension bridge, with the free margin of the tear corresponding to the cable and the anterior and posterior attachments of the tear corresponding to the supports at each end of the cable's span. By this model, the supraspinatus muscle, even with a supraspinatus tendon tear, can still exert its compressive effect on the shoulder joint by means of its distributed load along the span of the suspension bridge configuration.
- Nervous anatomy
    - The axillary nerve is a terminal branch of the posterior cord.
    - It arises posterior to the coracoid and travels along the subscapularis passing inferior to it, 3 to 5 cm medial to the musculotendinous junction.[14]
    - The axillary nerve is then in intimate contact with the inferior capsule. The nerve is held in loose areolar tissue between the 5 and 7 o'clock positions.
    - Anterior to the long head of the triceps, the nerve branches into anterior and posterior branches:
        - The posterior branch divides into the following:
            - Superior lateral brachial cutaneous
            - Nerve to the teres minor (courses medially along posterior aspect of inferior glenoid rim for 18 mm before entering muscle)
            - The posterior branch is more at risk during arthroscopic procedures (especially thermal capsulorrhaphy or suture imbrication of the capsule).
            - Deficits of this branch cause sensory loss to the deltoid region and loss of teres minor function.
        - The anterior branch provides innervation to the lateral and anterior deltoid.
            - The anterior branch is more at risk during open procedures.
            - It passes with the posterior humeral circumflex artery through the quadrangular space (teres minor superiorly, teres major inferiorly, long head medially, humerus laterally).
            - The nerve then passes anteriorly on the undersurface of the deltoid, an average of 5.5 cm distal to posterolateral corner of the acromion but as close as 3.1 cm.
            - It is 5 cm from the anterolateral corner of the acromion. This distance narrows by almost 30% in abduction.
        - The suprascapular nerve arises from the upper trunk and passes below the transverse scapular ligament to innervate the supraspinatus.
            - The nerve is 3 cm from the supraglenoid tubercle as it passes below this ligament.
            - It then passes inferiorly and laterally around the spine of the scapula to innervate the infraspinatus and lies 1.8 cm from the posterior glenoid rim at this point.
        - The musculocutaneous nerve is a terminal branch of the lateral cord and courses obliquely to enter the coracobrachialis muscle about 5.6 cm from the tip of the coracoid.
            - The nerve may have more than one branch, with smaller branches entering the muscle about 3.1 cm from the tip.[26]
- GH skeletal anatomy

- The articular surface of the glenoid has a thin layer of cartilage in the center.
  - This area should not be mistaken for early osteoarthritis or chondromalacia.
- The anterior edge of the glenoid has a normal indentation just superior to the glenoid's midpoint, marking the point of fusion between the 2 ossific nuclei of the glenoid and gives the glenoid its inverted comma shape (pear shape).
- The supraglenoid tubercle serves as the origin of the LHBT.
- The infraglenoid tubercle serves as the origin of the long head of the triceps.
- The humeral head is devoid of articular cartilage at the posterolateral aspect and is termed the "bare area."
  - The bare area can appear quite irregular on inspection, but it has a smooth transition with the articular cartilage surface.

- Normal anatomic variants
  - Thirteen percent of shoulders have anatomic variants in the anterior or superior quadrant of the glenoid labrum, and the surgeon must be aware that normal variants exist in this anterosuperior quadrant.
  - Repair of a normal variant can result in shoulder stiffness.
    - Sublabral foramen
      - This is a normal variant found in 11% to 12% of people.
      - In 2% of patients, the anterosuperior labrum is absent.
    - Buford complex
      - The Buford complex was described by Williams et al.[27]
      - An absent anterosuperior labrum associated with a thickened, cordlike middle glenohumeral ligament is called a Buford complex.
      - It is seen in about 2% of people.
      - If the Buford complex is mistakenly reattached, painful restriction of rotation and elevation may result.

General Shoulder Examination

- Inspection
  - Symmetry
  - Scars
  - Gross deformity
- Palpation
  - AC joint
  - Greater tuberosity
  - Bicipital groove
  - Clavicle
  - Sternoclavicular joints
- ROM
  - Examine each plane of motion both in active and passive ROM.
    - Disruption of passive and active ROM: results from capsule pathology (eg, adhesive capsulitis) or GH joint arthritis
    - Disruption of active ROM only: results from rotator cuff pathology or nerve lesion (eg, suprascapular nerve palsy)

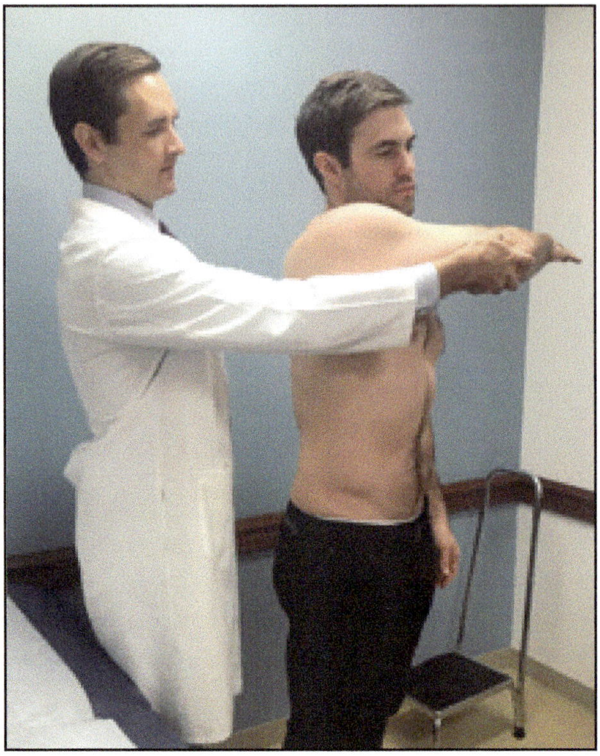

Figure 8-8. The crossover impingement test to assess AC joint arthritis vs AC joint separation.

- Normal shoulder ROM ranges include the following:
  - FF: 150 to 180 degrees
  - ER with arm at side: 30 to 60 degrees
  - ER with arm abducted to 90 degrees: 70 to 90 degrees
  - IR behind back: reaching (thoracic spine level) T4 to T8
    - Inferior angle of scapula is at T7 for reference
  - IR with arm abducted to 90 degrees: 50 to 70 degrees
  - Abduction: 150 to 180 degrees

Acromioclavicular Joint Examination

- Crossover Impingement Test (Figure 8-8)
  - This test assesses AC joint arthritis vs AC joint separation.
  - Adduct the arm across the chest, reaching for the opposite shoulder.
  - A positive test is determined by pain over the AC joint, indicating AC pathology.
    - Pain more anteriorly may be related to the following:
      - Supraspinatus
      - LHBT
      - Subscapularis
    - Pain posteriorly may indicate posterior rotator cuff (infraspinatus/teres minor) or posterior capsule.
- Acromioclavicular Joint Distraction Test: evaluation of the AC joint and CC ligaments

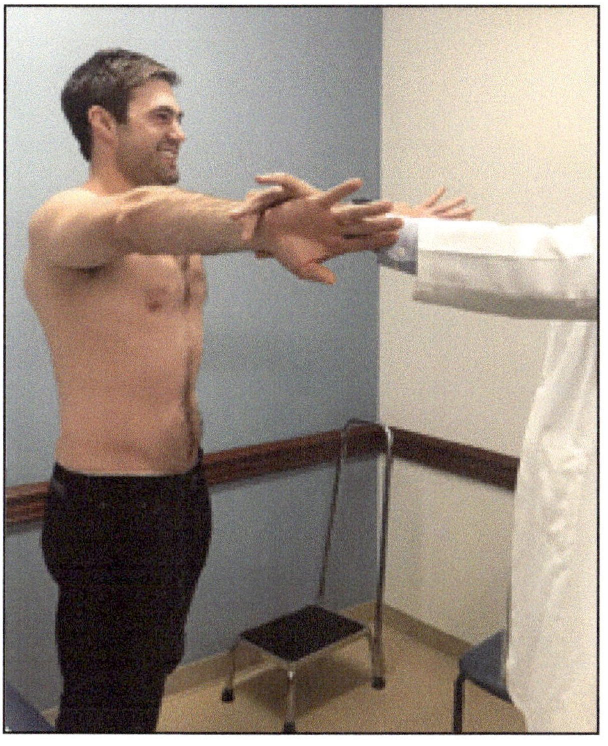

Figure 8-9. The Jobe Supraspinatus Test for supraspinatus pathology or subacromial impingement.

  - This test assesses AC joint separation.
  - With the patient sitting with arm at the side and at 90-degree elbow flexion, apply a gentle, downward force on humerus.
  - A positive test is determined by pain at the AC joint.
- AC Joint Compression Test
  - This test assesses AC joint separation.
  - With the patient in the same position as the distraction test, compress the joint to cause a grinding motion at the AC joint.
  - A positive test is determined by pain at the AC joint.
- Piano key sign
  - This test assesses AC joint separation.
  - Downward pressure is applied on the distal clavicle with the examiner's finger depressing the clavicle back to its normal location.
  - A positive test is determined by pain at the AC joint.

Rotator Cuff Examination

- Testing of rotator cuff integrity should be part of all shoulder examinations.
- There are 2 types of integrity tests:
  1. One kind determines whether movement can be undertaken actively.
  2. One kind determines whether a passive position can be maintained (lag signs).
- Jobe Supraspinatus Test[28] (Figure 8-9)
  - This test assesses for supraspinatus weakness and/or subacromial impingement.

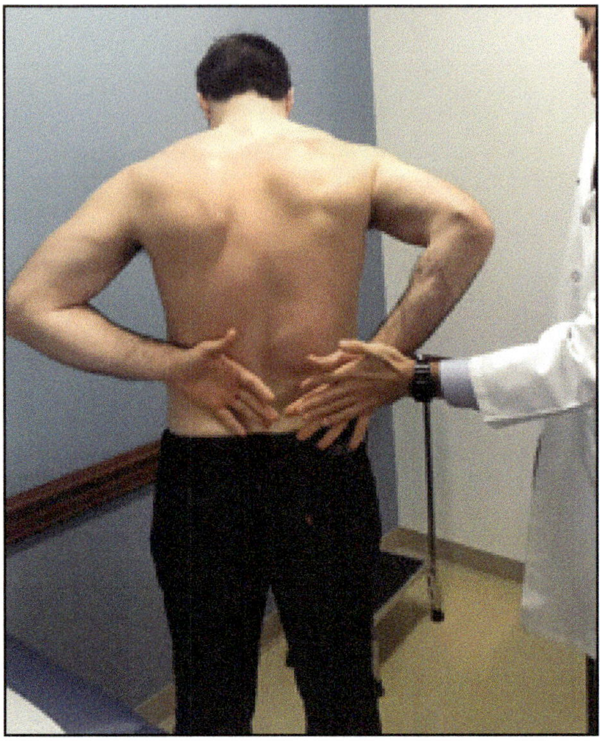

Figure 8-10. The Lift-Off Test for subscapularis pathology.

- The hand is held in abduction to 90 degrees in the plane of the scapula with arm IR (thumb down) to isolate the supraspinatus. Then the examiner presses down on the arm while the patient maintains arm position.
- Pain or weakness in the shoulder is associated with supraspinatus pathology and/or subacromial impingement. The examination is also referred to as the "empty can test" and the "supraspinatus test."

- Lift-Off Test[29] (Figure 8-10)
  - This test assesses the integrity of the subscapularis tendon.
  - The patient places a hand behind the back to the lumbar spine with the palm facing away from body; then test patient's ability to lift the hand off or away from the lumbar spine.
  - Inability to lift hand off lumbar spine indicates subscapularis pathology.
    - Weakness of IR is most easily demonstrated at the limit of amplitude of contraction of the muscle (when the arm is fully extended and internally rotated).
    - Electromyography study showed other internal rotators (especially the pectoralis major) was minimally active in this position of maximum IR.
- Lift-Off Test (Lag Sign)[30]
  - This test evaluates for isolated rupture of the subscapularis tendon.
  - Bringing the arm passively into maximum IR (behind the back), palm away from the body, and ask patient to hold the position off the lower back once released by the examiner.
  - Inability to hold the hand off the lower back indicates a positive test.

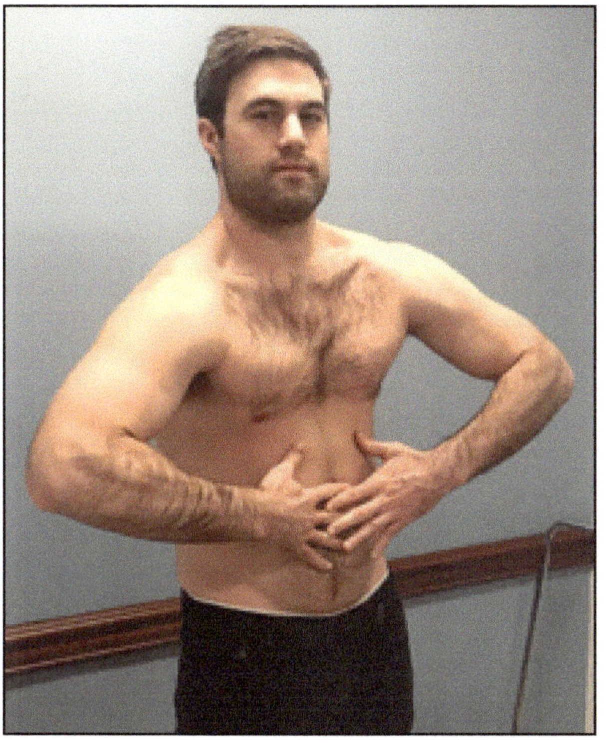

Figure 8-11. The Belly Press Test for subscapularis pathology.

- Belly Press Test[30] (Figure 8-11)
    - This test evaluates for subscapularis insufficiency.
    - The patient presses the abdomen with the palm of the hand and attempts to keep the arm in maximum IR. If active IR is strong, the elbow does not drop backward, meaning that it remains in front of the trunk.
    - If the elbow drops behind the trunk, then the subscapularis is weak or torn.
- Hornblower's sign[31]
    - This test assesses for teres minor pathology.
    - Abduct the shoulder to 90 degrees, with the elbow flexed to 90 degrees, ask the patient to ER against resistance.
    - If the hand falls in front of the patient's face from the ER position, this is considered a positive hornblower's sign.
        - The teres minor is responsible for up to 45% of ER power but is commonly ignored or factored in with the infraspinatus.
        - In chronic teres minor tears older than 1 year, the hornblower's sign had a sensitivity of 100% and specificity of 93% for the presence of stage 3 or stage 4 fatty degeneration of teres minor on computed tomography scan and indicates an irrepairable tear of the teres minor.
- Dropping sign[31]
    - This test assesses for infraspinatus insufficiency.
    - Place the patient's arm at 0-degrees abduction (at the side) and the elbow at 90 degrees of flexion, then ER the shoulder to 45 degrees and ask patient to hold that position.
    - If the patient is unable to maintain the ER position and the arm drops back to the neutral position, the test is positive.

Figure 8-12. The ER lag sign to assess integrity of supraspinatus and infraspinatus tendons.

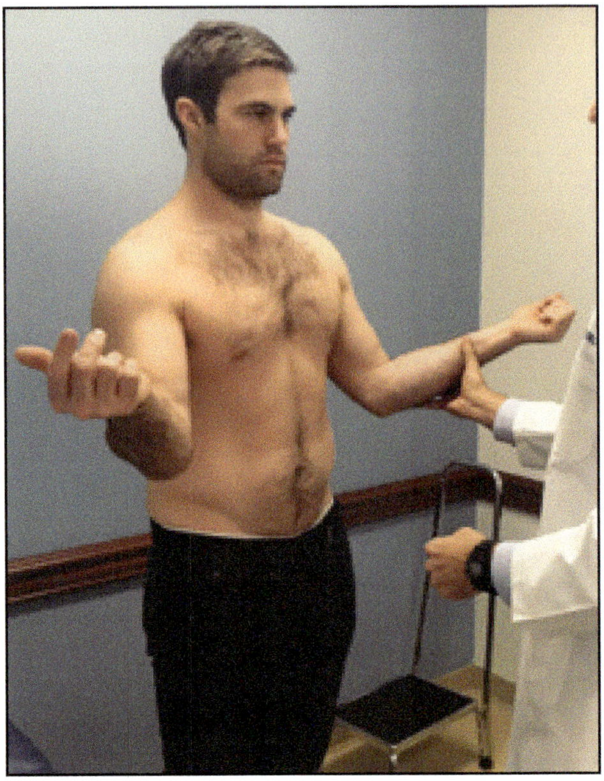

- In chronic infraspinatus tears older than 1 year, the dropping sign had a sensitivity and specificity of 100% for the presence of stage 3 or stage 4 fatty degeneration of the infraspinatus on computed tomography scan and indicates an irrepairable tear of the infraspinatus.

Lag Signs

- Hertel et al described lag signs in the diagnosis of rotator cuff tears.[32] *Recommended reading for historical context*
- ER lag sign (Figure 8-12)
    - This test assesses the integrity of the supraspinatus and infraspinatus tendons.
    - The maneuver is performed as follows:
        - The physician flexes the patient's elbow to 90 degrees, and the shoulder is held at 20-degrees elevation (in scapular plane) and near maximum ER (minus 5 degrees to avoid elastic recoil in the shoulder).
        - Ask the patient to hold this position, and release the hand while supporting the elbow.
    - The sign is positive when a lag, or angular drop, occurs. The magnitude of the lag sign is recorded to the nearest 5 degrees.
- Drop sign
    - This test assesses the integrity of the infraspinatus tendon.
    - The maneuver is performed as follows:

        - Physician has the patient flex the elbow to 90 degrees and hold the arm at 90 degrees of elevation (in the scapular plane) and almost full ER. Tell the patient to hold this position.
        - Then, the examiner supports elbow and releases the wrist.
    - The sign is positive when a lag or angular drop occurs. The magnitude of the lag sign is recorded to the nearest 5 degrees.
- IR lag sign
    - This test assesses the integrity of the subscapularis tendon.
    - The maneuver is performed as follows:
        - Flex the elbow to 90 degrees, hold the shoulder at 20 degrees of elevation and 20 degrees of extension with the arm in maximum IR, and hold the hand elevated off the back.
        - Ask the patient to maintain this position while releasing the patient's hand.
    - The sign is positive when a lag or angular drop occurs.
        - A slight lag indicates a partial tear of the upper-border part of the subscapularis tendon. This is more sensitive than the lift-off sign.
        - Very similar to the Gerber lift-off test lag sign.

Impingement Tests

- The Neer Impingement Sign and Impingement Test[33,34]
    - Purpose: This test assesses for impingement of the rotator cuff at the anterior edge of the acromion.
    - Maneuver: Scapular rotation is prevented with one hand as the other raises the arm in forced forward elevation (somewhere between flexion and abduction), causing the greater tuberosity to impinge against the acromion.
    - Positive impingement sign: pain elicited at anterior edge of acromion with greater tuberosity impinging on acromion.
        - Pain elicited in patients with the following:
            - Impingement lesions
            - Rotator cuff tendinitis/bursitis
            - Stiffness (eg, partial frozen shoulder/adhesive capsulitis)
            - Instability (eg, anterior subluxation)
            - Arthritis
            - Calcium deposits (calcific tendinitis)
            - Bone lesions
    - Positive Impingement Test: Pain can be eliminated or markedly reduced by the injection of 10 mL of 1% xylocaine beneath the anterior acromion if pain is due to one of the above causes.
        - An anatomic study[35] revealed soft-tissue contact with the medial aspect of the acromion in all specimens when the shoulder was in the "Neer position."
        - In an arthroscopic study, there was no significant difference in the rate of internal impingement seen arthroscopically for those with and without positive impingement tests (Neer and Hawkins), raising doubt as to its significance.[36]

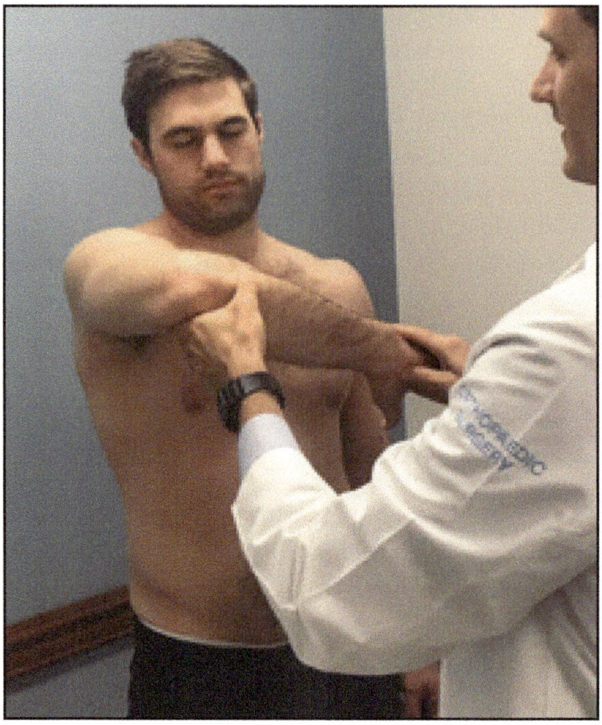

Figure 8-13. The Hawkins-Kennedy Test for subacromial impingement.

- Hawkins-Kennedy Test[37] (Figure 8-13)
  - Purpose: used to assess for impingement of the rotator cuff against acromion or CA ligament
  - Maneuver: the patient's arm is placed in 90-degree abduction in the scapular plane, with the elbow flexed at 90 degrees, examiner IR shoulder
  - Positive test: pain elicited with IR as greater tuberosity impinges against acromion and/or CA ligament
    - Pain elicited in patients with the following:
      - Subacromial bursitis
      - Rotator cuff pathology
      - Bankart lesions
      - SLAP lesions
      - AC joint arthritis
    - In an anatomic study, all specimens demonstrated contact between the CA ligament and either the rotator cuff or the biceps tendon.[35] There was also contact between the articular surface of the rotator cuff and the anterosuperior glenoid rim.
    - Not as reliable as the Neer Test.
- IR Resistance Stress Test[38]
  - Purpose: This test is used to differentiate between intra-articular (internal impingement) and classic subacromial (outlet) impingement syndromes.
  - Maneuver: The patient is standing and the arm is in 90 degrees of abduction and 80 degrees ER (pitching position). Manual isometric muscle testing for ER and IR are performed.
  - Positive test: Good strength in ER in this position and apparent weakness in IR indicate internal impingement.
    - Etiologies of internal (intra-articular) impingement include the following:

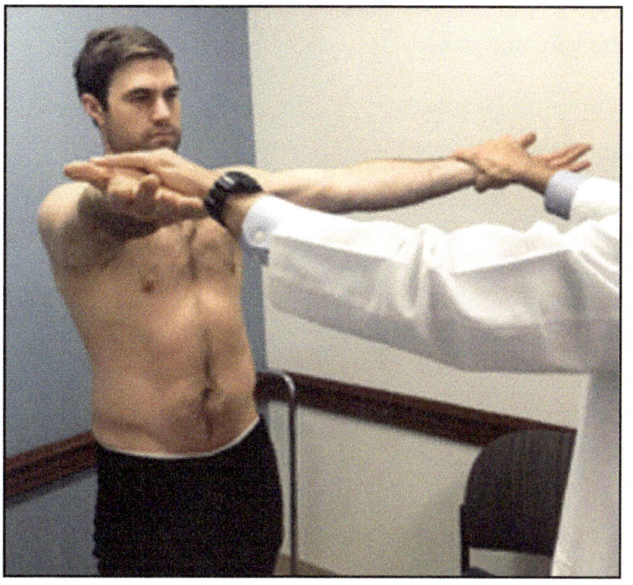

Figure 8-14. The Speed Test to assess for LHBT tendon pathology.

        - Anterior glenoid erosions or Bankart lesion (instability)
        - Posterosuperior labral or SLAP lesions
        - MGHL tearing
        - Partial-thickness articular-sided rotator cuff tears
    - Negative test: More weakness in ER is suggestive of classic subacromial (outlet) impingement (external impingement)
- Gerber Subcoracoid Impingement Test[39]
    - Purpose: This test is used to assess for subcoracoid impingement of the rotator cuff.
    - Maneuver: FF to 90 degrees with IR
        - This position results in the smallest CHL distance and causes entrapment of the rotator cuff between the humeral head and the coracoid process.
    - Positive test: This test is positive if pain is experienced at the front of the shoulder with or without radiation to the upper arm and forearm.
        - FF with IR is the most sensitive at detecting impingement produced as a result of iatrogenic or traumatic change in anatomy between the coracoid process and humeral head.
        - Although uncommon, it has been described in patients with a long or laterally placed coracoid process and should be considered in patients with negative classic impingement signs that describe anterior or lateral pain with overhead activities and have subjective complaints similar to those with classic outlet impingement.

Biceps Tendon Tests

- Speed Test[40] (Figure 8-14)
    - Purpose: This test is used to assess pathology to the LHBT.
    - Maneuver: Flexion of the shoulder to 90 degrees is performed while the elbow is extended and the forearm is supinated. The patient attempts to forward elevate the shoulder against resistance.
    - Positive test: Pain is localized to the bicipital groove.

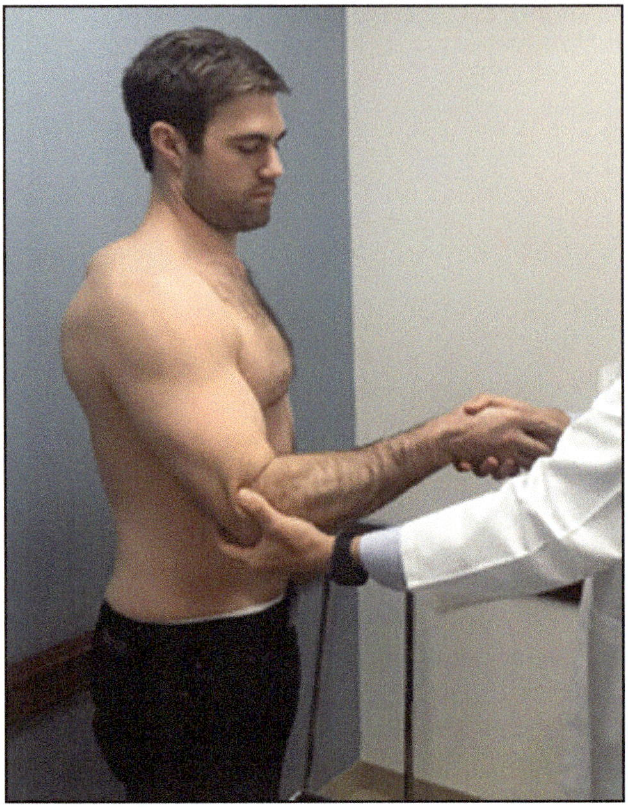

Figure 8-15. The Yergason Test for LHBT pathology.

        - Pain can occur in patients with the following:
            - LHBT inflammation
            - SLAP lesions
- The Yergason Test[41] (Figure 8-15)
    - Purpose: This test is used to assess pathology to the LHBT.
    - Maneuver: The elbow is flexed at 90 degrees, the forearm is pronated, and the examiner prevents resisted supination.
    - Positive test: pain localized to bicipital groove
    - Also known as the "supination sign."

Laxity Tests

- Increased joint laxity has been associated with instability.
- These tests indicate joint laxity only and should not be interpreted as indicating instability.
- Sulcus sign[42]
    - Purpose: This test is used to assess multidirectional instability and IGHL laxity.
    - Maneuver: The patient is relaxed, with the arm at the side, then inferior subluxation is produced by the examiner grabbing the arm and applying downward traction.
    - Positive test: The test is positive if a depression (sulcus) is seen between the lateral edge of the acromion and the humeral head on gentle downward traction of the humerus.
    - Sulcus grading is based on the gap between the lateral acromion and humeral head.

- Grade +1: gap is less than 1 cm
- Grade +2: gap is 1 to 2 cm
- Grade +3: gap is greater than 2 cm

Translation Tests

- Load and Shift Test[43]
  - Purpose: This test is used to classify and diagnose shoulder instability.
  - Maneuver: The patient is seated with the examiner behind the patient, with one hand on the shoulder and scapula to stabilize and the other hand on the humeral head. As the head is loaded, both anterior and posterior stresses are applied and the amount of translation is noted.
  - Positive test: This test is positive when there is increased translation compared to the contralateral side.
  - Grading of translation
    - A translation of more than 25% of the diameter of the humeral head is positive and graded as follows:
      - Grade I: 25% to 50% translation
      - Grade II: greater than 50% translation with reduction
      - Grade III: greater than 50% translation without reduction
  - Faber et al described an alternative version of the Load and Shift Test as part of a comparison of the effects of anesthesia on the results of the test in their article.[44]

Instability Tests

- Apprehension Test[45] (Figure 8-16)
  - Purpose: This test is used to assess anterior or posterior GH instability.
  - Maneuver:
    - Anterior: The shoulder is abducted to 90 degrees and moved passively into maximum ER, then forward pressure is applied to the posterior aspect of the humeral head.
    - Posterior: Place the patient supine, forward flexing to 90 degrees, IR, and applying a downward force to push the humeral head out the back
  - Positive test: The test is positive if the patient suddenly becomes apprehensive (feeling of instability) and complains of pain in the shoulder.
- The Jobe Apprehension-Relocation Test[46] (Figure 8-17)
  - Purpose: This test is used to assess anterior GH instability.
  - Maneuver: After performing the Apprehension Test as described above, with the shoulder abducted at 90 degrees and maximum ER, administer a posteriorly directed force on the humeral head.
  - Positive test: The test is positive if the patient experiences relief of pain and the sensation of instability.
    - Fowler sign is the same as a positive Jobe Relocation Test, representing diminution of apprehension with the posteriorly directed force in the Jobe Relocation Test.

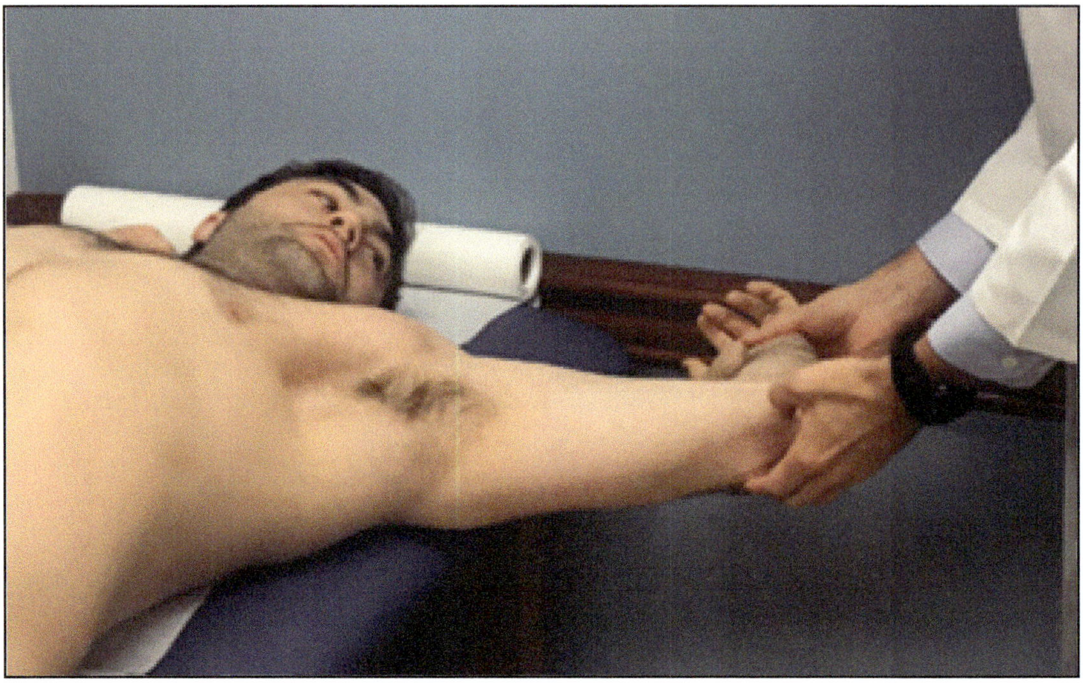

Figure 8-16. The Apprehension Test for anterior GH instability.

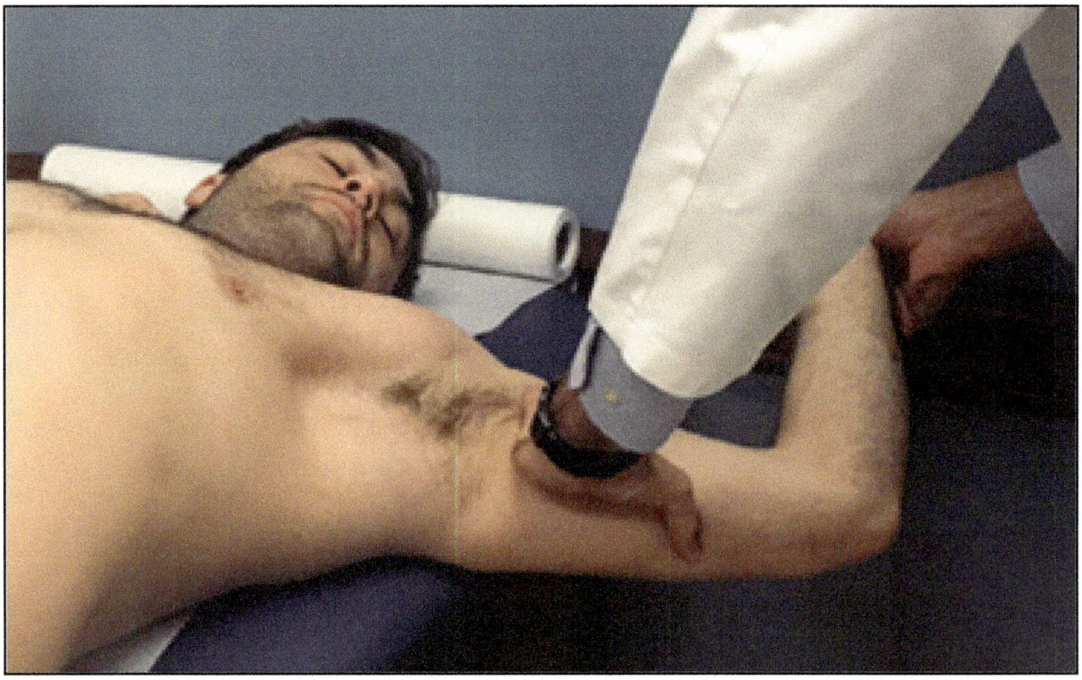

Figure 8-17. The Jobe Apprehension-Relocation Test to assess anterior GH instability.

Glenoid Labrum Tests

- Grind Test
  - Purpose: This test is used to assess glenoid labral tears.
  - Maneuver: With the patient supine with 90 degrees of abduction and elbow flexed to 90 degrees, and one hand on the elbow and one hand on the proximal humerus, apply a compressive load while circumducting the humeral head 360 degrees around the glenoid.
  - Positive test: A clunk or grind may indicate a labrum tear.
- Clunk Test
  - Purpose: This test is used to assess glenoid labral tears.
  - Maneuver: With the patient supine, with one hand posterior to the humeral head and other hand proximal to the elbow joint, passively abduct the arm and ER (or IR) the arm overhead and apply an anterior force to the humerus. The humeral head is then circumducted around the glenoid.
  - Positive test: A clunk or grind may indicate a labrum tear.

Superior Labrum Anterior and Posterior Tests

- SLAP tears were first described by Andrews and colleagues[47] in 1985 and were later classified by Snyder et al[48] in 1990.
- Snyder Biceps Tension Test
  - Purpose: This test is used to assess for a SLAP lesion.
  - Maneuver: The patient forward flexes to 90 degrees at the shoulder with the elbow extended and forearm supinated, and examiner applies downward resistance (similar to the speed test).
  - Positive test: Pain deep in the shoulder suggests possible a SLAP lesion.
    - Pain that is more superficial and anterior may indicate an LHBT lesion.
    - Field and Savoie observed that the Snyder Biceps Tension Test was positive in 20 consecutive patients with a diagnosis of SLAP lesion.[49]
- Snyder Compression-Rotation Test
  - Purpose: This test is used to assess for a SLAP lesion.
  - Maneuver: The patient's shoulder is placed in 90 degrees abduction with the elbow flexed to 90 degrees. A compression force is applied to the humerus, which is rotated, in an attempt to trap the torn labrum.
  - Positive test: Labral tears may be felt to catch and snap during the test.
- The Crank Test[50]
  - Purpose: This test is used to assess for a SLAP lesion.
  - Maneuver: The patient is seated upright with the arm elevated to 160 degrees in the scapular plane. Joint load is applied along the axis of the humerus with one hand while the other performs humeral rotation (ER/IR).
  - Positive test: A positive test is indicated by pain during the maneuver (usually during ER) and reproduction of symptoms with or without a click.

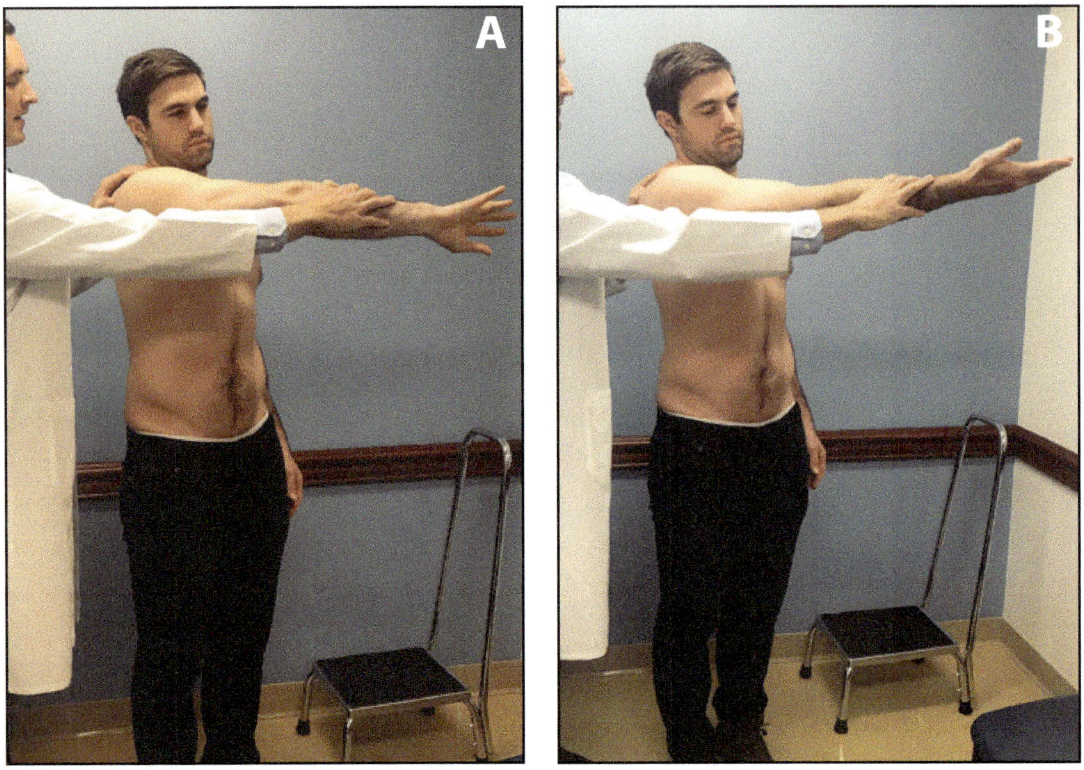

Figure 8-18. (A) The first part of the O'Brien Active Compression Test with the hand in pronation with thumb to ground (shoulder IR). (B) The second part of the O'Brien Active Compression Test with the hand in supination (shoulder ER). Both parts of the test are used to distinguish between AC abnormalities and SLAP lesions.

- The O'Brien Active Compression Test[51] (Figure 8-18)
  - Purpose: This test is used to distinguish between AC abnormalities and SLAP lesions.
  - Maneuver:
    - The patient forward flexes the affected arm to 90 degrees with the elbow in full extension. The patient then adducts the arm 10 to 15 degrees medially (across the chest). The arm is IR so that the thumb is pointing downward, and the examiner applies a uniform downward force to the arm.
    - The arm is then fully supinated and the examiner then reapplies the same force.
  - Positive test: A positive test is indicated when pain is elicited deep in the shoulder with the arm in the IR position and relieved in the supinated position.
    - Pain localized to the AC joint or on top of the shoulder is often seen with AC joint abnormality.
- Biceps Load Test[52]
  - Purpose: This test is used to assess SLAP tears in patients with recurrent anterior dislocations.
  - Maneuver:
    - The patient is supine while his or her wrist and elbow are gently grasped. The arm is abducted to 90 degrees, with the elbow in 90 degrees flexion, with the forearm in the supinated position.

- The patient is allowed to relax and an anterior apprehension test is performed. When the patient becomes apprehensive during ER, the ER is stopped and the patient is then asked to flex the elbow while the examiner resists flexion with one hand and asks how the apprehension has changed, if at all.
  - Positive test: If the apprehension has not changed, or if the shoulder becomes more painful, the test is positive for a SLAP tear.
  - Negative test: If the apprehension is lessened or if the patient feels more comfortable than before the test, the test is negative for a SLAP tear.
- Biceps Load Test II[53]
  - Purpose: This test is used to assess for SLAP tears in shoulders without recurrent dislocation.
  - Maneuver:
    - The patient is supine and the patient's wrist and elbow are gently grasped. The arm is elevated to 120 degrees and ER to its maximum point, with the elbow in 90 degrees flexion and the forearm supinated.
    - The patient is asked to flex the elbow while resisting the elbow flexion.
  - Positive test: The test is positive if the patient complains of shoulder pain during the resisted elbow flexion.
    - The test is also considered positive if the patient complains of more pain from the resisted elbow flexion regardless of the degree of pain before the elbow flexion maneuver.

References

1. Matsen FI, Lippitt S, DeBartolo S. *Shoulder Surgery: Principles and Procedures*. Philadelphia, PA: Saunders Elsevier; 2004.
2. Mohammed H, Skalski MR, Patel DB, et al. Coracoid process: the lighthouse of the shoulder. *Radiographics*. 2016;36(7):2084-2101. doi:10.1148/rg.2016160039.
3. von Schroeder HP, Kuiper SD, Botte MJ. Osseous anatomy of the scapula. *Clin Orthop Relat Res*. 2001;(383):131-139. doi:10.1097/00003086-200102000-00015.
4. Mallon WJ, Brown HR, Vogler JB III, Martinez S. Radiographic and geometric anatomy of the scapula. *Clin Orthop Relat Res*. 1992;(277):142-154.
5. Bigliani LU, Morrison DS, April EW. The morphology of the acromion and its relationship to rotator cuff tears. *Orthop Trans*. 1986;10:228.
6. Codman EA. *The Shoulder, Rupture of the Supraspinatus Tendon and Other Lesions in or About the Subacromial Bursa*. Malabar, FL: Krieger Publishing; 1934:313-331.
7. Neer CS II. Displaced proximal humeral fractures. I. Classification and evaluation. *J Bone Joint Surg Am*. 1970;52(6):1077-1089.
8. Lippitt SB, Vanderhooft JE, Harris SL, Sidles JA, Harryman DT, Matsen FA. Glenohumeral stability from concavity-compression: a quantitative analysis. *J Shoulder Elbow Surg*. 1993;2(1):27-35. doi:10.1016/S1058-2746(09)80134-1.
9. Howell SM, Galinat BJ. The glenoid-labral socket. A constrained articular surface. *Clin Orthop Relat Res*. 1989;(243):122-125.
10. Boehm TD, Kirschner S, Fischer A, Gohlke F. The relation of the coracoclavicular ligament insertion to the acromioclavicular joint: a cadaver study of relevance to lateral clavicle resection. *Acta Orthop Scand*. 2003;74(6):718-721. doi:10.1080/00016470310018261.
11. Gerber C, Schneeberger AG, Vinh TS. The arterial vascularization of the humeral head. An anatomical study. *J Bone Joint Surg Am*. 1990;72(10):1486-1494.
12. Laing PG. The arterial supply of the adult humerus. *J Bone Joint Surg Am*. 1956;38-A(5):1105-1116.
13. Hettrich CM, Boraiah S, Dyke JP, Neviaser A, Helfet DL, Lorich DG. Quantitative assessment of the vascularity of the proximal part of the humerus. *J Bone Joint Surg Am*. 2010;92(4):943-948. doi:10.2106/JBJS.H.01144.
14. Burkhead WZ, Scheinberg RR, Box G. Surgical anatomy of the axillary nerve. *J Shoulder Elbow Surg*. 1992;1(1):31-36. doi:10.1016/S1058-2746(09)80014-1.

15. Davidson PA, Tibone JE. Anterior-inferior (5 o'clock) portal for shoulder arthroscopy. *Arthroscopy.* 1995;11(5):519-525. doi:10.1016/0749-8063(95)90126-4.
16. Mehta VM. Clinical safety of the 5 o'clock portal in shoulder arthroscopy: a prospective study. *Shoulder Elbow.* 2010;2(1):17-19. doi:10.1111/j.1758-5740.2009.00043.x.
17. Davidson PA, Rivenburgh DW. The 7-o'clock posteroinferior portal for shoulder arthroscopy. *Am J Sports Med.* 2002;30(5):693-696. doi:10.1177/03635465020300051101.
18. Habermeyer P, Kaiser E, Knappe M, Kreusser T, Wiedemann E. Functional anatomy and biomechanics of the long biceps tendon [in German]. *Unfallchirurg.* 1987;90(7):319-29.
19. Vangsness CT Jr, Jorgenson SS, Watson T, Johnson DL. The origin of the long head of the biceps from the scapula and glenoid labrum. An anatomical study of 100 shoulders. *J Bone Joint Surg Br.* 1994;76-B(6):951-954.
20. Jost B, Koch PP, Gerber C. Anatomy and functional aspects of the rotator interval. *J Shoulder Elbow Surg.* 2000;9(4):336-341. doi:10.1067/mse.2000.106746.
21. Tetro AM, Bauer G, Hollstien SB, Yamaguchi K. Arthroscopic release of the rotator interval and coracohumeral ligament: an anatomic study in cadavers. *Arthroscopy.* 2002;18(2):145-150. doi:10.1053/jars.2002.30438.
22. Uhthoff HK, Piscopo M. Anterior capsular redundancy of the shoulder: congenital or traumatic? An embryological study. *J Bone Joint Surg Br.* 1985;67(3):363-366.
23. Wolf EM, Cheng JC, Dickson K. Humeral avulsion of glenohumeral ligaments as a cause of anterior shoulder instability. *Arthroscopy.* 1995;11(5):600-607. doi:10.1016/0749-8063(95)90139-6.
24. Mochizuki T, Sugaya H, Uomizu M, et al. Humeral insertion of the supraspinatus and infraspinatus. New anatomical findings regarding the footprint of the rotator cuff. Surgical technique. *J Bone Joint Surg Am.* 2009;91(suppl 2 pt 1):1-7. doi:10.2106/JBJS.H.01426.
25. Burkhart SS, Esch JC, Jolson RS. The rotator crescent and rotator cable: an anatomic description of the shoulder's "suspension bridge." *Arthroscopy.* 1993;9(6):611-616. doi:10.1016/s0749-8063(05)80496-7.
26. Flatow EL, Bigliani LU, April EW. An anatomic study of the musculocutaneous nerve and its relationship to the coracoid process. *Clin Orthop Relat Res.* 1989;(244):166-171. doi:10.1097/00003086-198907000-00014.
27. Williams MM, Snyder SJ, Buford D Jr. The Buford complex—the "cord-like" middle glenohumeral ligament and absent anterosuperior labrum complex: a normal anatomic capsulolabral variant. *Arthroscopy.* 1994;10(3):241-247. doi:10.1016/s0749-8063(05)80105-7.
28. Jobe FW, Jobe CM. Painful athletic injuries of the shoulder. *Clin Orthop Relat Res.* 1983;(173):117-124.
29. Gerber C, Krushell RJ. Isolated rupture of the tendon of the subscapularis muscle. Clinical features in 16 cases. *J Bone Joint Surg Br.* 1991;73(3):389-394. doi:10.1302/0301-620X.73B3.1670434.
30. Gerber C, Hersche O, Farron A. Isolated rupture of the subscapularis tendon. *J Bone Joint Surg Am.* 1996;78(7):1015-1023. doi:10.2106/00004623-199607000-00005.
31. Walch G, Boulahia A, Calderone S, Robinson AH. The "dropping" and "hornblower's" signs in evaluation of rotator-cuff tears. *J Bone Joint Surg Br.* 1998;80(4):624-628. doi:10.1302/0301-620x.80b4.8651.
32. Hertel R, Ballmer FT, Lambert SM, Gerber Ch. Lag signs in the diagnosis of rotator cuff rupture. *J Shoulder Elbow Surg.* 1996;5(4):307-313. doi:10.1016/S1058-2746(96)80058-9.
33. Neer CS II. Anterior acromioplasty for the chronic impingement syndrome in the shoulder: a preliminary report. *J Bone Joint Surg Am.* 1972;54(1):41-50.
34. Neer CS II. Impingement lesions. *Clin Orthop Relat Res.* 1983;(173):70-77.
35. Valadie AL III, Jobe CM, Pink MM, Ekman EF, Jobe FW. Anatomy of provocative tests for impingement syndrome of the shoulder. *J Shoulder Elbow Surg.* 2000;9(1):36-46. doi:10.1016/S1058-2746(00)90008-9.
36. McFarland EG, Hsu CY, Neira C, O'Neil O. Internal impingement of the shoulder: a clinical and arthroscopic analysis. *J Shoulder Elbow Surg.* 1999;8(5):458-460. doi:10.1016/S1058-2746(99)90076-9.
37. Hawkins RJ, Kennedy JC. Impingement syndrome in athletes. *Am J Sports Med.* 1980;8(3):151-158. doi:10.1177/036354658000800302.
38. Zaslav KR. Internal rotation resistance strength test: a new diagnostic test to differentiate intra-articular pathology from outlet (Neer) impingement syndrome in the shoulder. *J Shoulder Elbow Surg.* 2001;10(1):23-27. doi:10.1067/mse.2001.111960.
39. Gerber C, Terrier F, Ganz R. The role of the coracoid process in the chronic impingement syndrome. *J Bone Joint Surg Br.* 1985;67(5):703-708. doi:10.1302/0301-620X.67B5.4055864.
40. Crenshaw AH, Kilgore WE. Surgical treatment of bicipital tenosynovitis. *J Bone Joint Surg Am.* 1966;48(8):1496-1502. doi:10.2106/00004623-196648080-00003.
41. Yergason RM. Supination sign. *J Bone Joint Surg Br.* 1931;13(1):160.
42. Neer CS II, Foster CR. Inferior capsular shift for involuntary inferior and multidirectional instability of the shoulder. A preliminary report. *J Bone Joint Surg Am.* 1980;62(6):897-908. doi:10.2106/00004623-198062060-00004.
43. Silliman JF, Hawkins RJ. Classification and physical diagnosis of instability of the shoulder. *Clin Orthop Relat Res.* 1993;(291):7-19.

44. Faber KJ, Homa K, Hawkins RJ. Translation of the glenohumeral joint in patients with anterior instability: awake examination versus examination with the patient under anesthesia. *J Shoulder Elbow Surg.* 1999;8(4):320-323. doi:10.1016/s1058-2746(99)90153-2.
45. Rowe CR, Zarins B. Recurrent transient subluxation of the shoulder. *J Bone Joint Surg Am.* 1981;63(6):863-872.
46. Jobe FW, Kvitne RS, Giangarra CE. Shoulder pain in the overhand or throwing athlete. The relationship of anterior instability and rotator cuff impingement. *Orthop Rev.* 1989;18(9):963-975.
47. Andrews JR, Carson WG Jr, McLeod WD. Glenoid labrum tears related to the long head of the biceps. *Am J Sports Med.* 1985;13(5):337-341. doi:10.1177/036354658501300508.
48. Snyder SJ, Karzel RP, Del Pizzo W, Ferkel RD, Friedman MJ. SLAP lesions of the shoulder. *Arthroscopy.* 1990;6(4):274-279. doi:10.1016/0749-8063(90)90056-j.
49. Field LD, Savoie FH. Arthroscopic suture repair of superior labral detachment lesions of the shoulder. *Am J Sports Med.* 1993;21(6):783-790; discussion 790. doi:10.1177/036354659302100605.
50. Liu SH, Henry MH, Nuccion SL. A prospective evaluation of a new physical examination in predicting glenoid labral tears. *Am J Sports Med.* 1996;24(6):721-725. doi:10.1177/036354659602400604.
51. O'Brien SJ, Pagnani MJ, Fealy S, McGlynn SR, Wilson JB. The active compression test: a new and effective test for diagnosing labral tears and acromioclavicular joint abnormality. *Am J Sports Med.* 1998;26(5):610-613. doi:10.1177/03635465980260050201.
52. Kim SH, Ha KI, Han KY. Biceps load test: a clinical test for superior labrum anterior and posterior lesions in shoulders with recurrent anterior dislocations. *Am J Sports Med.* 1999;27(3):300-303. doi:10.1177/03635465990270030501.
53. Kim SH, Ha KI, Ahn JH, Kim SH, Choi HJ. Biceps load test II: A clinical test for SLAP lesions of the shoulder. *Arthroscopy.* 2001;17(2):160-164. doi:10.1053/jars.2001.20665.

9

Rotator Cuff Disease

Michael A. Stone, MD and Reza Omid, MD

Pathophysiology

Rotator Cuff Composition

- Basic science
  - Rotator cuff (RC) tendons are composed of type I collagen (85% of dry weight), type III collagen (increased with tendon degeneration), glycosaminoglycans, proteoglycans (decorin, biglycan, aggrecan), and water.
  - Chronically degenerated tendons have increased levels of type III collagen, increased fat content, and are stiffer.
  - Tendon enthesis
    - Zone 1: well-aligned type I collagen fibers and a small amount of decorin
    - Zone II: fibrocartilage composed of type II and III collagen with small amounts of type I, IX, and X collagen
      - Also contains aggrecan and decorin
    - Zone III: mineralized fibrocartilage; composed mostly of type II collagen with high amounts of type X collagen and aggrecan
    - Zone IV: bone; predominantly type I collagen
      - The tendon enthesis is not restored with RC repair. Histologically, the tissue is composed of primarily type I and II collagen, and is biomechanically inferior to intact RC tissue.[1]
- Anatomy (see Chapter 8 for more comprehensive discussion)
  - Subscapularis
    - The superior two-third inserts as a tendon onto the lesser tuberosity and the inferior one-third as a direct muscular insertion along the surgical neck of the humerus.

Namdari S, Zmistowski B, Omid R, eds.
The Foundations of Shoulder and Elbow Surgery (pp 175-189).

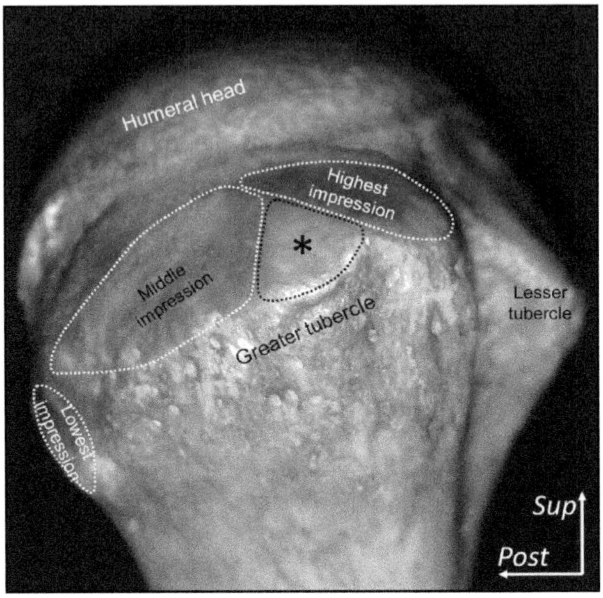

Figure 9-1. Lateral impression. (Reprinted with permission from Nozaki T, Nimura A, Fujishiro H, et al. The anatomic relationship between the morphology of the greater tubercle of the humerus and the insertion of the infraspinatus tendon. *J Shoulder Elbow Surg.* 2015;24[4]:555-560. doi:10.1016/j.jse.2014.09.038.)

- The anterior humeral circumflex vessels approximate this separation between the muscular and the tendinous insertion.

- Supraspinatus
  - Large anterior fusiform muscle belly with smaller unipennate posterior muscle belly
  - The anterior portion of the tendon (rotator cable) is thicker and more important in repair.
- Infraspinatus
  - Bipennate muscle belly
  - The "lateral impression" of the greater tuberosity is triangle shaped, and this delineates the point of insertion of the infraspinatus and the insertion of the supraspinatus at the highest impression (Figure 9-1).[2,3]
- Teres minor
  - Fusiform muscle belly with a tendinous insertion supplemented by a direct muscular attachment to the surgical neck
- Rotator cable
  - Thickened capsular structure of the RC and fibers of the rotator interval (coracohumeral ligament)
- Rotator crescent
  - Thin central portion of RC tissue lateral to the rotator cable
  - Considered a hypovascular zone of the RC tendon, where most degenerative RC tears begin
- Rotator interval
  - The area between the anterior surface of the supraspinatus and the superior border of the subscapularis.
  - Composed of the coracohumeral ligament, superior glenohumeral (GH) ligament, upper portions of the middle GH ligament, and contains within it the long head of the biceps tendon (LHBT)

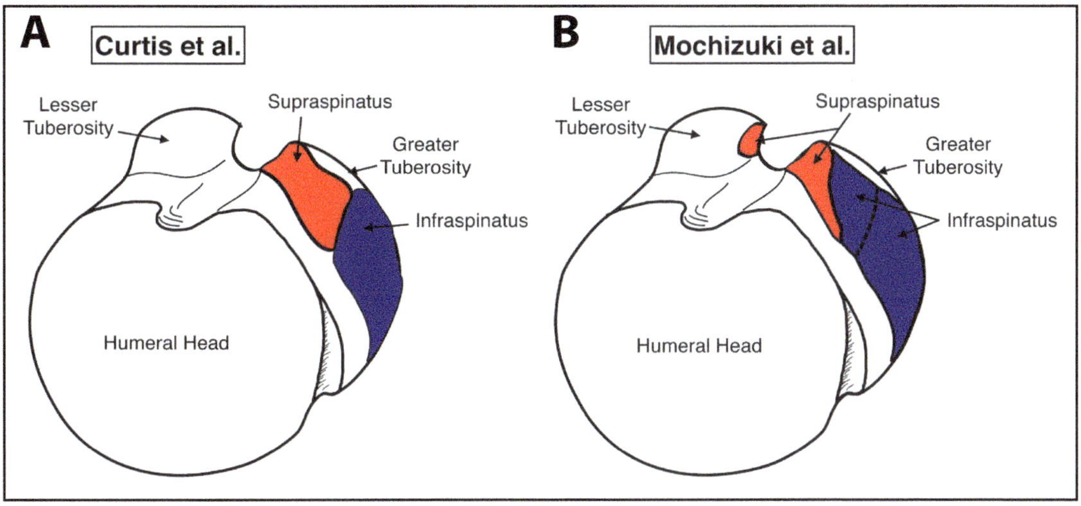

Figure 9-2. RC insertion anatomy. (A) Diagram of the original description of the attachment site of the supraspinatus and infraspinatus. (B) Diagram of the more current understanding of the attachment of the supraspinatus and infraspinatus. (Adapted from Mochizuki T, Sugaya H, Uomizu M, et al. Humeral insertion of the supraspinatus and infraspinatus. New anatomical findings regarding the footprint of the rotator cuff. *J Bone Joint Surg Am*. 2008;90[5]:962-969. doi:10.2106/JBJS.G.00427.)

- Footprint anatomy: Curtis initially described the anatomy of the RC footprint.[4] This was later refuted in another cadaveric study that demonstrated that the insertion of the supraspinatus was more anterior than previously thought, and the infraspinatus occupied more surface area of the greater tuberosity (Figure 9-2).[3]
- Superior GH joint capsule (Figure 9-3)
  - The width of the capsule ranges from 5.6 mm at the anterior margin of the greater tuberosity, to 3.5 mm at the midportion, and 9.1 mm posteriorly.[5]
  - The proximity of the anatomy of the superior capsule to the supraspinatus tendon may play a role in the progression of rotator cuff tears (RCTs).
  - The superior capsule is critically important for superior stability of the shoulder, as well as anterior-inferior stability.[6]

Biomechanics

- Force couples: Burkhart described the force-couple concept of the RC after performing fluoroscopic evaluations of patients with massive RCTs.
  - Normal shoulder function is possible as long as there are balanced forces between the 2 force couples; ie, the first force couple in the transverse plane (subscapularis and teres minor/infraspinatus), and the second force couple in the coronal plane (deltoid and inferior cuff).[7]
- Biomechanics of RC-deficient shoulders
  - The RC creates concavity compression of the GH joint (maintains the humeral head in the center of the glenoid), which allows the periscapular muscles and deltoid to function properly and elevate the arm.
  - In massive RCT, the force required for humeral abduction increases incrementally with the size of the tear. A 6 to 8 cm defect increases the required force of the subscapularis by 30% to 85%, infraspinatus/teres minor by 32% to 86%, and deltoid by 22% to 45%, respectively.[8]

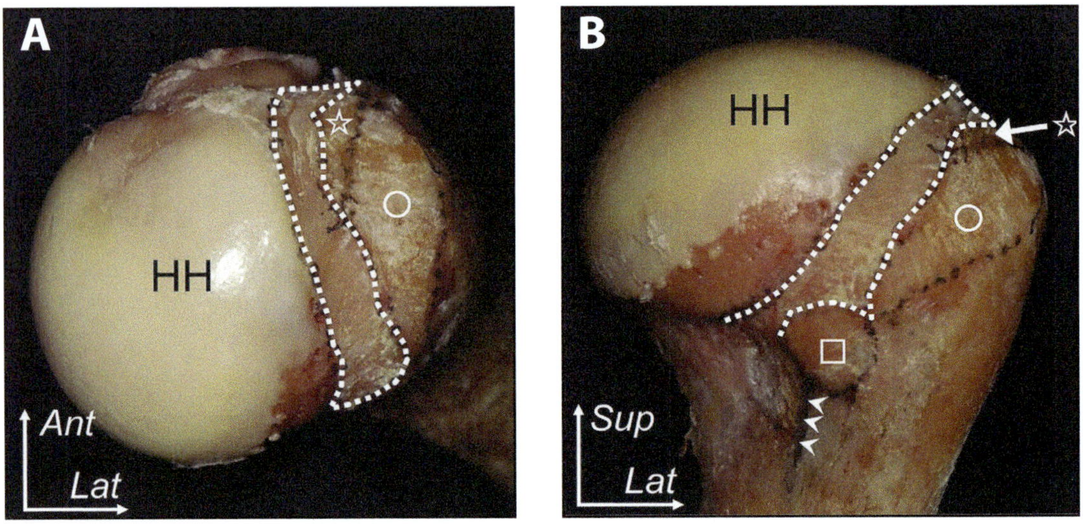

Figure 9-3. Superior capsule anatomy. Abbreviation: HH, humeral head. (Reprinted with permission from Nimura A, Kato A, Yamaguchi K, et al. The superior capsule of the shoulder joint complements the insertion of the rotator cuff. *J Shoulder Elbow Surg*. 2012;21[7]:867-872. doi:10.1016/j.jse.2011.04.034.)

- Complete tear of the supraspinatus decreases the capability of GH joint abduction, and involvement of 50% of the infraspinatus yields the critical tear size that alters GH kinematics. As the RCTs progress, the pectoralis major and latissimus become important secondary stabilizers to GH stability[9] and some patients, even with massive tears, are able to compensate well enough to generate overhead elevation.
- As previously mentioned, the superior capsule is very important for passive stability to the shoulder. Full-thickness RCTs will cause disruption of the superior capsule as well, which leads to abnormal shoulder kinematics.[6]

Diagnosis

- Physical examination
  - There are 2 types of integrity testing: active (movement against examiner resistance) and passive position testing (ie, lag signs)
  - RCTs typically lead to deficiency in active motion and preservation of passive range of motion.
  - Limitations in passive motion can result from concomitant adhesive capsulitis.
- Imaging
  - XR: Four standard x-rays determine the position of the humeral head and measure humeral head migration.
    - Standard anteroposterior (AP), true AP (Grashey): beam directed 30 degrees externally toward GH joint, axillary view, scapular-Y
  - Magnetic resonance imaging (MRI): T1-weighted sagittal oblique is useful for determining fatty degeneration/infiltration of the RC, especially on the sagittal cuts.
    - A normal RC tendon should demonstrate low signal intensity on all sequences. T2-weighted sequencing may show an increased signal of the tendon in cases of tendinopathy, and high signal intensity in cases of partial or full-thickness RCTs.

- A wavy or kinked tendon with muscle edema and a tendon stump still attached to greater tuberosity are suggestive of an acute RCT on MRI.
- Ultrasound: highly operator dependent
  - High-frequency transducers (10 to 18 MHz) should be used for the shoulder.
  - Ultrasound has comparable accuracy to MRI for detecting and measuring size of full-thickness and partial-thickness RCTs.[10,11]

Epidemiology, Classification, and Treatment

Rotator Cuff Tears

- Partial-thickness rotator cuff tears (PTRCTs)
  - Epidemiology
    - Twenty percent of asymptomatic individuals had a PTRCT with up to 26% occurring in patients older than 60 years old, and 4% in those younger than 40 years old.[12]
  - Etiology and natural history
    - PTRCTs can progress to full-thickness tears. Kartus et al showed that 35% of patients with PTRCTs will go on to develop full-thickness tears by 5 years.[13]
    - Fifty-one percent of asymptomatic PTRCTs will progress to symptomatic tears by 2.8 years[14] *Recommended reading for understanding progression of asymptomatic tears*
    - Although numerous studies have failed to show a benefit of subacromial decompression,[15-17] this may still be of benefit in patients with bursal-sided tears.[18]
  - Classification
    - Ellmann classification of partial-thickness tears
      - Tear thickness
        - Less than 3 mm or less than 25%
        - 3 to 6 mm or 25% to 50%
        - Greater than 6 mm or greater than 50%
      - Tear location
        - Articular
        - Bursal
        - Intratendinous
      - Greater than 50% (grade 3) carries a high risk of progression, and surgery is indicated if failed nonoperative trial for 3 to 6 months
  - Treatment
    - Bursal-sided tears greater than 6 mm or greater than 50%: complete tear and perform full-thickness repair
      - Do not complete the tear if it is less than 50%.
      - Tear completion with single-row repair has a 13% to 20% retear rate,[19] and a 9.5% retear rate when a suture bridge construct was used[20]; another study reported a 12% retear rate when performing tear completion and repair with either single-row or double-row.[21]
    - Articular-sided tears greater than 6 mm or greater than 50%: complete tear and perform full-thickness repair or in situ repair (Figure 9-4)[22]
      - Symptomatic: articular/bursal/intratendinous

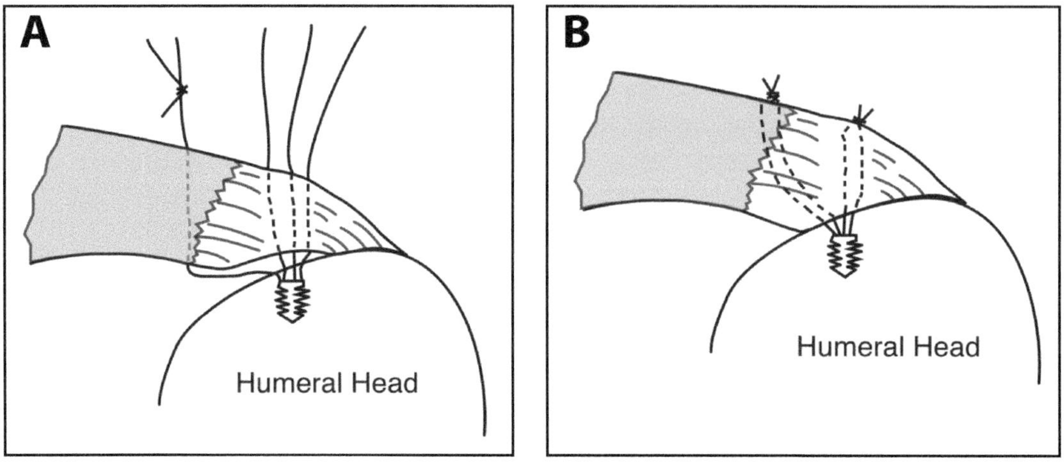

Figure 9-4. Partial tear in situ repair technique. (A) Placement of suture anchors through the articular side of the tendon. (B) Final fixation with transtendinous sutures.

- Twenty percent progress to full-thickness tears.
- Nonoperative: 91% satisfaction at 4 years; improved outcomes in small tears in the nondominant arm[23]
  - The first-line treatment for degenerative partial thickness tears is nonoperative.
- Operative
  - Debridement ± subacromial decompression is appropriate if there is less than a 50% thickness tear; 90% good outcome. Bursal-sided tears treated with only debridement had a high failure rate (29%) compared to articular-sided tears (3%).[18]
  - Repair should be considered in the young patient with a traumatic, greater than 50% tear,[24] or less than 50% tear if bursal-sided; may need to convert to a full-thickness tear for better repair.[18]
  - Transtendon repair has an improved biomechanical advantage but there is no clinical difference.[25]
  - A good candidate is young with a partial articular supraspinatus tendon avulsion lesion.
  - Conversion to full-thickness tear showed similar satisfaction outcomes, but higher strength measured on dynamometer than transtendon repair.[26]
  - Intratendinous repair is used for partial-thickness articular surface tears with intratendinous extension lesions. Usually performed only in athletes.[27]

- Biomechanical study showed increased strain at the articular side if tear is greater than a 50% thickness, and strain is decreased with in situ repair.[28]

- Full-thickness rotator cuff tears (FTRCTs)
  - FTRCTs result in altered GH kinematics and contact pressures. This may be due to tearing of the superior capsule and may be the first step in the pathophysiology of RCT arthropathy.[6]
  - Epidemiology
    - The incidence of FTRCTs is around 17% according to one cadaveric study dissecting shoulders in those 27 to 102 years old.[29]

        - Patients with a symptomatic FTRCT have a 35% prevalence of an asymptomatic FTRCT on the contralateral side.[30] *Recommended reading for understanding characteristics of asymptomatic tears*
    - Etiology and natural history
        - Acute traumatic tears
            - Rare in younger individuals; however, usually traumatic in etiology
            - Commonly associated with traumatic anterior shoulder dislocation[31]
            - Consider acute on chronic injury; determination of preinjury function is crucial in the history taking
            - Commonly repaired acutely, regardless of age
        - Degenerative tears
            - Tears start most commonly 15 mm posterior to the biceps tendon[32] and continue to propagate with time
                - Tear size increases in asymptomatic shoulders with increasing age.
                - Twenty percent in 60 to 69 year olds
                - Forty percent in those older than 70 years old[33]
                - Fifty percent likelihood of bilateral tears after 66 years old[30]
            - Tear size correlates strongly with proximal humeral migration, and a size of 175 mm^2 (approximately 1.5 cm) was found to be the critical size tear for superior migration.[34]
            - Asymptomatic tears tend to progress in size, increase in fatty degeneration, and become symptomatic.[35,36]
            - Large tears (greater than 15 mm), tears that progressively enlarge (greater than 9 mm), and tears involving the anterior cable (tears located closer to the LHBT) are associated with increased progression of fatty degeneration of the RC.[37,38]
    - Classification
        - DeOrio and Cofield based their classification on tear size,[39] measured anterior to posterior distance of the tear:
            - Small: less than 1 cm
            - Medium: 1 to 3 cm
            - Large: 3 to 5 cm
            - Massive: greater than 5 cm
                - The more common classification for massive tears is the European definition, which is described as involving 2 or more tendons.[40]
        - RC fatty degeneration or infiltration

          The Goutallier classification is based on computed tomography scan and assessed on a parasagittal cut.
            - Stage 0: normal muscle without fatty streaks
            - Stage 1: fatty streaking
            - Stage 2: more muscle than fat
            - Stage 3: equal amounts of fat to muscle
            - Stage 4: more fat than muscle
                - Later validated with shoulder MRI[41]
        - Tangent sign (Figure 9-5): A line is drawn from the coracoid to the superior border of the scapular spine. If the supraspinatus muscle belly fails to intersect this line, then atrophy is present.[42] The tangent sign is the predictor of whether a RCT will be repairable.

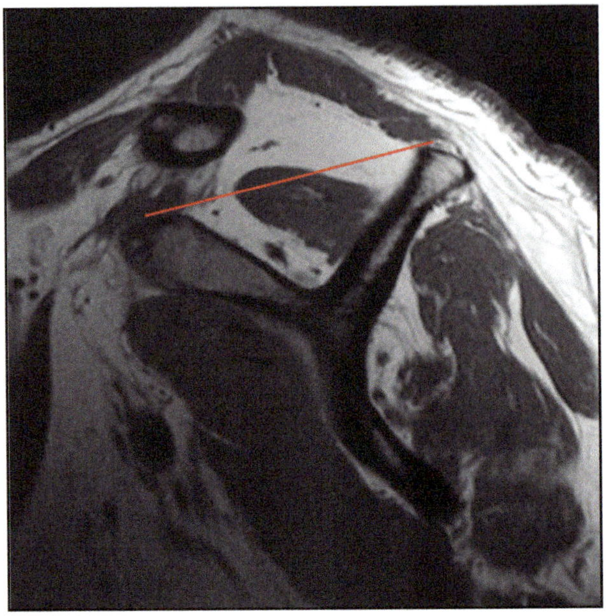

Figure 9-5. Tangent sign. Line drawn from superior border of the coracoid process to the superior border of the scapular spine.

- Occupation ratio: The cross-sectional area of the supraspinatus muscle belly is measured in relation to the supraspinatus fossa on the sagittal oblique cut. A measurement of 0.6 to 1 is normal or slight atrophy, 0.4 to 0.6 is moderate atrophy, and less than 0.4 is severe atrophy.[43]

- Treatment
  - Full-thickness degenerative tears (Figure 9-6)
    - A trial of nonoperative treatment for at least 3 months is essential, and includes pain control, stretching, and strengthening.[44]
    - There are higher rates of retears in patients older than 60 years old, even with suture bridge technique.[45]
- Primary repair
  - Single-row: The anchors are placed in a linear fashion at the tendon footprint. The most common mode of failure is cutout at the suture-tendon interface.
  - Double-row: Biomechanical studies have shown double-row repair to be superior to single-row repair with stronger fixation and better footprint restoration.[46] *Recommended reading for understanding single- vs double-row repair* However, clinical studies have shown equivalent functional outcomes and similar retear rates for most tear types, except massive tears.[47]
  - Transosseous equivalent (TOE): In a biomechanical study, TOE was superior to double-row repair with ultimate failure loads; however, gap formation was similar between the 2 techniques[48]; there is a trend toward a lower retear rate with double-row or TOE compared to single-row; however, no statistically significant functional difference.[49] *Recommended reading for understanding single-row vs TOE benefits*
  - Tension band: The tension band had improved constant scores but an overall 25% retear rate.[50]
- Retears
  - Retears after RC repair are common; however, they are not necessarily associated with poor outcomes.[51] *Recommended reading for study design and understanding RC repair failure*

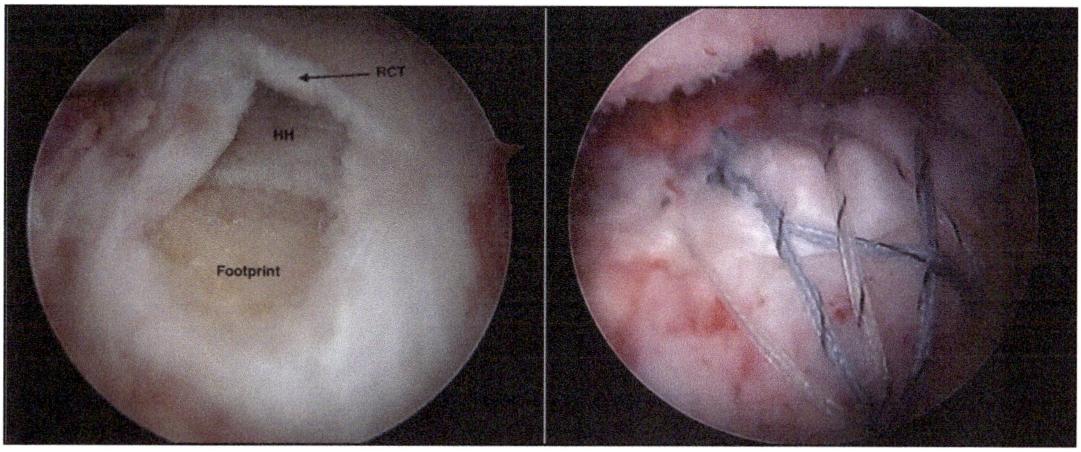

Figure 9-6. TOE RC repair. Abbreviation: HH, humeral head.

        - The mean time to retear after RC repair is 19.2 weeks (most occurring within 3 to 6 months from repair), with an overall 17% retear rate up to 1 year.[51]
        - Repairs should be protected for at least 6 months.
    - Graft use
        - Augment: acellular dermal matrix, small intestinal submucosa xenograft (high rates of failure and graft rejection)[52]
            - May be used as augment to primary repair, or interpositional tissue to "bridge" the gap.[53,54] There are high rates of retear in massive cuff tears when used as interpositional tissue.[55]
        - Superior capsule reconstruction (SCR; Figure 9-7): SCR was described in a biomechanical study in 2012, using fascia lata autograft tissue. The superior capsule is reconstructed and secured with suture anchors from the glenoid to the supraspinatus footprint.
            - Acellular dermal matrix is more widely used in the United States than fascia lata graft because of avoidance of donor-site morbidity.
            - Concerns over graft stretching, healing rates, and long-term functional outcomes have been expressed.
        - Vascularized dermal autograft (SCA flap): described in cadavers with a proposed benefit of stimulating vascular ingrowth using a pedicled flap; however, this technique has not yet been implemented clinically.[56]
- Irreparable rotator cuff tears (IRCTs)[57]
    - IRCT is poorly defined: a tendon that is unable to be repaired to the tuberosity footprint despite adequate mobilization techniques
    - The acromiohumeral distance is a measurement of the distance from the lower border of the acromion to the top of the humeral head on the true AP view, which gives an indication of proximal humeral migration. With an acromiohumeral distance less than 7 mm, static proximal humeral migration is associated with IRCT.[34]
    - Goutallier stage 3 or 4[58]
    - Treatment
        - When tendon repair to bone is not possible, other treatment options usually become necessary, such as graft augmentation ("bridging" or SCR), partial repair with debridement,[59] tendon transfer, or arthroplasty.

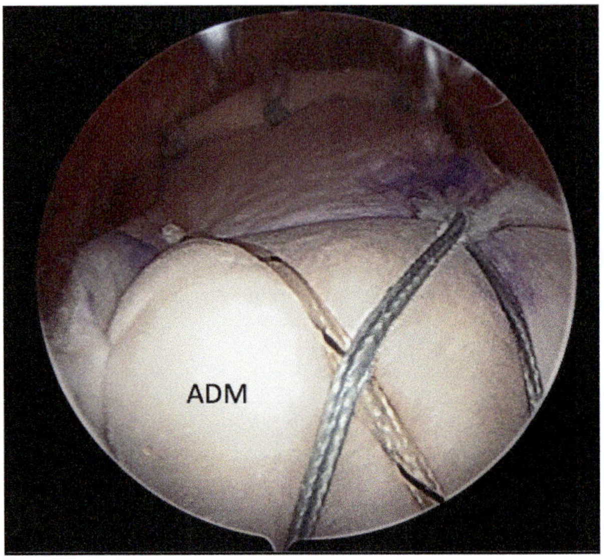

Figure 9-7. SCR. Abbreviation: ADM, acellular dermal matrix.

- Tendon transfer: Indications include a patient with an IRCT with maintained active forward flexion, loss of external rotation (ER), and no GH arthritis.
  - High morbidity and rigorous rehabilitation
- Latissimus dorsi: used for irreparable posterosuperior RCTs[60,61]
  - The deltoid and subscapularis tendon must be intact to add as a force couple.
  - There is a 64% to 73% satisfaction rate.
  - Preoperative weakness, female sex, and poor preoperative function are all risk factors for poor outcome.[62,63]
- Lower trapezius: The fibers of the lower border of the trapezius have a more direct line of pull to improve ER.[64,65]
  - Allograft tissue is required to improve excursion of the tendon.
- Pectoralis major: may help to restore internal rotation in subscapularis-deficient shoulders, without anterosuperior escape[66]
  - The sternal head or the entire tendon may be transferred depending on the size of the tear and the amount of muscle atrophy.
  - Pectoralis major transfers should not be performed for the treatment of anterior instability of the shoulder.

- Rotator cuff tear arthropathy (RCTA)[67]
  - Epidemiology
    - The prevalence of RCTA is around 32% in the setting of an RCT.[68]
  - Etiology and natural history
    - There are many hypotheses as to the pathogenesis of RCTA. A degenerative RCT generally increases in size over time, leading to proximal humeral migration. Once this has occurred, GH arthritis progresses more rapidly.[69]
    - RCTA pathogenesis: RCT → abnormal GH kinematics → edge-loading at the superior glenoid → tear and degeneration of the superior capsule → worsening GH kinematics and extravasation of synovial fluid into surrounding tissues → accelerated progression of arthritis

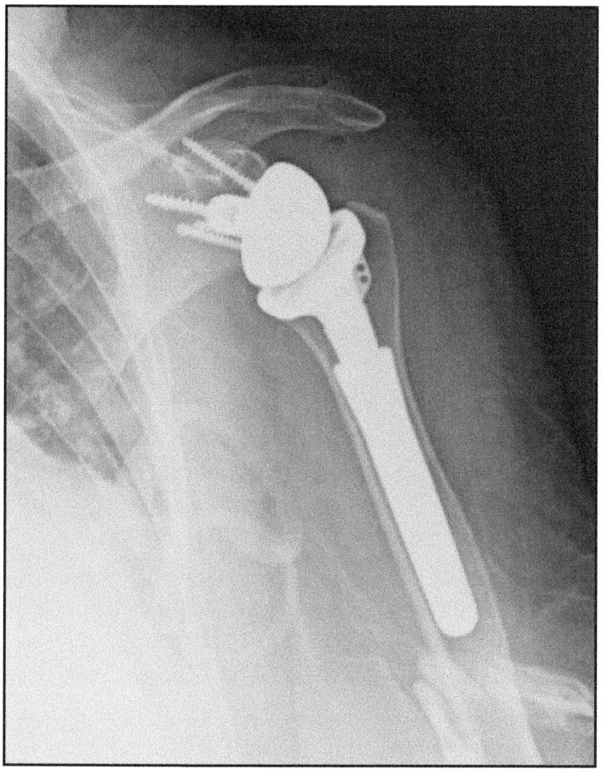

Figure 9-8. Reverse shoulder arthroplasty.

- "Femoralization" of the proximal humerus and "acetabularization" of the acromion in advanced stages
- Classification
  - Hamada classification
    - Grade 1: acromiohumeral interval (AHI) greater than or equal to 6 mm
    - Grade 2: AHI less than or equal to 5 mm
    - Grade 3: AHI less than 5 mm with acetabularization of the acromion
    - Grade 4: grade 3 with GH arthritis
    - Grade 5: grade 4 with humeral head collapse
- Treatment
  - Arthroplasty
    - Reverse total shoulder arthroplasty (Figure 9-8): The center of rotation is shifted medially, which decreases shear forces on the glenoid. The deltoid is tensioned, which improves the lever arm of the shoulder, and the articulation has increased constraint by matching the radius of curvature between the polyethylene and glenosphere.[70]
    - These alterations in the biomechanics of the shoulder allow the prosthesis to effectively bypass the RC and allow the deltoid to function.
  - Reverse total shoulder arthroplasty plus tendon transfer
    - Latissimus transfer is used to improve ER in cases of a positive hornblower's sign, indicating teres minor insufficiency.
    - Results in improved functional outcomes in patients with weak or absent ER[71]

Other Causes of Rotator Cuff Dysfunction

- Paralabral cysts
  - These cysts generally arise in the setting of a labral tear. Fluid escapes the joint and gets sealed off to form a cyst.
  - They may cause impingement on the suprascapular nerve at the spinoglenoid notch, resulting in infraspinatus weakness and/or pain.
  - Arthroscopic decompression and debridement may be performed.
- Calcific tendinitis
  - Calcific tendinitis has an unknown etiology characterized by cyclical progression of intratendinous hydroxyapatite crystal deposition.
  - It occurs at 30 to 50 years old, more often in women.
  - Calcific tendinitis occurs 1 to 2 cm proximal to the insertion site (in the watershed area of the tendon), whereas dystrophic calcification (the degenerative process seen in RCT) occurs at the insertion site of the tendon.
  - It occurs in 3 stages:
    1. Precalcific stage: Fibrocartilaginous metaplasia (tenocytes are converted to chondrocytes) occurs with no pain but progresses to the formative phase, which may be painful.
    2. Calcific stage: Once the calcium is formed, pain is possible, but this is a "resting phase" and will progress to a resorptive phase. The resorptive phase is associated with an abrupt onset of severe pain that limits function.
    3. Postcalcific stage: At this stage the tendon reconstitutes, and pain is possible but decreases from the resorptive phase.
  - Needle lavage is often extremely useful during the resorptive phase to decrease intratendinous pressure.
  - Arthroscopic surgery to perform a debridement, and calcium excision is also an option for recalcitrant calcific tendinopathy. If a defect in the tendon is created after removal of the calcified tissue, a repair of the tendon is commonly performed.

References

1. Galatz LM, Sandell LJ, Rothermich SY, et al. Characteristics of the rat supraspinatus tendon during tendon-to-bone healing after acute injury. *J Orthop Res.* 2006;24(3):541-550. doi:10.1002/jor.20067.
2. Nozaki T, Nimura A, Fujishiro H, et al. The anatomic relationship between the morphology of the greater tubercle of the humerus and the insertion of the infraspinatus tendon. *J Shoulder Elbow Surg.* 2015;24(4):555-560. doi:10.1016/j.jse.2014.09.038.
3. Mochizuki T, Sugaya H, Uomizu M, et al. Humeral insertion of the supraspinatus and infraspinatus. New anatomical findings regarding the footprint of the rotator cuff. *J Bone Joint Surg Am.* 2008;90(5):962-969. doi:10.2106/JBJS.G.00427.
4. Curtis AS, Burbank KM, Tierney JJ, Scheller AD, Curran AR. The insertional footprint of the rotator cuff: an anatomic study. *Arthroscopy.* 2006;22(6):609.e1. doi:10.1016/j.arthro.2006.04.001.
5. Nimura A, Kato A, Yamaguchi K, et al. The superior capsule of the shoulder joint complements the insertion of the rotator cuff. *J Shoulder Elbow Surg.* 2012;21(7):867-872. doi:10.1016/j.jse.2011.04.034.
6. Nguyen L, Park KJ, McGarry MH, et al. Role of the superior shoulder capsule in passive stability of the glenohumeral joint. *J Shoulder Elbow Surg.* 2014;23(5):642-648. doi:10.1016/j.jse.2013.09.025.
7. Burkhart SS. Arthroscopic treatment of massive rotator cuff tears. Clinical results and biomechanical rationale. *Clin Orthop Relat Res.* 1991(267):45-56. doi:10.1097/00003086-199106000-00006.
8. Hansen ML, Otis JC, Johnson JS, Cordasco FA, Craig EV, Warren RF. Biomechanics of massive rotator cuff tears: implications for treatment. *J Bone Joint Surg Am.* 2008;90(2):316-325. doi:10.2106/JBJS.F.00880.

9. Oh JH, Jun BJ, McGarry MH, Lee TQ. Does a critical rotator cuff tear stage exist? A biomechanical study of rotator cuff tear progression in human cadaver shoulders. *J Bone Joint Surg Am.* 2011;93(22):2100-2109. doi:10.2106/JBJS.J.00032.
10. Teefey SA, Rubin DA, Middleton WD, Hildebolt CF, Leibold RA, Yamaguchi K. Detection and quantification of rotator cuff tears. Comparison of ultrasonographic, magnetic resonance imaging, and arthroscopic findings in seventy-one consecutive cases. *J Bone Joint Surg Am.* 2004;86-A(4):708-716.
11. Wall LB, Teefey SA, Middleton WD, et al. Diagnostic performance and reliability of ultrasonography for fatty degeneration of the rotator cuff muscles. *J Bone Joint Surg Am.* 2012;94(12):e83. doi:10.2106/JBJS.J.01899.
12. Sher JS, Uribe JW, Posada A, Murphy BJ, Zlatkin MB. Abnormal findings on magnetic resonance images of asymptomatic shoulders. *J Bone Joint Surg Am.* 1995;77(1):10-15.
13. Kartus J, Kartus C, Rostgard-Christensen L, Sernert N, Read J, Perko M. Long-term clinical and ultrasound evaluation after arthroscopic acromioplasty in patients with partial rotator cuff tears. *Arthroscopy.* 2006;22(1):44-49. doi:10.1016/j.arthro.2005.07.027.
14. Yamaguchi K, Tetro AM, Blam O, Evanoff BA, Teefey SA, Middleton WD. Natural history of asymptomatic rotator cuff tears: a longitudinal analysis of asymptomatic tears detected sonographically. *J Shoulder Elbow Surg.* 2001;10(3):199-203. doi:10.1067/mse.2001.113086.
15. Coghlan JA, Buchbinder R, Green S, Johnston RV, Bell SN. Surgery for rotator cuff disease. *Cochrane Database Syst Rev.* 2008(1):CD005619. doi:10.1002/14651858.CD005619.pub2.
16. Gartsman GM, O'Connor D P. Arthroscopic rotator cuff repair with and without arthroscopic subacromial decompression: a prospective, randomized study of one-year outcomes. *J Shoulder Elbow Surg.* 2004;13(4):424-426. doi:10.1016/S1058274604000527.
17. Milano G, Grasso A, Salvatore M, Zarelli D, Deriu L, Fabbriciani C. Arthroscopic rotator cuff repair with and without subacromial decompression: a prospective randomized study. *Arthroscopy.* 2007;23(1):81-88. doi:10.1016/j.arthro.2006.10.011.
18. Cordasco FA, Backer M, Craig EV, Klein D, Warren RF. The partial-thickness rotator cuff tear: is acromioplasty without repair sufficient? *Am J Sports Med.* 2002;30(2):257-260. doi:10.1177/03635465020300021801.
19. Iyengar JJ, Porat S, Burnett KR, Marrero-Perez L, Hernandez VH, Nottage WM. Magnetic resonance imaging tendon integrity assessment after arthroscopic partial-thickness rotator cuff repair. *Arthroscopy.* 2011;27(3):306-313. doi:10.1016/j.arthro.2010.08.017.
20. Kim KC, Shin HD, Cha SM, Park JY. Repair integrity and functional outcome after arthroscopic conversion to a full-thickness rotator cuff tear: articular- versus bursal-side partial tears. *Am J Sports Med.* 2014;42(2):451-456. doi:10.1177/0363546513512770.
21. Kamath G, Galatz LM, Keener JD, Teefey S, Middleton W, Yamaguchi K. Tendon integrity and functional outcome after arthroscopic repair of high-grade partial-thickness supraspinatus tears. *J Bone Joint Surg Am.* 2009;91(5):1055-1062. doi:10.2106/JBJS.G.00118.
22. Ide J, Maeda S, Takagi K. Arthroscopic transtendon repair of partial-thickness articular-side tears of the rotator cuff: anatomical and clinical study. *Am J Sports Med.* 2005;33(11):1672-1679. doi:10.1177/0363546505277141.
23. Denkers M, Pletsch K, Boorman R, Hollinshead R, Lo KY. Partial thickness rotator cuff tears: observe or operative. Presented at: Annual Meeting of the American Academy of Orthopaedic Surgeons; February 7-11, 2012; San Francisco, CA.
24. Weber SC. Arthroscopic debridement and acromioplasty versus mini-open repair in the treatment of significant partial-thickness rotator cuff tears. *Arthroscopy.* 1999;15(2):126-131. doi:10.1053/ar.1999.v15.0150121.
25. Gonzalez-Lomas G, Kippe MA, Brown GD, et al. In situ transtendon repair outperforms tear completion and repair for partial articular-sided supraspinatus tendon tears. *J Shoulder Elbow Surg.* 2008;17(5):722-728. doi:10.1016/j.jse.2008.01.148.
26. Castagna A, Borroni M, Garofalo R, et al. Deep partial rotator cuff tear: transtendon repair or tear completion and repair? A randomized clinical trial. *Knee Surg Sports Traumatol Arthrosc.* 2015;23(2):460-463. doi:10.1007/s00167-013-2536-6.
27. Conway JE. Arthroscopic repair of partial-thickness rotator cuff tears and SLAP lesions in professional baseball players. *Orthop Clin North Am.* 2001;32(3):443-456. doi:10.1053/otsm.2000.17778.
28. Mazzocca AD, Rincon LM, O'Connor RW, et al. Intra-articular partial-thickness rotator cuff tears: analysis of injured and repaired strain behavior. *Am J Sports Med.* 2008;36(1):110-116. doi:10.1177/0363546507307502.
29. Lehman C, Cuomo F, Kummer FJ, Zuckerman JD. The incidence of full thickness rotator cuff tears in a large cadaveric population. *Bull Hosp Jt Dis.* 1995;54(1):30-31.
30. Yamaguchi K, Ditsios K, Middleton WD, Hildebolt CF, Galatz LM, Teefey SA. The demographic and morphological features of rotator cuff disease. A comparison of asymptomatic and symptomatic shoulders. *J Bone Joint Surg Am.* 2006;88(8):1699-1704. doi:10.2106/JBJS.E.00835.
31. Sonnabend DH. Treatment of primary anterior shoulder dislocation in patients older than 40 years of age. Conservative versus operative. *Clin Orthop Relat Res.* 1994(304):74-77.
32. Kim HM, Dahiya N, Teefey SA, et al. Location and initiation of degenerative rotator cuff tears: an analysis of three hundred and sixty shoulders. *J Bone Joint Surg Am.* 2010;92(5):1088-1096. doi:10.2106/JBJS.I.00686.

33. Kim HM, Teefey SA, Zelig A, Galatz LM, Keener JD, Yamaguchi K. Shoulder strength in asymptomatic individuals with intact compared with torn rotator cuffs. *J Bone Joint Surg Am.* 2009;91(2):289-296. doi:10.2106/JBJS.H.00219.
34. Keener JD, Wei AS, Kim HM, Steger-May K, Yamaguchi K. Proximal humeral migration in shoulders with symptomatic and asymptomatic rotator cuff tears. *J Bone Joint Surg Am.* 2009;91(6):1405-1413. doi:10.2106/JBJS.H.00854.
35. Keener JD, Galatz LM, Teefey SA, et al. A prospective evaluation of survivorship of asymptomatic degenerative rotator cuff tears. *J Bone Joint Surg Am.* 2015;97(2):89-98. doi:10.2106/JBJS.N.00099.
36. Mall NA, Kim HM, Keener JD, et al. Symptomatic progression of asymptomatic rotator cuff tears: a prospective study of clinical and sonographic variables. *J Bone Joint Surg Am.* 2010;92(16):2623-2633. doi:10.2106/JBJS.I.00506.
37. Hebert-Davies J, Teefey SA, Steger-May K, et al. Progression of Fatty Muscle Degeneration in Atraumatic Rotator Cuff Tears. *J Bone Joint Surg Am.* 2017;99(10):832-839. doi:10.2106/JBJS.16.00030.
38. Kim HM, Dahiya N, Teefey SA, Keener JD, Galatz LM, Yamaguchi K. Relationship of tear size and location to fatty degeneration of the rotator cuff. *J Bone Joint Surg Am.* 2010;92(4):829-839. doi:10.2106/JBJS.H.01746.
39. DeOrio JK, Cofield RH. Results of a second attempt at surgical repair of a failed initial rotator-cuff repair. *J Bone Joint Surg Am.* 1984;66(4):563-567.
40. Zumstein MA, Jost B, Hempel J, Hodler J, Gerber C. The clinical and structural long-term results of open repair of massive tears of the rotator cuff. *J Bone Joint Surg Am.* 2008;90(11):2423-2431. doi:10.2106/JBJS.G.00677.
41. Fuchs B, Weishaupt D, Zanetti M, Hodler J, Gerber C. Fatty degeneration of the muscles of the rotator cuff: assessment by computed tomography versus magnetic resonance imaging. *J Shoulder Elbow Surg.* 1999;8(6):599-605. doi:10.1016/S1058-2746(99)90097-6.
42. Zanetti M, Gerber C, Hodler J. Quantitative assessment of the muscles of the rotator cuff with magnetic resonance imaging. *Invest Radiol.* 1998;33(3):163-170. doi:10.1097/00004424-199803000-00006.
43. Bassett RW, Cofield RH. Acute tears of the rotator cuff. The timing of surgical repair. *Clin Orthop Relat Res.* 1983(175):18-24. doi:10.1097/00003086-198305000-00003.
44. Kuhn JE, Dunn WR, Sanders R, et al. Effectiveness of physical therapy in treating atraumatic full-thickness rotator cuff tears: a multicenter prospective cohort study. *J Shoulder Elbow Surg.* 2013;22(10):1371-1379. doi:10.1016/j.jse.2013.01.026.
45. Voigt C, Bosse C, Vosshenrich R, Schulz AP, Lill H. Arthroscopic supraspinatus tendon repair with suture-bridging technique: functional outcome and magnetic resonance imaging. *Am J Sports Med.* 2010;38(5):983-991. doi:10.1177/0363546509359063.
46. Kim DH, Elattrache NS, Tibone JE, et al. Biomechanical comparison of a single-row versus double-row suture anchor technique for rotator cuff repair. *Am J Sports Med.* 2006;34(3):407-414. doi:10.1177/0363546505281238.
47. Koh KH, Kang KC, Lim TK, Shon MS, Yoo JC. Prospective randomized clinical trial of single- versus double-row suture anchor repair in 2- to 4-cm rotator cuff tears: clinical and magnetic resonance imaging results. *Arthroscopy.* 2011;27(4):453-462. doi:10.1016/j.arthro.2010.11.059.
48. Park MC, Tibone JE, ElAttrache NS, Ahmad CS, Jun BJ, Lee TQ. Part II: biomechanical assessment for a footprint-restoring transosseous-equivalent rotator cuff repair technique compared with a double-row repair technique. *J Shoulder Elbow Surg.* 2007;16(4):469-476. doi:10.1016/j.jse.2006.09.011.
49. DeHaan AM, Axelrad TW, Kaye E, Silvestri L, Puskas B, Foster TE. Does double-row rotator cuff repair improve functional outcome of patients compared with single-row technique? A systematic review. *Am J Sports Med.* 2012;40(5):1176-1185. doi:10.1177/0363546511428866.
50. Boileau P, Brassart N, Watkinson DJ, Carles M, Hatzidakis AM, Krishnan SG. Arthroscopic repair of full-thickness tears of the supraspinatus: does the tendon really heal? *J Bone Joint Surg Am.* 2005;87(6):1229-1240. doi:10.2106/JBJS.D.02035.
51. Iannotti JP, Deutsch A, Green A, et al. Time to failure after rotator cuff repair: a prospective imaging study. *J Bone Joint Surg Am.* 2013;95(11):965-971. doi:10.2106/JBJS.L.00708.
52. Sclamberg SG, Tibone JE, Itamura JM, Kasraeian S. Six-month magnetic resonance imaging follow-up of large and massive rotator cuff repairs reinforced with porcine small intestinal submucosa. *J Shoulder Elbow Surg.* 2004;13(5):538-541. doi:10.1016/S1058274604001193.
53. Bond JL, Dopirak RM, Higgins J, Burns J, Snyder SJ. Arthroscopic replacement of massive, irreparable rotator cuff tears using a GraftJacket allograft: technique and preliminary results. *Arthroscopy.* 2008;24(4):403-409.e1. doi:10.1016/j.arthro.2007.07.033.
54. Snyder SJ, Arnoczky SP, Bond JL, Dopirak R. Histologic evaluation of a biopsy specimen obtained 3 months after rotator cuff augmentation with GraftJacket Matrix. *Arthroscopy.* 2009;25(3):329-333. doi:10.1016/j.arthro.2008.05.023.
55. Gupta AK, Hug K, Berkoff DJ, et al. Dermal tissue allograft for the repair of massive irreparable rotator cuff tears. *Am J Sports Med.* 2012;40(1):141-147. doi:10.1177/0363546511422795.
56. Stone MA, Carre A, Trasolini N, Minneti M, Omid R. Vascularized dermal autograft for the treatment of irreparable rotator cuff tears. *J Shoulder Elbow Surg.* 2018;27(9):1664-1671. doi:10.1016/j.jse.2018.02.069.

57. Omid R, Lee B. Tendon transfers for irreparable rotator cuff tears. *J Am Acad Orthop Surg.* 2013;21(8):492-501. doi:10.5435/JAAOS-21-08-492.
58. Goutallier D, Postel JM, Bernageau J, Lavau L, Voisin MC. Fatty muscle degeneration in cuff ruptures. Pre- and postoperative evaluation by CT scan. *Clin Orthop Relat Res.* 1994(304):78-83.
59. Rockwood CA Jr, Williams GR Jr, Burkhead WZ Jr. Débridement of degenerative, irreparable lesions of the rotator cuff. *J Bone Joint Surg Am.* 1995;77(6):857-866. doi:10.2106/00004623-199506000-00006.
60. Gerber C. Latissimus dorsi transfer for the treatment of irreparable tears of the rotator cuff. *Clin Orthop Relat Res.* 1992(275):152-160.
61. Gerber C, Vinh TS, Hertel R, Hess CW. Latissimus dorsi transfer for the treatment of massive tears of the rotator cuff. A preliminary report. *Clin Orthop Relat Res.* 1988(232):51-61.
62. Warner JJ, Parsons IM IV. Latissimus dorsi tendon transfer: a comparative analysis of primary and salvage reconstruction of massive, irreparable rotator cuff tears. *J Shoulder Elbow Surg.* 2001;10(6):514-521. doi:10.1067/mse.2001.118629.
63. Iannotti JP, Hennigan S, Herzog R, et al. Latissimus dorsi tendon transfer for irreparable posterosuperior rotator cuff tears. Factors affecting outcome. *J Bone Joint Surg Am.* 2006;88(2):342-348. doi:10.2106/JBJS.D.02996.
64. Omid R, Heckmann N, Wang L, McGarry MH, Vangsness CT Jr, Lee TQ. Biomechanical comparison between the trapezius transfer and latissimus transfer for irreparable posterosuperior rotator cuff tears. *J Shoulder Elbow Surg.* 2015;24(10):1635-1643. doi:10.1016/j.jse.2015.02.008.
65. Hartzler RU, Barlow JD, An KN, Elhassan BT. Biomechanical effectiveness of different types of tendon transfers to the shoulder for external rotation. *J Shoulder Elbow Surg.* 2012;21(10):1370-1376. doi:10.1016/j.jse.2012.01.026.
66. Wirth MA, Rockwood CA Jr. Operative treatment of irreparable rupture of the subscapularis. *J Bone Joint Surg Am.* 1997;79(5):722-731. doi:10.2106/00004623-199705000-00012.
67. Ecklund KJ, Lee TQ, Tibone J, Gupta R. Rotator cuff tear arthropathy. *J Am Acad Orthop Surg.* 2007;15(6):340-349. doi:10.5435/00124635-200706000-00003.
68. Ranebo MC, Björnsson Hallgren HC, Adolfsson LE. Patients with a long-standing cuff tear in one shoulder have high rates of contralateral cuff tears: a study of patients with arthroscopically verified cuff tears 22 years ago. *J Shoulder Elbow Surg.* 2018;27(3):e68-e74. doi:10.1016/j.jse.2017.10.007.
69. Jensen KL, Williams GR Jr, Russell IJ, Rockwood CA Jr. Rotator cuff tear arthropathy. *J Bone Joint Surg Am.* 1999;81(9):1312-1324. doi:10.2106/00004623-199909000-00013.
70. Grammont PM, Baulot E. Delta shoulder prosthesis for rotator cuff rupture. *Orthopedics.* 1993;16(1):65-68. doi:10.3928/0147-7447-19930101-11.
71. Boileau P, Chuinard C, Roussanne Y, Neyton L, Trojani C. Modified latissimus dorsi and teres major transfer through a single delto-pectoral approach for external rotation deficit of the shoulder: as an isolated procedure or with a reverse arthroplasty. *J Shoulder Elbow Surg.* 2007;16(6):671-682. doi:10.1016/j.jse.2007.02.127.

10

Shoulder Instability

Vahid Entezari, MD, MMSc and Mark D. Lazarus, MD

Pathoanatomy

- Shoulder stability[1] *Recommended reading for understanding the role of static and dynamic stabilizers in shoulder stability*
    - Static stabilizers
        - Glenohumeral (GH) articulation
            - Articular congruity[2]
            - Negative intra-articular pressure[3]
            - Glenoid retroversion and superior tilt[4]
        - Glenoid labrum
            - The labrum is the attachment site for the capsule and the long head of the biceps tendon (LHBT).
            - At any given time, only 25% to 30% of the humeral head is in contact with the glenoid face.[5]
            - Loss of labrum results in a 50% decrease in glenoid depth and a 20% reduction in the translational force required for anterior dislocation.[6]
        - Capsuloligamentous structures[7,8]
            - The superior GH ligament is the primary stabilizer to inferior translation with the arm in neutral abduction (0 degrees).
            - The middle GH ligament is the primary stabilizer to anterior translation and external rotation (ER) with the arm in midabduction (45 to 60 degrees).
            - The inferior glenohumeral ligament (IGHL) is the primary stabilizer to anterior translation with arm in full abduction (90 degrees).

Namdari S, Zmistowski B, Omid R, eds.
The Foundations of Shoulder and Elbow Surgery (pp 191-214).

- The anterior band of the IGHL is the principal static anterior stabilizer of the shoulder with the arm in the abducted and externally rotated position.[9]
- The coracohumeral ligament is the primary restraint to posterior subluxation with the arm in forward flexion and internal rotation (IR).
- The rotator interval (RI) consists of soft tissue extending from the base of the coracoid to the anterior edge of the supraspinatus and the superior edge of the subscapularis, which consists of coracohumeral ligament (superficial), LHBT (in the middle), and superior GH ligament (deep).[10]
  - Surgical tightening of the RI leads to loss of ER and inferior and posterior translation of the humeral head.[11]
- Dynamic stabilizers[12]
  - Rotator cuff muscles create concavity compression, especially in midrange when capsule and ligaments are relaxed.[13]
    - A cadaveric model showed that creation of anteroinferior chondrolabral defect results in loss of concavity and instability and simulated reconstruction of the defect results in normalization of concavity compression.[14]
  - The LHBT acts as a humeral head depressor and shoulder stabilizer in all directions, based on cadaveric studies. This is a function that has yet to be confirmed in vivo.[15]
  - Deltoid and humerothoracic muscle contributions.[16]
  - Scapulothoracic rhythm is the coordinated contraction of muscles around the shoulder during range of motion to maintain stable GH relationships.[17]
  - Proprioception

Definitions[18]

- Instability is a subjective phenomenon by which “unwanted translation of the humeral head on the glenoid compromises the comfort and function of the shoulder.”[19]
- Laxity is the objective clinical finding of passive GH translation.
- Thrower’s shoulder is the developmental bony and soft-tissue adaptation (commonly seen between 13 and 14 years old) in the dominant shoulder to accommodate throwing, resulting in decreased total rotational arc of motion, increased ER, and decreased IR.
- Pathology of anterior instability
  - A Bankart lesion is the avulsion of the capsule and labrum from the anterior glenoid rim with or without a bony fragment, commonly resulting from an anterior shoulder dislocation. The Bankart lesion is associated with complete periosteal disruption and floating of the capsulolabral complex (Figure 10-1A).[20]
  - A Perthes lesion is an anterior GH labral tear with an intact capsule and periosteal attachment to the glenoid neck. It usually does not result in detachment of the IGHL and anterior capsule (Figure 10-1B).
  - An anterior ligamentous periosteal sleeve avulsion (ALPSA) is similar to the Bankart lesion but the periosteal sleeve is intact, usually associated with medial displacement of the labroligamentous complex. This lesion usually heals and results in incompetency of the capsule and the IGHL (Figure 10-1C).[21]
  - A glenoid labrum articular defect is the superficial loss of articular cartilage from the anterior rim of the glenoid. This lesion does not have associated capsular and periosteal stripping.[22]

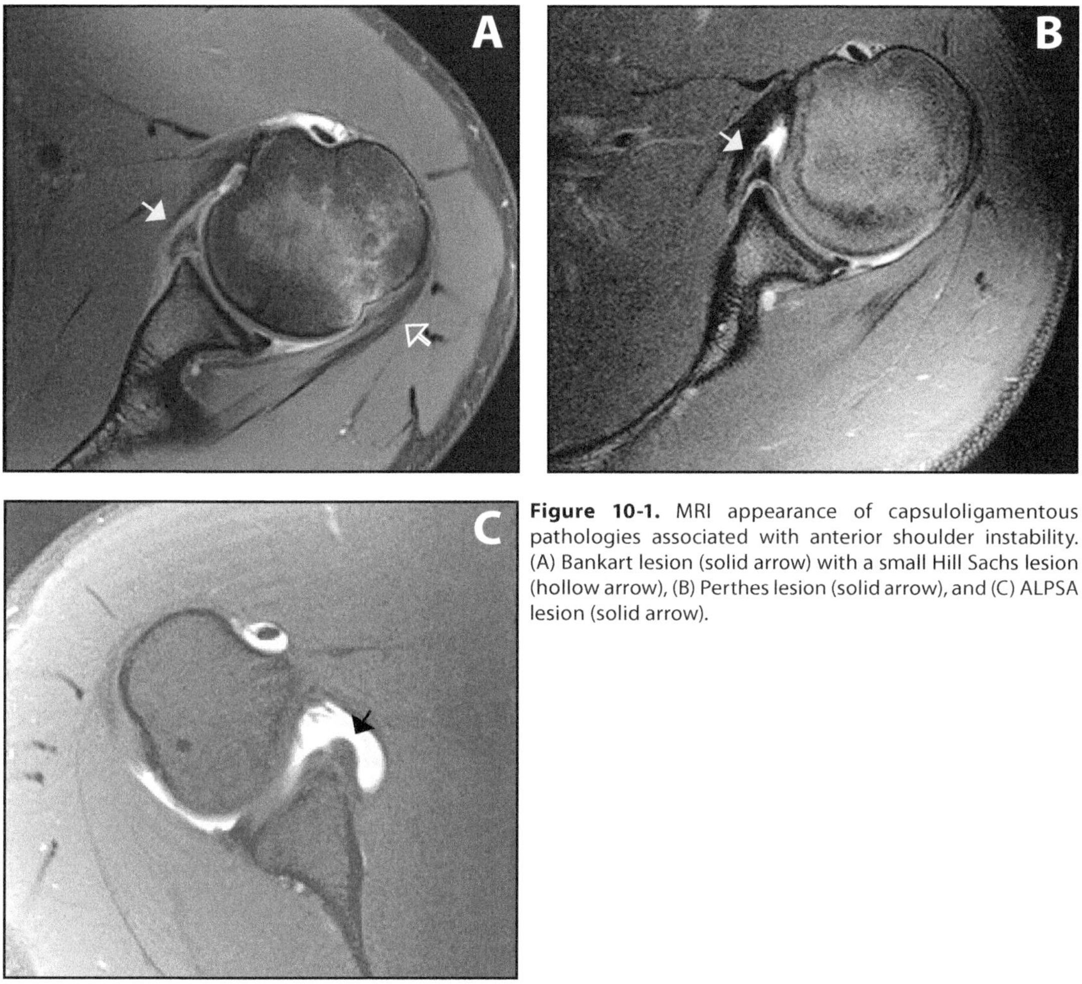

Figure 10-1. MRI appearance of capsuloligamentous pathologies associated with anterior shoulder instability. (A) Bankart lesion (solid arrow) with a small Hill Sachs lesion (hollow arrow), (B) Perthes lesion (solid arrow), and (C) ALPSA lesion (solid arrow).

  - A Hill-Sachs lesion is a chondral or osteochondral compression fracture in the anterosuperior aspect of the humeral head against the bony glenoid rim as a result of posterior shoulder dislocation.
- Pathology of posterior instability
  - A reverse Bankart lesion is the disruption of the posteroinferior glenoid labrum, along with the posterior band of the IGHL, in a patient with posterior instability.
  - A Kim lesion is a concealed and incomplete avulsion of the posteroinferior labrum, which can be a source of persistent posterior or multidirectional shoulder instability.[23,24]
  - A reverse Hill-Sachs lesion is a chondral or osteochondral compression fracture in the posterolateral aspect of the humeral head as a result of anterior shoulder dislocation.[25]
- Inferior pathology
  - Humeral avulsion of glenohumeral ligaments (HAGL) is avulsion of the IGHL from its humeral attachment site, commonly associated with high-energy dislocations and typical "J sign" of the inferior capsular pouch on magnetic resonance imaging (MRI).[26]

Classification[27]

- Shoulder instability can be classified based on the following:
  - Etiology
    - Traumatic
    - Atraumatic (voluntary or involuntary)
    - Acquired (microtrauma)
    - Congenital (glenoid dysplasia, Ehlers-Danlos syndrome)
  - Severity
    - Dislocation (commonly requires formal reduction)
    - Subluxation (commonly is self-reduced)
    - Microinstability (commonly associated with repetitive or sport-type activity)
  - Direction
    - Anterior
    - Posterior
    - Inferior (luxatio erecta)
    - Multidirectional
  - Time[28]
    - Acute (less than 1 week)
    - Chronic
      - Early (1 to 3 weeks)
      - Late (greater than 3 weeks)
  - Frequency
    - Single
    - Recurrent (greater than 1 incident)

Anterior Instability

- The incidence of shoulder dislocation is estimated to be 24 per 100,000 person-years while the majority occur in young males. More than 85% of them are anterior dislocations.[29,30]
- Mechanism of injury (MOI) is anteriorly directed force applied to the shoulder with the arm in abduction and ER, such as arm tackling in football, falling while skiing, or sliding into a base.
- Almost all dislocations are subcoracoid unless the coracoid is fractured.
- A younger patient is likely to have a ligamentous injury involving the labrum and capsule.
- In patients older than 40 years old, the rotator cuff, proximal humerus, and surrounding neurovascular structures are at higher risk of associated injury.
- Associated pathology
  - Bankart lesion
    - Historically the Bankart lesion is called an "essential lesion" of recurrent anterior instability (Figure 10-2).
    - A Bankart lesion is found in 85% to 97% of traumatic anterior dislocations. It is also present in close to 70% of traumatic subluxations.[5,31]
    - Cadaveric study of a simulated Bankart lesion showed that although creating a Bankart lesion results in a small increase in humeral translation, it does not result in dislocation, suggesting that additional capsular injuries may be required to lead to true shoulder instability.[32]

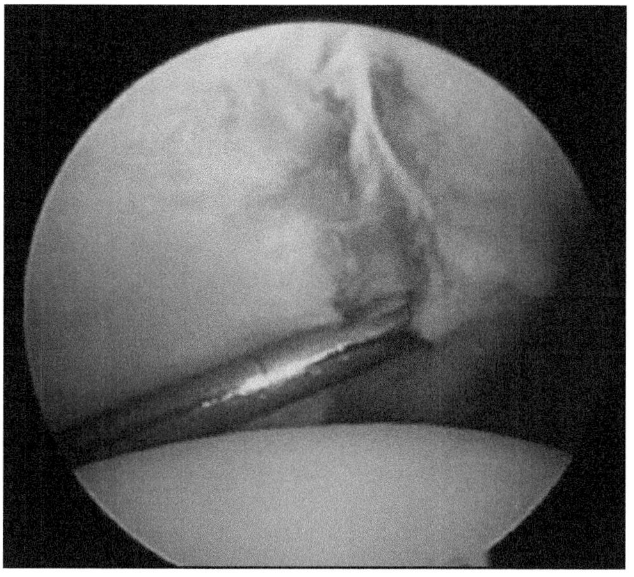

Figure 10-2. Arthroscopic image of a Bankart lesion in a young patient with recurrent anterior instability.

- Capsular tearing or stretching
  - Plastic deformation of the IGHL may occur during anterior subluxation or dislocation and may be an important factor contributing to instability.
  - Congenital collagen disorders (eg, Ehlers-Danlos and Marfan syndromes) can cause structural collagen alterations that affect capsular biomechanics.
- Osseous glenoid insufficiency
  - Glenoid bone loss has been reported after 22% of initial dislocation and in up to 90% of patients with recurrent dislocation.[33]
  - The normal pear-shaped glenoid takes on an "inverted pear" configuration in the presence of a glenoid deficiency.[34]
  - Eighty percent of glenoid defects occur at the 3 o'clock (range, the 2:30 to 4:20 clock) position. Anterior tilting of the scapula in vivo explains why this pattern of bone defect corresponds to the common anteroinferior path for shoulder dislocation.[35]
  - If the greatest length of the glenoid defect exceeds the radius of the glenoid at its maximum diameter, the force necessary for anterior dislocation is reduced by 30%.[27]
  - Milano et al evaluated predictors of glenoid bone loss after first anterior shoulder dislocation. They found glenoid defect in 72% of their cohort and number of dislocations and age at the time of first dislocation were the most significant predictors of glenoid bone loss.[36]
- Superior labrum anterior and posterior (SLAP) tear
  - The superior portion of the labrum may be important for GH stability.
  - A complete SLAP lesion is associated with destabilization of the LHBT and results in increased anteroposterior (AP) translation of the humerus on the glenoid in the lower ranges of elevation in cadaveric models.[37]
- In an ALPSA lesion, the anterior IGHL, labrum, and the anterior scapular periosteum are stripped and displaced in a sleeve-type fashion medially on the glenoid neck. In a chronic situation, a cursory inspection of the anterior-inferior quadrant of the glenoid may not reveal evidence of trauma.

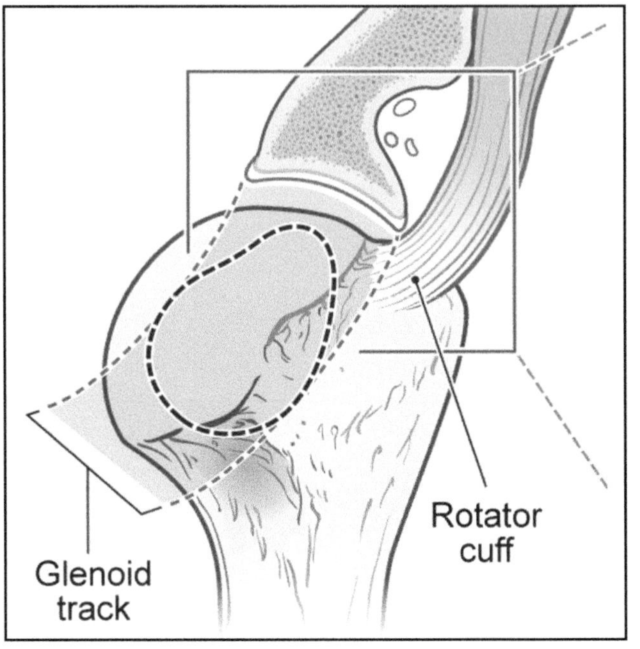

Figure 10-3. Depiction of glenoid track defined by the contact zone of glenoid face on the humeral head. (Reprinted with permission from Patel RM, Amin NH, Lynch TS, Miniaci A. Management of bone loss in glenohumeral instability. *Orthop Clin North Am.* 2014;45[4]:523-539. doi:10.1016/j.ocl.2014.06.005.)

- A HAGL lesion is caused by forceful abduction and appears as thickened or rolled edges of the capsule, typically in the inferior recess during arthroscopy and can be associated with bony avulsion in less than 10% of cases.[26]
- A rotator cuff tear is uncommon in a patient younger than 40 years old, but it should be suspected if pain and weakness persist 3 to 4 weeks after the injury.[38]
  - If present, a posterosuperior rotator cuff is avulsed with anterior dislocation. Avulsion of the subscapularis may also be present.
- Fracture
  - Hill-Sachs lesion
    - They occur in 90% of anterior dislocations and 25% of anterior subluxations.
    - The size and location of the Hill-Sachs lesion relative to the glenoid bone defect ("on-track" vs "off-track" lesion) may determine its effect on recurrent shoulder instability.[39]
    - The on-track vs off-track concept was introduced by Itoi et al. As the arm moves along the various degrees of abduction and ER, the glenoid contact zone with the humeral head creates a "glenoid track" (Figure 10-3). If a Hill-Sachs lesion stays on glenoid track (on-track lesion), it will not engage with the glenoid rim and will not result in dislocation as opposed to lesions that are out of the glenoid track (off-track lesion) that will engage with the glenoid and result in dislocation.[40,41]
  - Greater tuberosity fractures occur in approximately 15% to 20% of anterior GH dislocations.[42,43]
  - Coracoid fractures are rare and usually involve the tip of the coracoid process.
- Nerve injury
  - Nerve injuries are seen in 32% to 65% of patients with dislocations and are more common in older patients and patients with an associated fracture.

- Axillary nerve injury is the most commonly injured nerve, especially in anterior dislocation, and may present as a droopy shoulder on examination or a mildly subluxated joint after reduction due to a weakened deltoid.[44]
- Brachial plexus and musculocutaneous nerve injuries have also been reported.[45]

Posterior Instability

- Posterior instability accounts for 2% to 4% of all shoulder dislocations.
- The MOI is a posteriorly directed force with the arm forward elevated and adducted in high-energy trauma, such as a car accident or pass blocking in football. Also, seizure or electrocution can produce a traumatic posterior shoulder dislocation due to muscle imbalance, with internal rotator muscles overpowering external rotators.
- Glenoid dysplasia is a congenital deformity of the glenoid associated with deficient posterior glenoid rim, excessive retroversion, and hypertrophy of the posterior cartilage and labrum and can be associated with posterior instability.[46,47]
- Associated pathology
  - A reverse Bankart lesion involves a disruption of the posteroinferior glenoid labrum, along with the posterior band of the IGHL.
  - A SLAP lesion involves a superior extension of the labral pathology that can extend posteriorly and should be investigated during arthroscopy.
  - A Kim lesion can be concealed by intact superficial layers of the labrum. Thorough arthroscopic evaluation of the posteroinferior labrum is required. If present, completion of the lesion and labroplasty is required to restore normal labral height and tension of the posterior capsule.[23]
  - In fractures, lesser tuberosity fractures or avulsion are seen with posterior GH dislocation.
  - In rotator cuff tears, subscapularis tendon can be avulsed with posterior dislocation.

Inferior Instability

- Inferior instability accounts for less than 1% of all shoulder dislocations.[48]
- The MOI is an axial force applied to an already abducted shoulder or forceful hyperabduction of the shoulder.
- Patients classically present with the elbow flexed and the forearm pronated with the hand either positioned over the patient's forehead or behind their head ("luxatio erecta").
- Associated pathology
  - Inferior dislocation is associated with a high number of greater tuberosity fractures (30%), glenoid fractures (7%), and nerve (29%) and vascular injuries (10%).[49]

Multi-Directional Instability

- Multi-directional instability (MDI) was popularized by Neer and Foster and is consistent with increased global laxity in the shoulder. They defined it as having signs of inferior laxity and concurrent symptoms in at least one other direction.[50]
- Incidence is greatest in the second and third decades of life, and most patients are younger than 35 years old.
- Classification
  - Etiology
    - Congenital (primary)

        - Congenital MDI is inherited ligamentous laxity and patients frequently have a positive family history.
        - Congenital MDI presents with a high prevalence of collagen disorders such as Ehlers-Danlos and Marfan syndrome.
        - These patients tend to develop symptoms relatively early and are less likely to be successfully treated with surgery.
    - Acquired (secondary)
        - Acquired MDI is due to repetitive microtrauma to the shoulder.
        - It is commonly seen in swimmers, weight lifters, gymnasts, and athletes who participate in throwing or racket sports.
        - A previously asymptomatic patient may become symptomatic after a minor injury.
  - Direction
    - Anterior-inferior dislocation and posterior subluxation
    - Posterior-inferior dislocation and anterior subluxation
    - Instability in all 3 directions
- Associated pathology
  - RI insufficiency
    - Defects in RI can disrupt the normal negative intra-articular pressure and contribute to instability.
  - Redundant inferior capsular pouch
    - The IGHL, during humeral rotation, imparts AP stability.
    - A capacious inferior pouch can contribute to instability in the inferior, anterior, and posterior directions.

Clinical Evaluation

History and Physical Examination

- The patient with anterior instability reports pain and apprehension with the arm in abduction and ER.
- Patients with posterior instability initially present with severe pain but the pain subsides, allowing the patient to use the arm for waist-level activities, which leads to a false sense of improvement. The patient usually reports a dull discomfort in the posterior shoulder when reaching across the body with the arm in IR or attempting a bench press or push-up or apprehension with arm flexed, in IR, and adducted. Locked posterior shoulder dislocation has been misdiagnosed as frozen shoulder.
- A patient with a history of instability and apprehension at low degrees of abduction and ER should raise concern for significant glenoid bone loss.
- Instability during sleep or a seizure or after an earlier stabilization procedure also may indicate the presence of a bone defect.
- A patient with MDI may have a variety of symptoms, such as pain, instability, weakness, paresthesia, fatigue, popping, clicking, grinding, dead arm syndrome, and difficulty throwing, lifting, or sleeping.
- Signs of generalized laxity have been reported in 45% to 75% of patients undergoing surgery for MDI.

- Squaring of the shoulder is a common finding in MDI with inferior instability because the normally round contour of the deltoid is lost.

Provocative Examination Maneuvers

- Anterior instability
  - Apprehension test: The patient becomes apprehensive by slowly bringing the arm into the position of 90 degrees of abduction and 90 degrees of ER. The test is positive when the patient expresses a subjective sense of impending dislocation or tries to get into a more comfortable position by moving the body.
  - The relocation test is conducted in succession with the apprehension test. If applying posteriorly directed force by the examiner to the front of the shoulder resolves the patient's sense of apprehension and guarding, the relocation test is positive.
  - Load and shift test: The patient is supine and the examiner grabs the wrist to keep the arm relaxed at the patient's side. With the other arm, the examiner will load the joint by pushing the humeral head into the glenoid fossa and will apply an anteriorly directed force and assess the amount of anterior translation of the humeral head. Instead of classifying the examination as positive or negative, the amount of humeral head translation will be graded as 0 if there is minimal translation, 1 if the humeral head reaches the glenoid rim, 2 if the humeral head can be dislocated but spontaneously relocated back, and 3 if it does not reduce spontaneously.[51]
  - The hyperabduction test is performed by bringing both arms into maximum abduction and IR. Increased abduction more than 105 degrees in the shoulder or more than 10 degrees compared to the contralateral side suggests incompetence of the IGHL.[52]
- Posterior instability
  - The patient with posterior shoulder dislocation may present with posterior shoulder prominence and anterior flattening of the shoulder joint with coracoid prominence.
  - These patients usually have limited forward elevation and minimal ER. ER less than neutral and loss of supination due to extreme IR are significant examination findings that should provoke further imaging to rule out posterior shoulder dislocation.
  - The jerk test is very similar to the load and shift test but is applied for evaluating the posteroinferior instability of the shoulder. The arm is at 90 degrees of flexion and IR, and the examiner will stabilize the scapula and clavicle with one hand and apply posteriorly directed force to the humerus. The test is considered positive if the humeral head reduces from a posteriorly subluxated position with a noticeable clunk or jerk.[53]
- Inferior instability
  - The sulcus test is applied with the patient standing with the arm at the side and the elbow bent at 90 degrees. The examiner applies an inferiorly directed axial force to the elbow, and inferior translation of the humeral head at neutral arm rotation that does not get corrected by ER is considered positive and is suggestive of inferior instability due to incompetency of the RI or MDI. The sulcus sign is graded from I to III based on the amount of downward translation of the humerus: Grade I is less than 1 cm translation, grade II is 1 to 2 cm translation, and grade III is more than 2 cm translation.[54]

Imaging

- A standard shoulder trauma radiographic series includes the following:
  - A true AP (Grashey) view to assess the superior-inferior GH relationship
  - A scapular-Y view, axillary lateral, or Velpeau view to assess the AP GH relationship

- The West Point view assesses bony Bankart lesions.
- The Stryker notch view assesses for Hill-Sachs lesions.
  - X-rays findings of posterior shoulder dislocation are commonly subtle and more than 60% are missed at the initial evaluation (because of normal-appearing AP views of the shoulder).
  - It usually presents as rounding of the proximal humerus, commonly referred to as the "light-bulb sign." The scapular-Y view is crucial for diagnosis.

- Computed tomography assesses glenoid deficiency or humeral head involvement and is useful in revision setting.
  - Computed tomography arthrogram is an alternative for patients who cannot undergo MRI and allows assessment both of bony and soft-tissue pathology.
  - By dividing the arc of the impacted surface of the humeral head with the arc of intact articular surface, one can measure the area of impaction in a percentage.
    - Less than 25% is considered minimal and closed reduction is all that is necessary.
    - More than 25% of humeral head involvement will likely require a surgical procedure.
- MRI assesses soft-tissue pathology, including a Bankart lesion, rotator cuff tear, ALPSA, or HAGL.
  - Magnetic resonance arthrography, especially in the abduction and externally rotated position, has been shown to be more accurate than noncontrast MRI in detecting labral lesions with intact capsular periosteum (Perthes lesions).[55]
  - MRI and magnetic resonance arthrogram have low sensitivity for panlabral tears that involve anterior, superior, and posterior labrum.[56]
- Examination under anesthesia
  - Examination under anesthesia is an important evaluation tool to assess patients' passive range of motion, abnormal translation in all directions, and overall shoulder laxity, and to recreate instability.[57]

Treatment

- Acute anterior shoulder dislocation
  - Acute closed reduction
    - The goal of the treatment is to disengage the humeral head from the glenoid rim and to guide the humeral head back to the glenoid fossa.
    - As long as adequate relaxation and sufficient analgesia are provided, close reduction has a greater than 95% chance of success with a very low rate of complications.
      - Close reduction using intra-articular lidocaine injection has shown to be as successful as intravenous analgesics, without increased complications and a significantly shortened overall visit.[58]
      - Before attempting a closed reduction, the physician should perform a thorough neurovascular examination and review radiographic studies to rule out associated fractures.
      - Having control of the scapula during any reduction technique is crucial because it is difficult to reduce the humeral head on a moving target.
    - Common techniques[59]
      - In the Hippocratic method, the patient is in a supine position, and axial traction is applied to the abducted arm with countertraction through direct force to the anterior shoulder or a sheet wrapped around the body.

- In the Milch method, the patient is in a supine position, and axial traction, abduction, and ER is applied to the arm while supporting the humeral head.
- In the Stimpson method, the patient is in a prone position and traction is applied to the arm in hanging position through a 10-pound (4.5-kg) sand bag.
- The scapular manipulation method has the patient in a prone position and the arm is in a hanging position with a 5- to 10-pound (2.3- to 4.5-kg) weight. The scapula is IR to disengage it from the humeral head.
    - One study showed that despite a high overall success rate of closed reduction (92%), delay in presentation and longer time to reduction was associated with a high chance of failed reduction in the emergency department.[60]
    - Complications
        - Closed reduction in a controlled emergency room environment with standard techniques has a very low complication rate.
        - One study retrospectively reviewed 92 patients older than 40 years old who underwent closed reduction for first-time anterior shoulder dislocations. The researchers reported iatrogenic humeral neck fractures in 5 patients, all of whom had greater tuberosity fracture on their prereduction x-rays.[61]

- Nonoperative treatment
    - Nonsurgical management after first-time shoulder dislocation should focus on strengthening dynamic shoulder stabilizers, including rotator cuff and periscapular muscles.
    - A prospective, nonrandomized study of first-time dislocations in patients with an average age of 21 years old (range, 17 to 27 years old) found that 94.5% of patients treated nonoperatively had redislocations, whereas only 4.0% of patients who underwent arthroscopic stabilization had a recurrence.[62]
    - Risk of recurrence after first-time dislocation is high in patients who are young (less than 25 years old), engaged in contact sports, and have Bankart lesions on their MRI images.
    - Itoi et al[63] advocated immobilization in ER to increase tension on the capsule and reduce the labrum to its original position. They showed in a randomized clinical trial of 198 patients with first-time anterior dislocation that the rate of redislocation in a minimum of 2 years was significantly lower after 3 weeks' immobilization in ER than regular sling (26% vs 42%, $P = .03$).
    - Day and colleagues[64] performed a meta-analysis on patients who had first-time anterior shoulder dislocation and analyzed predictors of recurrent dislocation. Being younger than 30 years old was highly predictive of recurrent dislocation, but they found no benefit in conventional sling immobilization of more than 1 week.
- Surgical treatment: Most patients with recurrent traumatic anterior instability require surgical stabilization.
    - Rates of overall recurrence of instability following surgical stabilization range from 15% to 33%.[65]
    - Soft-tissue procedure (Bankart repair)
        - Open stabilization
            - Features
                - Some studies suggest that open Bankart repair results in lower recurrence rates and possibly worse shoulder range of motion compared with arthroscopic Bankart repair.[66,67]
                - Subscapularis takedown may compromise results. Sachs et al reported 23% abnormal lift-off tests after open stabilization with subscapularis

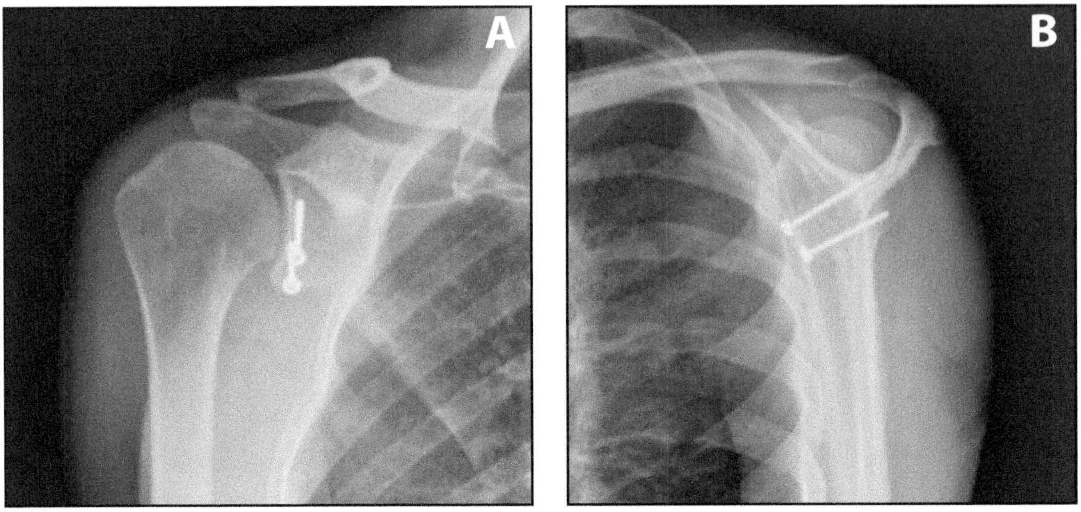

Figure 10-4. X-ray images of a coracoid transfer (Latarjet) procedure for anterior glenoid bone loss.

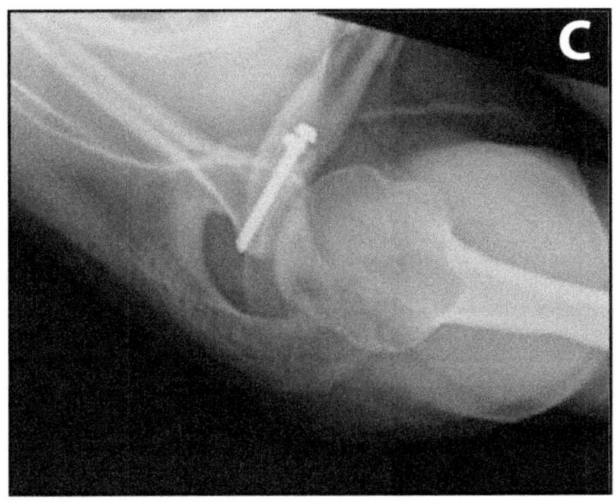

takedown.[68] Scheibel and colleagues[69] were not able to confirm any rupture of subscapularis with MRI after open stabilization, but they showed atrophy of the superior portion and hypertrophy of the inferior portion of the subscapularis muscle. Pagnani and Dome[70] showed a low rate of subscapularis incompetency after open stabilization and suggested that repair technique, especially freeing the anterior capsule from the subscapularis tendon and meticulous tensioning and repair of the tendon and capsule, might have contributed to their success.

- Indications
  - Bone deficiency remains the primary indication for open procedures, including coracoid transfer and bone grafting (for inverted pear-shaped glenoid).
    - Glenoid defects involving less than 15% of the anterior or anteroinferior glenoid margin are likely to be insignificant in most patients and can be addressed with a Bankart repair.
    - Glenoid defects of 15% to 30% represent an intermediate area within which the level of the patient activity dictates the importance of bone restoration (younger, more active individuals need more aggressive treatment).
    - Glenoid defects of more than 30% require a bony augmentation procedure such as Latarjet, allograft, or iliac crest bone grafting (ICBG) (Figure 10-4).

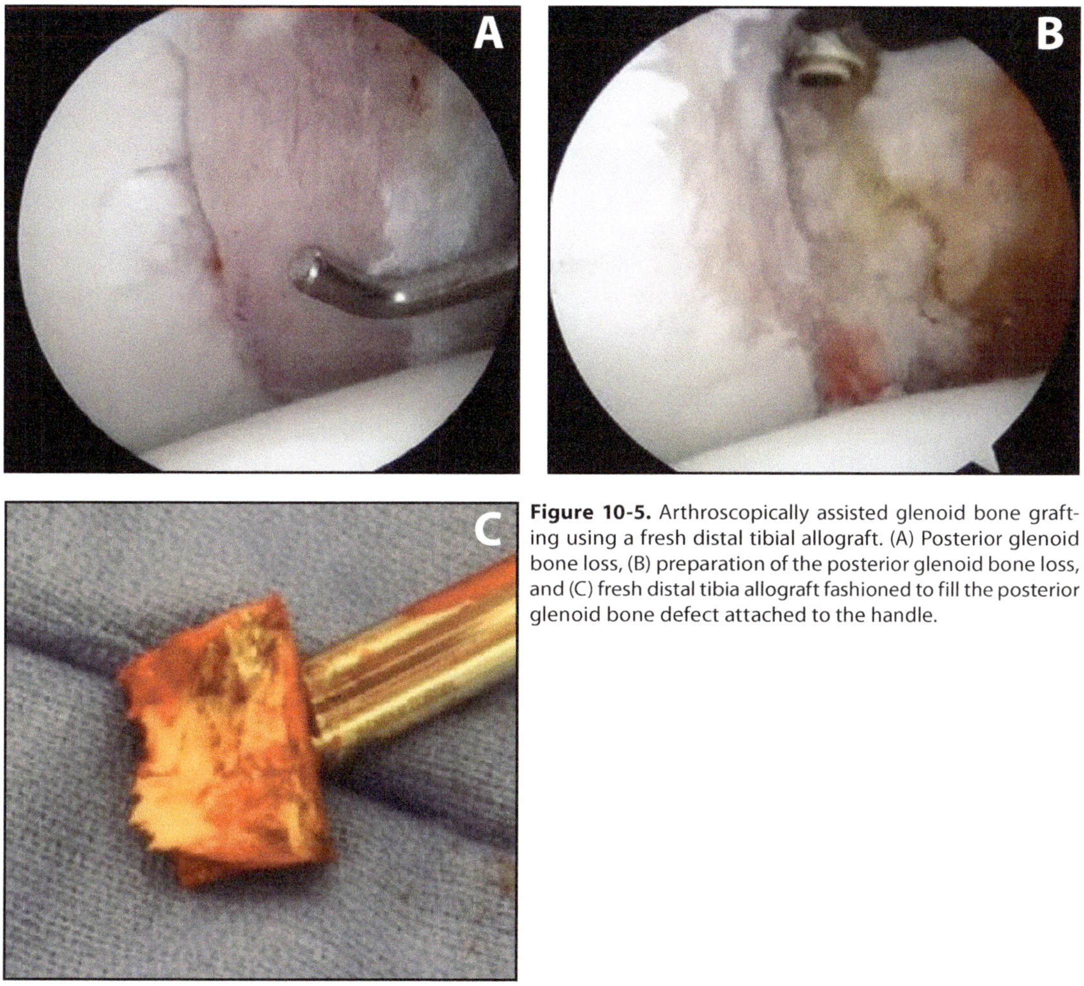

Figure 10-5. Arthroscopically assisted glenoid bone grafting using a fresh distal tibial allograft. (A) Posterior glenoid bone loss, (B) preparation of the posterior glenoid bone loss, and (C) fresh distal tibia allograft fashioned to fill the posterior glenoid bone defect attached to the handle.

- Conventionally, bone graft augmentation is performed though open surgery, but some authors have advocated arthroscopic-assisted or all-arthroscopic techniques with comparable results (Figure 10-5).
- HAGL lesion
- Midsubstance capsular rupture
- Engaging Hill-Sachs lesion
- Revision surgery
- Capsular deficiency
- Collision athletes
  - Recently arthroscopic stabilization has been used in collision and contact athletes with good results.[71]
  - This topic remains controversial.
- Posterior instability
  - Arthroscopic reconstruction of the posterior capsulolabral structures has been shown to be superior to the open-repair technique.[72]
- Arthroscopic stabilization
  - Feature

- › Arthroscopic stabilization may have possible higher recurrence rates for osseous glenoid defects and collision athletes.
- › It is less invasive and no subscapularis takedown is needed.
- › It has enhanced ability to address associated pathology (SLAP lesion, pan labral tear, Hill-Sachs lesion, rotator cuff tear).

- Open vs arthroscopic stabilization (still controversial)
  - The results of early arthroscopic instability surgery were worse than those of open surgery.[73,74]
  - In more recent comparisons, open and arthroscopic anterior stabilization were found to be equivalent,[75] with arthroscopic repair potentially providing faster recovery and better range of motion.[76]
  - Several recent meta-analyses have suggested that the results of open-stabilization procedures may be superior to those of arthroscopic procedures.[77-78]
  - The rate of recurrent instability after arthroscopic anterior stabilization is now less than 10%, although the rate may be higher among high-demand athletes, particularly those in collision sports.
  - Recent studies suggest that postsurgical subscapularis muscle function is critical in determining patients' perception of success.[68]
  - If the subscapularis is deficient or irreparable, a pectoralis major muscle transfer can be used to augment or replace the subscapularis.[79]
- Capsular plication
  - Suture plication alone achieved an average volume reduction of 19%, and thermal capsulorrhaphy alone achieved an average reduction of 33%; combining the 2 results in the greatest volume reduction, at an average of 41%.[80]
  - The following was noted in a cadaver model[81]:
    - › Anteroinferior plication reduced both abduction and ER by approximately 20 degrees, anterior translation by 61%, posterior translation by 13%, and inferior translation by 3%.
    - › Anterosuperior plication reduced ER of the adducted arm by approximately 30 degrees.
    - › Posterosuperior plication reduced IR of the adducted arm by 16 degrees.
  - The proximity of the axillary nerve to capsular placation sutures is concerning.
    - › One cadaveric study showed that the anteroinferior (12.5 mm) and inferior (14.4 mm) suture locations were closest to the axillary nerve.[82]
  - Throughout the course of the axillary nerve, its average distance from the IGHL was 2.5 mm.[83]
  - A more recent study found that the axillary nerve and the glenoid rim were closest to each other at the 6 o'clock position.[84]
  - Capsular deficiency is usually the result of multiple earlier surgeries or thermal capsulorrhaphy.
  - The tissue may be reconstructed using other local tissue or distant autograft vs allograft:
    - › Hamstring autograft
    - › Iliotibial band (Figure 10-6A)[85]
    - › Achilles autograft or allograft
    - › Semitendinosus/gracilis allograft (Figure 10-6B)[86]

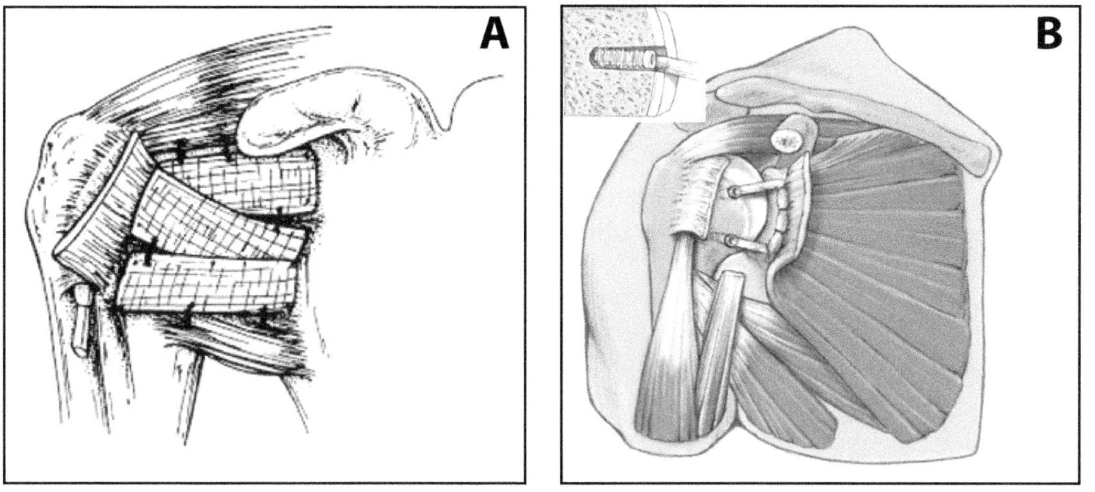

Figure 10-6. Soft-tissue augmentation for anterior shoulder instability with iliotibial band reconstruction of the anterior capsule. (Reprinted with permission from Iannotti JP, Antoniou J, Williams GR, Ramsey ML. Iliotibial band reconstruction for treatment of glenohumeral instability associated with irreparable capsular deficiency. *J Shoulder Elbow Surg*. 2002;11[6]:618-623. doi:10.1067/mse.2002.126763 and Braun S, Horan MP, Millett PJ. Open reconstruction of the anterior glenohumeral capsulolabral structures with tendon allograft in chronic shoulder instability. *Oper Orthop Traumatol*. 2011;23[1]:29-36.)

      - Pectoralis major transfer may restore dynamic stability in a muscle-deficient shoulder with a subscapularis tear or attenuation.
  - Thermal capsulorrhaphy
    - Thermal capsulorrhaphy uses a radiofrequency device to reduce capsular volume.
    - A study of the histology of the capsule after unsuccessful thermal capsulorrhaphy found changes in the collagen, along with denuded synovium, in all shoulders; the capsule was thin in 71%.[87]
    - Even in shoulders that had a successful clinical result, the collagen structure was histologically abnormal for as long as 16 months after thermal capsulorrhaphy.
    - It has fallen out of favor because of high failure rates.
    - Complications
      - Axillary nerve palsy
      - Capsular ablation
      - Chondrolysis
- Bone grafting
  - Bony reconstruction is preferable to routine capsulolabral repair if the glenoid surface deficiency is 15% to 25% in a young patient playing contact sports and bone loss is greater than 25%.
  - Soft-tissue repair failed in more than 80% of those who had the inverted-pear morphology.[34]
  - Restoring articular congruity is important for the stability of a joint with a chondrolabral defect. A cadaveric study showed that proper positioning of the graft is crucial to extend the articular surface and achieve stability after bone grafting.[14]
  - Autograft
    - Bristow procedure

    - Transfer of only the tip of the coracoid
- Coracoid transfer (Latarjet) procedure
    - The entire coracoid process at its base is osteotomized with a portion of the coracoacromial ligament and is transferred to the anteroinferior rim of the glenoid while keeping the coracobrachialis muscle attached to the tip of the graft.
    - The Latarjet procedure is believed to provide the following:
        - Static bone block extending the articular surface
        - Sling effect of the conjoined tendon
        - Reattachment and reinforcement of the anterior capsule with the coracoacromial ligament
        - The Latarjet procedure has gained popularity mainly because of its high success rate in addressing anterior instability. Long-term results show very low rates of redislocation of 1% to 6%,[88,89] high patient satisfaction, and close to an 80% return to same level of sports.[90] *Recommended reading for long-term outcome of the Latarjet procedure*
    - The position of the graft relative to the capsule may be described as follows:
        - Intra-articular (the capsule is repaired to the edge of the graft and the glenoid-graft junction remains within the joint)
        - Extra-articular (the capsule is repaired to the rim of the glenoid and the graft remains outside of the joint)
    - Orientation of the graft relative to the glenoid fossa may be described as follows:
        - Conventional (the lateral border of the coracoid becomes part of the GH joint)[91,92]
        - Congruent arc (inferior surface of the coracoid becomes part of the GH joint)[93,94]
    - Open vs arthroscopic
        - Despite an excellent clinical outcome, the complication rate is high in open Latarjet procedures (15% to 25% of patients have a complication) and includes graft malposition, graft fracture, neurovascular injuries, graft nonunion or resorption, late arthritis, and screw breakage.[95,96]
        - Open Latarjet procedures also result in an average 15-degree loss of ER, and 60% of patients develop mild to moderate GH arthritis.[90]
        - All-arthroscopic Latarjet was first introduced by Lafosse et al,[97] with Boileau and colleagues[98] and Athwal et al[99] subsequently presenting their own modifications.
        - This procedure is technically demanding, with early studies showing a similar short-term complication profile[99,100] with mixed outcomes.[101,102]
- Putti-Platt procedure (historical significance only)
    - The subscapularis is cut approximately 2.5 cm medial from insertion, and the lateral stump is attached to the anterior glenoid or most convenient soft-tissue structure along the anterior rim of the glenoid cavity.
    - The medial muscle stump is lapped over the lateral stump to produce a substantial shortening of the capsule and subscapularis muscle.
    - Complications include significant loss of ER and excessive anterior tightening, leading to capsulorrhaphy arthropathy.

    - Magnuson-Stack procedure (historical significance only)
        - Transfers the subscapularis tendon from the lesser tuberosity across the bicipital groove to the greater tuberosity
        - Complications are the same as for the Putti-Platt procedure.
    - Eden-Hybbinette procedure
        - This procedure uses the ICBG to extend the anterior glenoid.[103]
  - Allograft
    - Bone loss of more than 30% of the glenoid can be treated with ICBG for structural bone stock with good or excellent results.[104,105]
- Complications of instability repair[106]
  - The most common complication is recurrence of instability, which can vary in extent from subtle recurrent subluxation to frank dislocation.
  - The overall recurrence rate varies significantly depending on the patient population and surgical technique.
  - An incorrect presurgical diagnosis is a common reason for the recurrence of instability after a GH stabilization procedure.
  - Glenoid or humeral bone loss is the most common risk factor for recurrence, and therefore it must be identified and quantified before surgical treatment.
  - Patients with psychological disorders, the ability to voluntarily dislocate the shoulder, or secondary gain issues should be identified because surgical failure rates are high in these groups.
  - Complications
    - Arthritis
        - With asymmetric capsular contractures (or tightening), increased translations are observed in the opposite direction (excessive anterior tightening leads to posterior translation of humeral head and resulting degenerative joint disease [DJD]).
        - A loss of ER of more than 30% compared with the contralateral shoulder increases the risk of capsulorrhaphy arthropathy.
        - A capsular release with or without subscapularis lengthening can be performed to correct this condition.
        - Degenerative arthritis can occur after any type of instability repair:
            - Early DJD is usually due to chondrolysis resulting from thermal capsulorrhaphy or a loose staple, anchor, or other implant.
            - Late DJD is usually due to overconstraint of the GH joint; this leads to excessive restriction of motion.
        - Patients who have undergone an open Bankart repair or a Bristow-Latarjet, Putti-Platt, or other procedure for anterior instability are at increased risk of developing GH arthritis.[107]
    - Neurovascular injury: The greatest risk of injury to the axillary and musculocutaneous nerves occurs during the Bristow-Latarjet procedures.
    - Stiffness: Limited ER can be expected after capsular reconstruction or revision surgery.
        - A loss of 10 degrees of ER may not be significant to most patients, but it can be devastating to high-level overhead athletes.
        - Posterior stabilization results in stiffness due to loss of IR.

- › Capsular deficiency is most often found during revision surgery or after thermal capsulorrhaphy. The soft-tissue deficiency may include the subscapularis, especially after open repair.
- Risk factors for poor outcome after revision anterior shoulder reconstruction include the following[108]:
  - GH arthritis
  - Older than 30 years old
  - History of 2 or more earlier instability surgeries
  - Glenoid bone loss
  - Diagnosis of MDI
- Chronic shoulder dislocation
  - Closed reduction is rarely performed in chronically dislocated shoulder because the risk of iatrogenic fracture and neurovascular injuries is high.
  - It is acceptable to perform no treatment for some patients, especially the older and lower-demand patients with long-standing dislocation and minimal pain.
- Posterior shoulder dislocation
  - Posterior shoulder dislocation accounts for only 2% to 5% of shoulder dislocations.
  - Most chronic locked dislocations are posterior dislocations.
  - A concomitant surgical neck fracture is sometimes found.
  - Nonoperative management
    - Closed reduction then arm immobilization for 4 to 6 weeks in 15 degrees of extension and ER using a gunslinger-type brace are recommended.
    - Patients with a long-standing posterior fracture or dislocation who do not have significant pain should not be treated with surgery.
  - Operative management
    - General algorithm
      - For 20% to 45% bone loss, disimpaction with bone grafting, transfer of subscapularis, lesser tuberosity transfer or osteochondral allograft is recommended.
      - For more than 50% bone loss, hemi-shoulder or total shoulder arthroplasty
    - McLaughlin procedure
      - Transfer of the subscapularis tendon was first described by McLaughlin.[109]
      - The goal is that by using the subscapularis to fill in the humeral head defect, recurrent dislocations would likely be prevented.
    - Modified McLaughlin[110]
      - This procedure does not alter the anatomy of the proximal humerus as much as conventional McLaughlin, but provides stability by anchoring the subscapularis into the humeral head defect.
      - It is indicated for patients who are less than 8 weeks dislocated and with a defect of less than 30%.
    - Lesser tuberosity transfer
      - Transfer of the subscapularis tendon via a lesser tuberosity transfer was described by Hawkins and colleagues in 1987.[111]
      - It features the same concept as the McLaughlin procedure; however, it allows for better filling of the defect with lesser tuberosity and potentially more reliable bony healing.

- Results of tuberosity transfer have been superior to those of subscapularis transfer (McLaughlin procedure).[111]
- Allograft bony reconstruction
  - Allograft bone reconstruction was first described by Gerber and Lambert.[112] They argued that transfer of the subscapularis and lesser tuberosity changed the anatomy of the proximal humerus, which would make revision to arthroplasty difficult. This procedure also maintains the full articular arc.
  - It is recommended for patients who are dislocated for at least 4 weeks with involvement of up to 50% of the humeral head.
  - Use of the contralateral shoulder (in bilateral locked posterior dislocations) as autograft has been described.
  - Prosthetic replacement
    - Prosthetic replacement in chronic posterior fracture-dislocation has results inferior to those of arthroplasty for GH osteoarthritis.[113]
- Recurrent posterior instability
  - A patient with voluntary posterior instability is usually considered a poor surgical candidate. However, a patient with voluntary positional posterior instability and no underlying psychiatric or secondary gain issues may respond well to surgery.
  - A fall or blow to the arm in an at-risk position can result in a posterior labral detachment (reverse Bankart lesion). Repetitive stress on the posterior capsule during sports or another activity can lead to acquired posterior subluxation. Football lineman are at particular risk.
  - Nonsurgical treatment
    - The first line of treatment for posterior shoulder instability is nonoperative, and at least 6 month of strengthening exercises is commonly advised.[114]
    - The goal of physical therapy is to strengthen the dynamic muscular stabilizers to compensate for damaged or deficient static stabilizers.
    - The exercises should focus on strengthening the posterior deltoid, the external rotators, and the periscapular muscles.
  - Surgical treatment
    - The open posteroinferior capsular shift procedure has been historically used to address soft-tissue abnormalities resulting in posterior instability. This requires dividing the posterior rotator cuff.
    - Arthroscopic repair for posterior instability has been demonstrated to be effective in the management of this condition.
    - A patient with a posterior Bankart lesion is an ideal candidate for either an open posteroinferior capsular shift or arthroscopic treatment.
    - The posteroinferior labral lesion associated with posterior instability has recently received increased attention. Four types have been identified:
      - Type I: an incomplete detachment
      - Type II: marginal crack (Kim lesion)
      - Type III: chondrolabral erosion
      - Type IV: a flap tear

- MDI
  - Principal: remember "AMBRI"
    - Atraumatic
    - Multidirectional
    - Bilateral

- Rehabilitation
- Inferior capsular plication and possible RI imbrication

- Nonsurgical: the first line of treatment is prolonged physical therapy
  - It should focus on strengthening of the rotator cuff and periscapular musculature.
  - The goal is to restore effective concavity compression and normal muscle-firing patterns.
  - Positive results appear within the first 3 months.
  - Close to 80% of patients respond to this regimen and are able to avoid surgery.
- Surgical treatment
  - Inferior capsular shift
    - This procedure is intended to reduce capsular volume and thicken the capsule on the side with the greatest instability.
  - In current arthroscopic techniques, multiple portals and suture anchors are used to reduce capsular volume and recreate the capsulolabral construct.
  - Closure of the RI is another treatment option for MDI.
  - Thermal capsulorrhaphy has fallen out of favor because of its high recurrence and complication rate.

References

1. Bigliani LU, Kelkar R, Flatow EL, Pollock RG, Mow VC. Glenohumeral stability. Biomechanical properties of passive and active stabilizers. *Clin Orthop Relat Res.* 1996;(330):13-30.
2. Soslowsky LJ, Flatow EL, Bigliani LU, Mow VC. Articular geometry of the glenohumeral joint. *Clin Orthop Relat Res.* 1992;(285):181-190.
3. Gibb TD, Sidles JA, Harryman DT II, McQuade KJ, Matsen FA III. The effect of capsular venting on glenohumeral laxity. *Clin Orthop Relat Res.* 1991;(268):120-127.
4. Saha AK. Dynamic stability of the glenohumeral joint. *Acta Orthop Scand.* 1971;42(6):491-505. doi:10.3109/17453677108989066.
5. Wilk KE, Arrigo CA, Andrews JR. Current concepts: the stabilizing structures of the glenohumeral joint. *J Orthop Sports Phys Ther.* 1997;25(6):364-379. doi:10.2519/jospt.1997.25.6.364.
6. Howell SM, Galinat BJ. The glenoid-labral socket. A constrained articular surface. *Clin Orthop Relat Res.* 1989;(243):122-125.
7. Warner JJ, Deng XH, Warren RF, Torzilli PA. Static capsuloligamentous restraints to superior-inferior translation of the glenohumeral joint. *Am J Sports Med.* 1992;20(6):675-685. doi:10.1177/036354659202000608.
8. Burkart AC, Debski RE. Anatomy and function of the glenohumeral ligaments in anterior shoulder instability. *Clin Orthop Relat Res.* 2002;(400):32-39. doi:10.1097/00003086-200207000-00005.
9. O'Brien SJ, Schwartz RS, Warren RF, Torzilli PA. Capsular restraints to anterior-posterior motion of the abducted shoulder: a biomechanical study. *J Shoulder Elbow Surg.* 1995;4(4):298-308.
10. Jost B, Koch PP, Gerber C. Anatomy and functional aspects of the rotator interval. *J Shoulder Elbow Surg.* 2000;9(4):336-341. doi:10.1067/mse.2000.106746.
11. Harryman DT II, Sidles JA, Harris SL, Matsen FA III. The role of the rotator interval capsule in passive motion and stability of the shoulder. *J Bone Joint Surg Am.* 1992;74(1):53-66.
12. Wuelker N, Korell M, Thren K. Dynamic glenohumeral joint stability. *J Shoulder Elbow Surg.* 1998;7(1):43-52.
13. Lippitt SB, Vanderhooft JE, Harris SL, Sidles JA, Harryman DT II, Matsen FA III. Glenohumeral stability from concavity-compression: a quantitative analysis. *J Shoulder Elbow Surg.* 1993;2(1):27-35. doi:10.1016/S1058-2746(09)80134-1.
14. Lazarus MD, Sidles JA, Harryman DT II, Matsen FA III. Effect of a chondral-labral defect on glenoid concavity and glenohumeral stability. A cadaveric model. *J Bone Joint Surg Am.* 1996;78(1):94-102. doi:10.2106/00004623-199601000-00013.
15. Elser F, Braun S, Dewing CB, Giphart JE, Millett PJ. Anatomy, function, injuries, and treatment of the long head of the biceps brachii tendon. *Arthroscopy.* 2011;27(4):581-592. doi:10.1016/j.arthro.2010.10.014.

16. Lee SB, An KN. Dynamic glenohumeral stability provided by three heads of the deltoid muscle. *Clin Orthop Relat Res.* 2002;(400):40-47. doi:10.1097/00003086-200207000-00006.
17. McClure PW, Michener LA, Sennett BJ, Karduna AR. Direct 3-dimensional measurement of scapular kinematics during dynamic movements in vivo. *J Shoulder Elbow Surg.* 2001;10(3):269-277. doi:10.1067/mse.2001.112954.
18. Somford MP, Van der Linde JA, Wiegerinck JI, Hoornenborg D, Van den Bekerom MPJ, Van Deurzen DFP. Eponymous terms in anterior shoulder stabilization surgery. *Orthop Traumatol Surg Res.* 2017;103(8):1257-1263. doi:10.1016/j.otsr.2017.07.017.
19. Matsen FA III, Harryman DT II, Sidles JA. Mechanics of glenohumeral instability. *Clin Sports Med.* 1991;10(4):783-788.
20. Bankart ASB. Recurrent or habitual dislocation of the shoulder-joint. *Br Med J.* 1923;2(3285):1132-1133. doi:10.1136/bmj.2.3285.1132.
21. Neviaser TJ. The anterior labroligamentous periosteal sleeve avulsion lesion: a cause of anterior instability of the shoulder. *Arthroscopy.* 1993;9(1):17-21. doi:10.1016/s0749-8063(05)80338-x.
22. Neviaser TJ. The GLAD lesion: another cause of anterior shoulder pain. *Arthroscopy.* 1993;9(1):22-23. doi:10.1016/s0749-8063(05)80339-1.
23. Kim SH, Ha KI, Yoo JC, Noh KC. Kim's lesion: an incomplete and concealed avulsion of the posteroinferior labrum in posterior or multidirectional posteroinferior instability of the shoulder. *Arthroscopy.* 2004;20(7):712-720. doi:10.1016/j.arthro.2004.06.012.
24. Antoniou J, Duckworth DT, Harryman DT II. Capsulolabral augmentation for the management of posteroinferior instability of the shoulder. *J Bone Joint Surg Am.* 2000;82(9):1220-1230. doi:10.2106/00004623-200009000-00002.
25. Hill HA, Sachs MD. The grooved defect of the humeral head. A frequently unrecognized complication of dislocations of the shoulder joint. *Radiology.* 1940;35(6):690-700. doi:10.1148/35.6.690.
26. Wolf EM, Cheng JC, Dickson K. Humeral avulsion of glenohumeral ligaments as a cause of anterior shoulder instability. *Arthroscopy.* 1995;11(5):600-607. doi:10.1016/0749-8063(95)90139-6.
27. Gerber C, Nyffeler RW. Classification of glenohumeral joint instability. *Clin Orthop Relat Res.* 2002;(400):65-76. doi:10.1097/00003086-200207000-00009.
28. Goga IE. Chronic shoulder dislocations. *J Shoulder Elbow Surg.* 2003;12(5):446-450. doi:10.1016/S1058274603000880.
29. Owens BD, Dawson L, Burks R, Cameron KL. Incidence of shoulder dislocation in the United States military: demographic considerations from a high-risk population. *J Bone Joint Surg Am.* 2009;91(4):791-796. doi:10.2106/JBJS.H.00514.
30. Zacchilli MA, Owens BD. Epidemiology of shoulder dislocations presenting to emergency departments in the United States. *J Bone Joint Surg Am.* 2010;92(3):542-549.
31. Taylor DC, Arciero RA. Pathologic changes associated with shoulder dislocations. Arthroscopic and physical examination findings in first-time, traumatic anterior dislocations. *Am J Sports Med.* 1997;25(3):306-311. doi:10.1177/036354659702500306.
32. Speer KP, Deng X, Borrero S, Torzilli PA, Altchek DA, Warren RF. Biomechanical evaluation of a simulated Bankart lesion. *J Bone Joint Surg Am.* 1994;76(12):1819-1826. doi:10.2106/00004623-199412000-00008.
33. Piasecki DP, Verma NN, Romeo AA, Levine WN, Bach BR Jr, Provencher MT. Glenoid bone deficiency in recurrent anterior shoulder instability: diagnosis and management. *J Am Acad Orthop Surg.* 2009;17(8):482-493. doi:10.5435/00124635-200908000-00002.
34. Burkhart SS, De Beer JF. Traumatic glenohumeral bone defects and their relationship to failure of arthroscopic Bankart repairs: significance of the inverted-pear glenoid and the humeral engaging Hill-Sachs lesion. *Arthroscopy.* 2000;16(7):677-694. doi:10.1053/jars.2000.17715.
35. Saito H, Itoi E, Sugaya H, Minagawa H, Yamamoto N, Tuoheti Y. Location of the glenoid defect in shoulders with recurrent anterior dislocation. *Am J Sports Med.* 2005;33(6):889-893. doi:10.1177/0363546504271521.
36. Milano G, Grasso A, Russo A, et al. Analysis of risk factors for glenoid bone defect in anterior shoulder instability. *Am J Sports Med.* 2011;39(9):1870-1876. doi:10.1177/0363546511411699.
37. Pagnani MJ, Deng XH, Warren RF, Torzilli PA, Altchek DW. Effect of lesions of the superior portion of the glenoid labrum on glenohumeral translation. *J Bone Joint Surg Am.* 1995;77(7):1003-1010. doi:10.2106/00004623-199507000-00005.
38. Murthi AM, Ramirez MA. Shoulder dislocation in the older patient. *J Am Acad Orthop Surg.* 2012;20(10):615-622. doi:10.5435/JAAOS-20-10-615.
39. Di Giacomo G, Itoi E, Burkhart SS. Evolving concept of bipolar bone loss and the Hill-Sachs lesion: from "engaging/non-engaging" lesion to "on-track/off-track" lesion. *Arthroscopy.* 2014;30(1):90-98. doi:10.1016/j.arthro.2013.10.004.
40. Itoi E. 'On-track' and 'off-track' shoulder lesions. *EFORT Open Rev.* 2017;2(8):343-351. doi:10.1302/2058-5241.2.170007.
41. Patel RM, Amin NH, Lynch TS, Miniaci A. Management of bone loss in glenohumeral instability. *Orthop Clin North Am.* 2014;45(4):523-539. doi:10.1016/j.ocl.2014.06.005.

42. Robinson CM, Kelly M, Wakefield AE. Redislocation of the shoulder during the first six weeks after a primary anterior dislocation: risk factors and results of treatment. *J Bone Joint Surg Am.* 2002;84(9):1552-1559. doi:10.2106/00004623-200209000-00007.
43. Mattyasovszky SG, Burkhart KJ, Ahlers C, et al. Isolated fractures of the greater tuberosity of the proximal humerus: a long-term retrospective study of 30 patients. *Acta Orthop.* 2011;82(6):714-720. doi:10.3109/17453674.2011.618912.
44. Liveson JA. Nerve lesions associated with shoulder dislocation; an electrodiagnostic study of 11 cases. *J Neurol Neurosurg Psychiatry.* 1984;47(7):742-744. doi:10.1136/jnnp.47.7.742.
45. Travlos J, Goldberg I, Boome RS. Brachial plexus lesions associated with dislocated shoulders. *J Bone Joint Surg Br.* 1990;72(1):68-71.
46. Hurley JA, Anderson TE, Dear W, Andrish JT, Bergfeld JA, Weiker GG. Posterior shoulder instability. Surgical versus conservative results with evaluation of glenoid version. *Am J Sports Med.* 1992;20(4):396-400. doi:10.1177/036354659202000405.
47. Smith SP, Bunker TD. Primary glenoid dysplasia. A review of 12 patients. *J Bone Joint Surg Br.* 2001;83(6):868-872. doi:10.1302/0301-620x.83b6.11649.
48. Perron AD, Ingerski MS, Brady WJ, Erling BF, Ullman EA. Acute complications associated with shoulder dislocation at an academic emergency department. *J Emerg Med.* 2003;24(2):141-145. doi:10.1016/s0736-4679(02)00717-5.
49. Nambiar M, Owen D, Moore P, Carr A, Thomas M. Traumatic inferior shoulder dislocation: a review of management and outcome. *Eur J Trauma Emerg Surg.* 2018;44(1):45-51. doi:10.1007/s00068-017-0854-y.
50. Neer CS II, Foster CR. Inferior capsular shift for involuntary inferior and multidirectional instability of the shoulder. A preliminary report. *J Bone Joint Surg Am.* 1980;62(6):897-908.
51. Tzannes A, Murrell GA. Clinical examination of the unstable shoulder. *Sports Med.* 2002;32(7):447-457. doi:10.2165/00007256-200232070-00004.
52. Gagey OJ, Gagey N. The hyperabduction test. *J Bone Joint Surg Br.* 2001;83(1):69-74. doi:10.1302/0301-620x.83b1.10628.
53. Lerat JL, Chotel F, Besse JL, Moyen B, Brunet Guedj E. Dynamic anterior jerk of the shoulder. A new clinical test for shoulder instability. Preliminary study [in French]. *Rev Chir Orthop Reparatrice Appar Mot.* 1994;80(6):461-467.
54. Lizzio VA, Meta F, Fidai M, Makhni EC. Clinical evaluation and physical exam findings in patients with anterior shoulder instability. *Curr Rev Musculoskelet Med.* 2017;10(4):434-441. doi:10.1007/s12178-017-9434-3.
55. Tian CY, Cui GQ, Zheng ZZ, Ren AH. The added value of ABER position for the detection and classification of anteroinferior labroligamentous lesions in MR arthrography of the shoulder. *Eur J Radiol.* 2013;82(4):651-657. doi:10.1016/j.ejrad.2012.11.038.
56. Ricchetti ET, Ciccotti MC, Ciccotti MG, Williams GR Jr, Lazarus MD. Sensitivity of preoperative magnetic resonance imaging and magnetic resonance arthrography in detection of panlabral tears of the glenohumeral joint. *Arthroscopy.* 2013;29(2):274-279. doi:10.1016/j.arthro.2012.10.005.
57. Cofield RH, Irving JF. Evaluation and classification of shoulder instability. With special reference to examination under anesthesia. *Clin Orthop Relat Res.* 1987;(223):32-43.
58. Matthews DE, Roberts T. Intraarticular lidocaine versus intravenous analgesic for reduction of acute anterior shoulder dislocations. A prospective randomized study. *Am J Sports Med.* 1995;23(1):54-58. doi:10.1177/036354659502300109.
59. Riebel GD, McCabe JB. Anterior shoulder dislocation: a review of reduction techniques. *Am J Emerg Med.* 1991;9(2):180-188. doi:10.1016/0735-6757(91)90187-o.
60. Kanji A, Atkinson P, Fraser J, Lewis D, Benjamin S. Delays to initial reduction attempt are associated with higher failure rates in anterior shoulder dislocation: a retrospective analysis of factors affecting reduction failure. *Emerg Med J.* 2016;33(2):130-133. doi:10.1136/emermed-2015-204746.
61. Atoun E, Narvani A, Even T, et al. Management of first-time dislocations of the shoulder in patients older than 40 years: the prevalence of iatrogenic fracture. *J Orthop Trauma.* 2013;27:190-193. doi:10.1097/BOT.0b013e31826576f8.
62. Larrain MV, Botto GJ, Montenegro HJ, Mauas DM. Arthroscopic repair of acute traumatic anterior shoulder dislocation in young athletes. *Arthroscopy.* 2001;17(4):373-377. doi:10.1053/jars.2001.23226.
63. Itoi E, Hatakeyama Y, Sato T, et al. Immobilization in external rotation after shoulder dislocation reduces the risk of recurrence. A randomized controlled trial. *J Bone Joint Surg Am.* 2007;89(10):2124-2131. doi:10.2106/JBJS.F.00654.
64. Day JW, Li P, Patterson JT, et al. Charge inversion at position 68 of the glucagon and glucagon-like peptide-1 receptors supports selectivity in hormone action. *J Pept Sci.* 2011;17(3):218-225. doi:10.1002/psc.1317.
65. Karlsson J, Magnusson L, Ejerhed L, Hultenheim I, Lundin O, Kartus J. Comparison of open and arthroscopic stabilization for recurrent shoulder dislocation in patients with a Bankart lesion. *Am J Sports Med.* 2001;29(5):538-542. doi:10.1177/03635465010290050201.

66. Wang L, Liu Y, Su X, Liu S. A meta-analysis of arthroscopic versus open repair for treatment of Bankart lesions in the shoulder. *Med Sci Monit.* 2015;21:3028-3035. doi:10.12659/MSM.894346.
67. Neviaser AS, Benke MT, Neviaser RJ. Open Bankart repair for revision of failed prior stabilization: outcome analysis at a mean of more than 10 years. *J Shoulder Elbow Surg.* 2015;24(6):897-901. doi:10.1016/j.jse.2014.11.036.
68. Sachs RA, Williams B, Stone ML, Paxton L, Kuney M. Open Bankart repair: correlation of results with postoperative subscapularis function. *Am J Sports Med.* 2005;33(10):1458-1462. doi:10.1177/0363546505275350.
69. Scheibel M, Tsynman A, Magosch P, Schroeder RJ, Habermeyer P. Postoperative subscapularis muscle insufficiency after primary and revision open shoulder stabilization. *Am J Sports Med.* 2006;34(10):1586-1593. doi:10.1177/0363546506288852.
70. Pagnani MJ, Dome DC. Surgical treatment of traumatic anterior shoulder instability in American football players. *J Bone Joint Surg Am.* 2002;84(5): 711-715. doi:10.2106/00004623-200205000-00002.
71. Mazzocca AD, Brown FM Jr, Carreira DS, Hayden J, Romeo AA. Arthroscopic anterior shoulder stabilization of collision and contact athletes. *Am J Sports Med.* 2005;33(1):52-60. doi:10.1177/0363546504268037.
72. Bradley JP, Baker CL III, Kline AJ, Armfield DR, Chhabra A. Arthroscopic capsulolabral reconstruction for posterior instability of the shoulder: a prospective study of 100 shoulders. *Am J Sports Med.* 2006;34(7):1061-1071. doi:10.1177/0363546505285585.
73. Guanche CA, Quick DC, Sodergren KM, Buss DD. Arthroscopic versus open reconstruction of the shoulder in patients with isolated Bankart lesions. *Am J Sports Med.* 1996;24(2):144-148. doi:10.1177/036354659602400204.
74. Steinbeck J, Jerosch J. Arthroscopic transglenoid stabilization versus open anchor suturing in traumatic anterior instability of the shoulder. *Am J Sports Med.* 1998;26(3):373-378. doi:10.1177/03635465980260030501.
75. Brophy RH, Marx RG. The treatment of traumatic anterior instability of the shoulder: nonoperative and surgical treatment. *Arthroscopy.* 2009;25(3):298-304. doi:10.1016/j.arthro.2008.12.007.
76. Lenters TR, Franta AK, Wolf FM, Leopold SS, Matsen FA III. Arthroscopic compared with open repairs for recurrent anterior shoulder instability. A systematic review and meta-analysis of the literature. *J Bone Joint Surg Am.* 2007;89(2):244-254. doi:10.2106/JBJS.E.01139.
77. Freedman KB, Smith AP, Romeo AA, Cole BJ, Bach BR Jr. Open Bankart repair versus arthroscopic repair with transglenoid sutures or bioabsorbable tacks for recurrent anterior instability of the shoulder: a meta-analysis. *Am J Sports Med.* 2004;32(6):1520-1527. doi:10.1177/0363546504265188.
78. Mohtadi NG, Bitar IJ, Sasyniuk TM, Hollinshead RM, Harper WP. Arthroscopic versus open repair for traumatic anterior shoulder instability: a meta-analysis. *Arthroscopy.* 2005;21(6):652-658. doi:10.1016/j.arthro.2005.02.021.
79. Resch H, Povacz P, Ritter E, Matschi W. Transfer of the pectoralis major muscle for the treatment of irreparable rupture of the subscapularis tendon. *J Bone Joint Surg Am.* 2000;82(3):372-382. doi:10.2106/00004623-200003000-00008.
80. Karas SG, Creighton RA, DeMorat GJ. Glenohumeral volume reduction in arthroscopic shoulder reconstruction: a cadaveric analysis of suture plication and thermal capsulorrhaphy. *Arthroscopy.* 2004;20(2):179-184. doi:10.1016/j.arthro.2003.11.004.
81. Alberta FG, Elattrache NS, Mihata T, McGarry MH, Tibone JE, Lee TQ. Arthroscopic anteroinferior suture plication resulting in decreased glenohumeral translation and external rotation. Study of a cadaver model. *J Bone Joint Surg Am.* 2006;88(1):179-187. doi:10.2106/JBJS.D.02974.
82. Eakin CL, Dvirnak P, Miller CM, Hawkins RJ. The relationship of the axillary nerve to arthroscopically placed capsulolabral sutures. An anatomic study. *Am J Sports Med.* 1998;26(4):505-509. doi:10.1177/03635465980260040501.
83. Price MR, Tillett ED, Acland RD, Nettleton GS. Determining the relationship of the axillary nerve to the shoulder joint capsule from an arthroscopic perspective. *J Bone Joint Surg Am.* 2004;86(10):2135-2142. doi:10.2106/00004623-200410000-00003.
84. Bokor DJ, Raniga S, Graham PL. Axillary nerve position in humeral avulsions of the glenohumeral ligament. *Orthop J Sports Med.* 2018;6(12):2325967118811044. doi:10.1177/2325967118811044.
85. Iannotti JP, Antoniou J, Williams GR, Ramsey ML. Iliotibial band reconstruction for treatment of glenohumeral instability associated with irreparable capsular deficiency. *J Shoulder Elbow Surg.* 2002;11(6):618-623. doi:10.1067/mse.2002.126763.
86. Lazarus MD, Harryman DT II. Open repair for anterior instability. In: Warner JJP, Iannotti JP, Gerber C, eds. *Complex and Revision Problems in Shoulder Surgery.* Philadelphia, PA: Lippincott-Raven; 1997:47-64.
87. McFarland EG, Kim TK, Banchasuek P, McCarthy EF. Histologic evaluation of the shoulder capsule in normal shoulders, unstable shoulders, and after failed thermal capsulorrhaphy. *Am J Sports Med.* 2002;30(5):636-642. doi:10.1177/03635465020300050201.
88. Burkhart SS, De Beer JF, Barth JR, Cresswell T, Roberts C, Richards DP. Results of modified Latarjet reconstruction in patients with anteroinferior instability and significant bone loss. *Arthroscopy.* 2007;23(10):1033-1041. doi:10.1016/j.arthro.2007.08.009.
89. Mizuno N, Denard PJ, Raiss P, Melis B, Walch G. Long-term results of the Latarjet procedure for anterior instability of the shoulder. *J Shoulder Elbow Surg.* 2014;23(11):1691-1699. doi:10.1016/j.jse.2014.02.015.
90. Allain J, Goutallier D, Glorion C. Long-term results of the Latarjet procedure for the treatment of anterior instability of the shoulder. *J Bone Joint Surg Am.* 1998;80(6):841-852. doi:10.2106/00004623-199806000-00008.

91. Hovelius L, Korner L, Lundberg B, et al. The coracoid transfer for recurrent dislocation of the shoulder. Technical aspects of the Bristow-Latarjet procedure. *J Bone Joint Surg Am.* 1983;65(7):926-934.
92. Ghodadra N, Gupta A, Romeo AA, et al. Normalization of glenohumeral articular contact pressures after Latarjet or iliac crest bone-grafting. *J Bone Joint Surg Am.* 2010;92(6):1478-1489. doi:10.2106/JBJS.I.00220.
93. de Beer JF, Roberts C. Glenoid bone defects—open Latarjet with congruent arc modification. *Orthop Clin North Am.* 2010;41(3):407-415. doi:10.1016/j.ocl.2010.02.008.
94. Montgomery SR, Katthagen JC, Mikula JD, et al. Anatomic and Biomechanical comparison of the classic and congruent-arc techniques of the Latarjet procedure. *Am J Sports Med.* 2017;45(6):1252-1260. doi:10.1177/0363546516685318.
95. Shah AA, Butler RB, Romanowski J, Goel D, Karadagli D, Warner JJ. Short-term complications of the Latarjet procedure. *J Bone Joint Surg Am.* 2012;94(6):495-501. doi:10.2106/JBJS.J.01830.
96. Gupta A, Delaney R, Petkin K, Lafosse L. Complications of the Latarjet procedure. *Curr Rev Musculoskelet Med.* 2015;8(1):59-66. doi:10.1007/s12178-015-9258-y.
97. Lafosse L, Lejeune E, Bouchard A, Kakuda C, Gobezie R, Kochhar T. The arthroscopic Latarjet procedure for the treatment of anterior shoulder instability. *Arthroscopy.* 2007;23(11):1242.e1-e5. doi:10.1016/j.arthro.2007.06.008.
98. Boileau P, Mercier N, Roussanne Y, Thélu CÉ, Old J. Arthroscopic Bankart-Bristow-Latarjet procedure: the development and early results of a safe and reproducible technique. *Arthroscopy.* 2010;26(11):1434-1450. doi:10.1016/j.arthro.2010.07.011.
99. Athwal GS, Meislin R, Getz C, Weinstein D, Favorito P. Short-term complications of the arthroscopic Latarjet procedure: a North American experience. *Arthroscopy.* 2016;32(10):1965-1970. doi:10.1016/j.arthro.2016.02.022.
100. Cunningham G, Benchouk S, Kherad O, Lädermann A. Comparison of arthroscopic and open Latarjet with a learning curve analysis. *Knee Surg Sports Traumatol Arthrosc.* 2016;24(2):540-545. doi:10.1007/s00167-015-3910-3.
101. Kordasiewicz B, Malachowski K, Kicinski M, Chaberek S, Pomianowski S. Comparative study of open and arthroscopic coracoid transfer for shoulder anterior instability (Latarjet)—clinical results at short term follow-up. *Int Orthop.* 2017;41(5):1023-1033. doi:10.1007/s00264-016-3372-3.
102. Randelli P, Fossati C, Stoppani C, Evola FR, De Girolamo L. Open Latarjet versus arthroscopic Latarjet: clinical results and cost analysis. *Knee Surg Sports Traumatol Arthrosc.* 2016;24(2):526-532. doi:10.1007/s00167-015-3978-9.
103. Fortun CM, Wong I, Burns JP. Arthroscopic iliac crest bone grafting to the anterior glenoid. *Arthrosc Tech.* 2016;5(4):e907-e912. doi:10.1016/j.eats.2016.04.011.
104. Montgomery WH Jr, Wahl M, Hettrich C, Itoi E, Lippitt SB, Matsen FA III. Anteroinferior bone-grafting can restore stability in osseous glenoid defects. *J Bone Joint Surg Am.* 2005;87(9):1972-1977. doi:10.2106/JBJS.D.02573.
105. Chen AL, Hunt SA, Hawkins RJ, Zuckerman JD. Management of bone loss associated with recurrent anterior glenohumeral instability. *Am J Sports Med.* 2005;33(6):912-925. doi:10.1177/0363546505277074.
106. Lazarus MD, Harryman DT II. Complications of open anterior stabilization of the shoulder. *J Am Acad Orthop Surg.* 2000;8(2):122-132. doi:10.5435/00124635-200003000-00006.
107. Kee YM, Kim HJ, Kim JY, Rhee YG. Glenohumeral arthritis after Latarjet procedure: Progression and it's [sic] clinical significance. *J Orthop Sci.* 2017;22(5):846-851. doi:10.1016/j.jos.2017.06.008.
108. Meehan RE, Petersen SA. Results and factors affecting outcome of revision surgery for shoulder instability. *J Shoulder Elbow Surg.* 2005;14(1):31-37. doi:10.1016/j.jse.2004.05.005.
109. McLaughlin HL. Posterior dislocation of the shoulder. *J Bone Joint Surg Am.* 1952;24 A(3):584-590.
110. Spencer EE Jr, Brems JJ. A simple technique for management of locked posterior shoulder dislocations: report of two cases. *J Shoulder Elbow Surg.* 2005;14(6):650-652. doi:10.1016/j.jse.2004.11.008.
111. Hawkins RJ, Neer CS II, Pianta RM, Mendoza FX. Locked posterior dislocation of the shoulder. *J Bone Joint Surg Am.* 1987;69(1):9-18.
112. Gerber C, Lambert SM. Allograft reconstruction of segmental defects of the humeral head for the treatment of chronic locked posterior dislocation of the shoulder. *J Bone Joint Surg Am.* 1996;78(3):376-382. doi:10.2106/00004623-199603000-00008.
113. Wooten C, Klika B, Schleck CD, Harmsen WS, Sperling JW, Cofield RH. Anatomic shoulder arthroplasty as treatment for locked posterior dislocation of the shoulder. *J Bone Joint Surg Am.* 2014;96(3):e19. doi:10.2106/JBJS.L.01588.
114. Tannenbaum E, Sekiya JK. Evaluation and management of posterior shoulder instability. *Sports Health.* 2011;3(3):253-263. doi:10.1177/1941738111400562.

11

Frozen Shoulder
Adhesive Capsulitis

Benjamin Zmistowski, MD and Surena Namdari, MD, MSc

Pathophysiology

- Terming this pathology has been controversial: "Frozen shoulder" is sometimes referred to as "adhesive capsulitis" (coined by Neviaser[1]). *Recommended reading for historical context*
  - Adhesive capsulitis denotes an inflammation of the shoulder capsule and joint adhesions, and therefore should be limited to such situations (eg, idiopathic).
  - Frozen shoulder is an applicable term for the description of pain with restricted motion (passive and active) regardless of underlying etiology (ie, all patients with adhesive capsulitis have frozen shoulder, but not all frozen shoulders are adhesive capsulitis).
- Definition (consensus)[2]: *Recommended reading for understanding classification and process of consensus definitions*
  - A condition characterized by functional restriction of both active and passive shoulder motion for which radiographs of the glenohumeral joint are essentially unremarkable except for the possible presence of osteopenia or calcific tendinitis.
  - No strict definition for extent of restricted motion
- Classification[2,3]
  - Primary (idiopathic): No underlying etiology or associated condition can be identified; the etiology of this disorder remains elusive.
  - Secondary
    - Systemic
      - Diabetes mellitus[4-9]
        - A review of more than 200,000 diabetic patients showed a 0.6% prevalence of frozen shoulder.[10] This same review demonstrated no association between frozen shoulder and hemoglobin A1C. Insulin-dependent patients (type 1) were 1.9 times more likely to get frozen shoulder than non–insulin-dependent (type 2) patients.

Namdari S, Zmistowski B, Omid R, eds.
The Foundations of Shoulder and Elbow Surgery (pp 215-221).

            - Patients with type 1 diabetes mellitus are more likely to require arthroscopic release than patients with type 2.[11]
        - Hypothyroidism[12,13]
        - Cardiac disease[14]
            - Bunker et al and Sung and colleagues have noted increased serum lipid levels in those patients with frozen shoulder compared to healthy controls.[15,16]
        - Hypoadrenalism[17]
    - Extrinsic (eg, humeral shaft fracture; Parkinson disease; cervical radiculopathy)
    - Intrinsic (eg, rotator cuff tendinitis; acromioclavicular arthritis)
  - Tertiary (postoperative or postfracture): not included in current definitions
    - Postoperative frozen shoulder is often more resistant both to nonoperative and operative treatment.[18]
- Idiopathic frozen shoulder phases
  - Three clinical phases[19]
    - Acute pain/inflammation (painful): 2 to 8 months
    - Severe stiffness/fibrosis (stiff): 4 to 12 months
    - Thawing/residual impairment (recovery): 5 to 26 months
    - Total duration: 12 to 42 months
  - Four arthroscopic stages[20]
    1. Stage I (preadhesive): fibrinous synovial inflammation; pain without motion limitations
    2. Stage II (acute adhesive synovitis): progressive synovitis with early adhesions; pain with early loss of motion
    3. Stage III (maturation): decreased synovitis with loss of the axillary fold and increased fibrosis; pain improved but motion restricted
    4. Stage IV (chronic): fully mature adhesions, with difficulty identifying intra-articular anatomic structures due to severe fibrosis; may be painless at rest, severe motion restrictions
- Contracture and thickening of the rotator interval (coracohumeral ligament [CHL] and superior glenohumeral ligament) is pathognomonic for frozen shoulder.[21-23] CHL contracture limits external rotation of the shoulder with the arm at the side (see Chapter 1),[24] which is very characteristic of frozen shoulder.
- Histologic analysis
  - Inflammatory involvement in idiopathic frozen shoulder is controversial
    - On histologic analysis of the CHL in 14 patients with an average of 21.8 months of symptoms, Bunker et al found active fibroblastic proliferation accompanied by some transformation to smooth-muscle myofibroblasts with histology indistinguishable from Dupuytren contracture of the hand.[25]
    - Lundberg (1969)[3] and Kay (1981)[26] described noninflammatory fibrosis on histologic analysis of capsular tissue in patients with frozen shoulder.
    - However, Neviaser has argued that histologic analysis during the first stages of "adhesive capsulitis" do suggest an inflammatory process and etiology.[1]
    - More recent analyses have suggested a combination of both these theories is more accurate; an inflammatory process leading to proliferative fibrosis.[27,28]
- An association between Dupuytren contracture of the hand and frozen shoulder has been repeatedly identified.[9,28-31]
  - Patients with a history of frozen shoulder had a 52% incidence of Dupuytren contracture compared to 6.2% in the general population.[29]

- When patients were treated for 1 month with a matrix metalloproteinase (MMP) inhibitor for gastric cancer, 50% (6/12) developed bilateral frozen shoulder and 3 of those developed Dupuytren contracture.[30]
  - Imbalance of MMP and MMP inhibitor ratios have been implicated as a potential pathway for frozen shoulder and Dupuytren contracture formation.[28,31]

Presentation and Diagnosis

- Demographics
  - Frozen shoulder affects 2% to 5% of the general population.[5,32]
  - It is most common in the following:
    - Women[27,33]
    - Individuals 40 to 60 years old[34]
    - Nondominant arm[27,35]
    - Those with family history[9]
  - Nonsimultaneous bilateral involvement occurs in 6% to 50%.[36-38]
  - Simultaneous bilateral involvement should prompt investigation for secondary cause.
- Patients report intense shoulder pain with restricted range of motion.
- Pain onset is often insidious but becomes disabling and difficult to control, with disabling night pain interfering with sleep during the acute pain phase. Pain may radiate to the neck or trapezius area.
- Physical examination
  - Global loss of active and passive range of motion of the glenohumeral joint, most notable in external rotation
  - The site is diffusely tender to palpation.
  - Scapular motion is dyskinetic, and non-neurologic scapular winging can be frequently seen.[39,40]
- Radiographic studies
  - In the case of idiopathic frozen shoulder, normal plain-film radiographic studies are seen.
  - For idiopathic frozen shoulder, magnetic resonance imaging may reveal diminished capsular volume and thickening of the CHL, with abnormalities similar to synovitis at the superior border of the subscapularis tendon.[41-43]
    - Magnetic resonance imaging should be used to rule out any secondary or tertiary causes of frozen shoulder if suspected or not following typical natural history.
  - Ultrasound may show CHL thickening, but is operator dependent.[44]

Treatment

- Exclusion of secondary or tertiary causes must be undertaken and treated if present.
- Classic teaching is that idiopathic frozen shoulder is self-limited, lasting 1 to 3 years.
  - However, follow-up studies have found that 50% of patients with frozen shoulder will suffer from residual pain and/or stiffness at least 2 years after initial symptom onset.[37]
  - In another long-term follow-up (average 4.3 years) of 223 patients, 41% had some extent of ongoing symptoms. Subjective severity at initial onset predicted long-term symptom persistence.[38]

- The principal treatment for frozen shoulder is physical therapy using gentle stretching, often requiring several months to 1 year of treatment.
  - The use of intensive formal physical therapy has been observed as having worse 1-year outcome measures and therefore some authors advocate "supervised neglect" (eg, home exercises).[45]
- Intra-articular injections in addition to physical therapy are helpful in decreasing pain better than physical therapy alone, at least in the short-term.[46]
- One study demonstrated that night pain was more rapidly relieved with a course of oral corticosteroids.[47]
- Brisement is a procedure designed to distend the shoulder capsule by an intra-articular injection (first with lidocaine and corticosteroid and then saline).[48] Hydrodilatation has been shown to provide faster improvement in pain and range of motion, with similar results at 6 months compared to intra-articular vs subacromial injectiona.[49] Dilatation may also be performed in conjunction with manipulation.[50]
- The motivated patient who has recalcitrant stiffness after 6 to 12 months of aggressive nonoperative management is a candidate for additional intervention with sedation.
  - Because of the high likelihood of resolution without intervention,[45] the risk of exacerbating the inflammatory reaction, and the lack of fibrosis formation,[20] frozen shoulder should not be treated surgically in the acute pain (inflammatory) phase.
  - MUA had previously been the mainstay of operative intervention.[51,52]
    - While stabilizing the scapula and using a short lever arm on the humerus, the shoulder should be taken through gradual flexion, abduction, external rotation, and internal rotation while feeling tearing of the capsular contractures.
    - A study reporting arthroscopic evaluation following manipulation under anesthesia (MUA) showed that 40% of patients had new damage, including superior labral anterior-posterior tears, labral detachments, partial subscapularis tears, or a medial glenohumeral ligament tear.[53]
    - MUA likely tears only the inferior capsular pouch and does not selectively release the rotator interval or CHL.[53]
  - Comparing MUA and arthroscopic release, a systematic review found no difference in shoulder range of motion or outcome scores.[54] However, arthroscopy does provide the advantage of diagnosis confirmation, release under direct visualization, and evaluation and treatment of concomitant shoulder pathology.
  - Arthroscopic release (Figure 11-1) is started in the rotator interval to release the CHL, anterior capsule, and medial glenohumeral ligament. If internal rotation contractures are present, posterior capsule release is necessary. Inferior capsule release puts the axillary nerve at risk and should be performed with vigilance (12.4 mm distal to the glenoid and only 2.5 mm deep to the inferior capsule).[55]
  - Open release is an alternative to arthroscopic release for those having failed manipulation with excision of the rotator interval.[56,57] A Z-plasty of the subscapularis may be useful if the subscapularis continues to be immobile. Open inferior and posterior capsulotomy may be necessary if abduction and internal rotation restrictions persist.

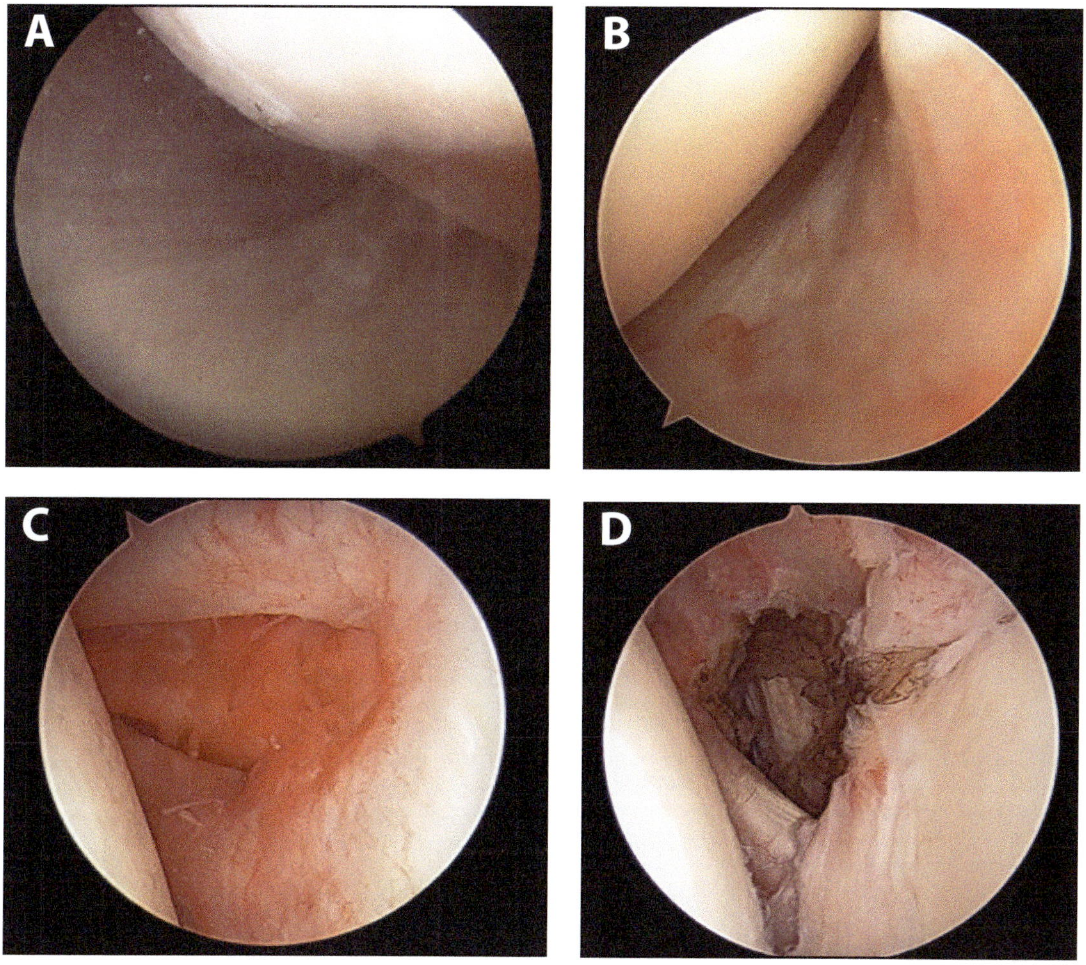

Figure 11-1. Arthroscopic view from the posterior portal of (A) normal inferior capsule, (B) contracted inferior capsule consistent with frozen shoulder, and contracted rotator interval (C) before and (D) after arthroscopic release.

References

1. Neviaser JS. Adhesive capsulitis of the shoulder. *J Bone Joint Surg Am.* 1945;27(2):211-222.
2. Zuckerman JD, Rokito A. Frozen shoulder: a consensus definition. *J Shoulder Elbow Surg.* 2011;20:322-325.
3. Lundberg BJ. The frozen shoulder. Clinical and radiographical observations the effect of manipulation under general anesthesia. Structure and glycosaminoglycan content of the joint capsule. Local bone metabolism. *Acta Orthop Scand.* 1969;40(suppl 119):1-59. doi:10.3109/ort.1969.40.suppl-119.01.
4. Huang YP, Fann CY, Chiu YH, et al. Association of diabetes mellitus with the risk of developing adhesive capsulitis of the shoulder: a longitudinal population-based followup study. *Arthritis Care Res (Hoboken).* 2013;65(7):1197-1202. doi:10.1002/acr.21938.
5. Thomas SJ, McDougall C, Brown ID, et al. Prevalence of symptoms and signs of shoulder problems in people with diabetes mellitus. *J Shoulder Elbow Surg.* 2007;16(6):748-751. doi:10.1016/j.jse.2007.02.133.
6. Pal B, Anderson J, Dick WC, Griffiths ID. Limitation of joint mobility and shoulder capsulitis in insulin- and non-insulin-dependent diabetes mellitus. *Br J Rheumatol.* 1986;25(2):147-151. doi:10.1093/rheumatology/25.2.147.
7. Arkkila PE, Kantola IM, Viikari JS, Rönnemaa T. Shoulder capsulitis in type I and II diabetic patients: association with diabetic complications and related diseases. *Ann Rheum Dis.* 1996;55(12):907-914. doi:10.1136/ard.55.12.907.
8. Austin DC, Gans I, Park MJ, Carey JL, Kelly JD IV. The association of metabolic syndrome markers with adhesive capsulitis. *J Shoulder Elbow Surg.* 2014;23(7):1043-1051. doi:10.1016/j.jse.2013.11.004.

9. Wang K, Ho V, Hunter-Smith DJ, Beh PS, Smith KM, Weber AB. Risk factors in idiopathic adhesive capsulitis: a case control study. *J Shoulder Elbow Surg.* 2013;22(7):e24-e29. doi:10.1016/j.jse.2012.10.049.
10. Yian EH, Contreras R, Sodl JF. Effects of glycemic control on prevalence of diabetic frozen shoulder. *J Bone Joint Surg.* 2012;94(10):919-923. doi:10.2106/JBJS.J.01930.
11. Massoud SN, Pearse EO, Levy O, Copeland SA. Operative management of the frozen shoulder in patients with diabetes. *J Shoulder Elbow Surg.* 2002;11(6):609-613. doi:10.1067/mse.2002.127301.
12. Huang SW, Lin JW, Wang WT, Wu CW, Liou TH, Lin HW. Hyperthyroidism is a risk factor for developing adhesive capsulitis of the shoulder: a nationwide longitudinal population-based study. *Sci Rep.* 2014;4:4183. doi:010.1038/srep04183.
13. Wohlgethan JR. Frozen shoulder in hyperthyroidism. *Arthritis Rheum.* 1987;30(8):936-939. doi:10.1002/art.1780300815.
14. Tuten HR, Young DC, Douoguih WA, Lenhardt KM, Wilkerson JP, Adelaar RS. Adhesive capsulitis of the shoulder in male cardiac surgery patients. *Orthopedics* 2000;23(7):693-696.
15. Bunker TD, Esler CN. Frozen shoulder and lipids. *J Bone Joint Surg Br.* 1995;77:684-686.
16. Sung CM, Jung TS, Park HB. Are serum lipids involved in primary frozen shoulder? *J Bone Joint Surg Am.* 2014;96:1828-1833. doi:10.2106/JBJS.M.00936.
17. Choy EH, Corkill MM, Gibson T, Hicks BH. Isolated ACTH deficiency presenting with bilateral frozen shoulder. *Br J Rheumatol.* 1991;30(3):226-227. doi:10.1093/rheumatology/30.3.226.
18. Wang JP, Huang TF, Hung SC, Ma HL, Wu JG, Chen TH. Comparison of idiopathic, post-trauma and post-surgery frozen shoulder after manipulation under anesthesia. *Int Orthop.* 2006;31(3):333. doi:10.1007/s00264-006-0195-7.
19. Reeves B. The natural history of the frozen shoulder syndrome. *Scand J Rheumat.* 1975;4(4):193-196. doi:10.3109/03009747509165255.
20. Neviaser RJ, Neviaser TJ. The frozen shoulder. Diagnosis and management. *Clin Orthop Relat Res.* 1987;(223):59-64.
21. Ozaki J, Nakagawa Y, Sakurai G, Tamai S. Recalcitrant chronic adhesive capsulitis of the shoulder. Role of contracture of the coracohumeral ligament and rotator interval in pathogenesis and treatment. *J Bone Joint Surg Am.* 1989;71(10):1511-1515.
22. DePalma AF. Loss of scapulohumeral motion (frozen shoulder). *Ann Surg.* 1952;135(2):193-204. doi:10.1097/00000658-195202000-00005.
23. Bunker TD. Frozen shoulder: unravelling the enigma. *Ann R Coll Surg Engl.* 1997;79(3):210-213.
24. Neer CS II, Satterlee CC, Dalsey RM, Flatow EL. The anatomy and potential effects of contracture of the coracohumeral ligament. *Clin Orthop Relat Res.* 1992;(280):182-185.
25. Bunker TD, Anthony PP. The pathology of frozen shoulder. A Dupuytren-like disease. *Bone Joint J* 1995;77(5):677-683.
26. Kay NRM, Slater DN. Fibromatoses and diabetes mellitus. *Lancet* 1981;2(8241):303. doi:10.1016/s0140-6736(81)90544-4.
27. Hand GC, Athanasou NA, Matthews T, Carr AJ. The pathology of frozen shoulder. *J Bone Joint Surg Br.* 2007;89(7):928-932.
28. Bunker TD, Reilly J, Baird KS, Hamblen DL. Expression of growth factors, cytokines and matrix metalloproteinases in frozen shoulder. *J Bone Joint Surg Br.* 2000;82(5):768-773. doi:10.1302/0301-620x.82b5.9888.
29. Smith SP, Devaraj VS, Bunker TD. The association between frozen shoulder and Dupuytren's disease. *J Shoulder Elbow Surg.* 2001;10(2):149-151.
30. Hutchinson JW, Tierney GM, Parsons SL, Davis TR. Dupuytren's disease and frozen shoulder induced by treatment with a matrix metalloproteinase inhibitor. *J Bone Joint Surg Br.* 1998;80(5):907-908. doi:10.1302/0301-620x.80b5.8464.
31. Baird KS, Crossan JF, Ralston SH. Abnormal growth factor and cytokine expression in Dupuytren's contracture. *J Clin Pathol.* 1993;46(5):425-428. doi:10.1136/jcp.46.5.425.
32. Bridgman JF. Periarthritis of the shoulder and diabetes mellitus. *Ann Rheum Dis.* 1972;31(1):69-71. doi:10.1136/ard.31.1.69.
33. White D, Choi H, Peloquin C, Zhu Y, Zhang Y. Secular trend of adhesive capsulitis. *Arthritis Care Res (Hoboken).* 2011;63(11):1571-1575. doi:10.1002/acr.20590.
34. Cho CH, Koo TW, Cho NS, et al. Demographic and clinical characteristics of primary frozen shoulder in a Korean population: a retrospective analysis of 1,373 cases. *Clin Should Elbow.* 2015;18(3):133-137. doi:10.5397/cise.2015.18.3.133.
35. Levine WN, Kashyap CP, Bak SF, Ahmad CS, Blaine TA, Bigliani LU. Nonoperative management of idiopathic adhesive capsulitis. *J Shoulder Elbow Surg.* 2007;16(5):569-573. doi:10.1016/j.jse.2006.12.007.
36. Balci N, Balci MK, Tüzüner S. Shoulder adhesive capsulitis and shoulder range of motion in type II diabetes mellitus: association with diabetic complications. *J Diabetes Complications.* 1999;13(3):135-140.
37. Shaffer B, Tibone JE, Kerlan RK. Frozen shoulder. A long-term follow-up. *J Bone Joint Surg Am.* 1992;74(5):738-746.
38. Hand C, Clipsham K, Rees JL, Carr AJ. Long-term outcome of frozen shoulder. *J Shoulder Elbow Surg.* 2008;17(2):231-236. doi:10.1016/j.jse.2007.05.009.

39. Vermeulen HM, Stokdijk M, Eilers PH, Meskers CG, Rozing PM, Vliet Vlieland TP. Measurement of three dimensional shoulder movement patterns with an electromagnetic tracking device in patients with a frozen shoulder. *Ann Rheum Dis.* 2002;61(2):115-120. doi:10.1136/ard.61.2.115.
40. Lin JJ, Wu YT, Wang SF, Chen SY. Trapezius muscle imbalance in individuals suffering from frozen shoulder syndrome. *Clin Rheumatol.* 2005;24(6):569-575. doi:10.1007/s10067-005-1105-x.
41. Mengiardi B, Pfirrmann CW, Gerber C, Hodler J, Zanetti M. Frozen shoulder: MR arthrographic findings. *Radiology.* 2004;233(2):486-492. doi:10.1148/radiol.2332031219.
42. Lee SY, Park J, Song SW. Correlation of MR arthrographic findings and range of shoulder motions in patients with frozen shoulder. *AJR Am J Roentgenol.* 2012;198(1):173-179. doi:10.2214/AJR.10.6173.
43. Song KD, Kwon JW, Yoon YC, Choi SH. Indirect MR arthrographic findings of adhesive capsulitis. *AJR Am J Roentgenol.* 2011;197(6):W1105-W1109. doi:10.2214/AJR.10.6099.
44. Homsi C, Bordalo-Rodrigues M, da Silva JJ, Stump XM. Ultrasound in adhesive capsulitis of the shoulder: is assessment of the coracohumeral ligament a valuable diagnostic tool? *Skeletal Radiol.* 2006;35(9):673-678. doi:10.1007/s00256-006-0136-y.
45. Diercks RL, Stevens M. Gentle thawing of the frozen shoulder: a prospective study of supervised neglect versus intensive physical therapy in seventy-seven patients with frozen shoulder syndrome followed up for two years. *J Shoulder Elbow Surg.* 2004;13(5):499-502. doi:10.1016/S1058274604000825.
46. Ranalletta M, Rossi LA, Bongiovanni SL, Tanoira I, Elizondo CM, Maignon GD. Corticosteroid injections accelerate pain relief and recovery of function compared with oral NSAIDs in patients with adhesive capsulitis: a randomized controlled trial. *Am J Sports Med.* 2016;44(2):474-481. doi:10.1177/0363546515616238.
47. Binder A, Hazleman BL, Parr G, Roberts S. A controlled study of oral prednisolone in frozen shoulder. *Br J Rheumatol.* 1986;25(3):288-292. doi:10.1093/rheumatology/25.3.288.
48. Simon WH. Soft tissue disorders of the shoulder. Frozen shoulder, calcific tendintis, and bicipital tendinitis. *Orthop Clin North Am.* 1975;6(2):521-539.
49. Yoon JP, et al. Intra-articular injection, subacromial injection, and hydrodilatation for primary frozen shoulder: a randomized clinical trial. *J Shoulder Elbow Surg.* 2016;25(3):376-383. doi:10.1016/j.jse.2015.11.009.
50. Quraishi NA, Johnston P, Bayer J, Crowe M, Chakrabarti AJ. Thawing the frozen shoulder. A randomised trial comparing manipulation under anaesthesia with hydrodilatation. *J Bone Joint Surg Br.* 2007;89(9):1197-1200. doi:10.1302/0301-620X.89B9.18863.
51. Farrell CM, Sperling JW, Cofield RH. Manipulation for frozen shoulder: long-term results. *J Shoulder Elbow Surg.* 2005;14(5):480-484. doi:10.1016/j.jse.2005.02.012.
52. Dodenhoff RM, Levy O, Wilson A, Copeland SA. Manipulation under anesthesia for primary frozen shoulder: effect on early recovery and return to activity. *J Shoulder Elbow Surg.* 2000;9(1):23-26.
53. Loew M, Heichel TO, Lehner B. Intraarticular lesions in primary frozen shoulder after manipulation under general anesthesia. *J Shoulder Elbow Surg.* 2005;14(1):16-21. doi:10.1016/j.jse.2004.04.004.
54. Grant JA, Schroeder N, Miller BS, Carpenter JE. Comparison of manipulation and arthroscopic capsular release for adhesive capsulitis: a systematic review. *J Shoulder Elbow Surg.* 2013;22(8):1135-1145. doi:10.1016/j.jse.2013.01.010.
55. Price MR, Tillett ED, Acland RD, Nettleton GS. Determining the relationship of the axillary nerve to the shoulder joint capsule from an arthroscopic perspective. *J Bone Joint Surg Am.* 2004;86(10):2135-2142. doi:10.2106/00004623-200410000-00003.
56. Omari A, Bunker TD. Open surgical release for frozen shoulder: surgical findings and results of the release. *J Shoulder Elbow Surg.* 2001;10(4):353-357. doi:10.1067/mse.2001.115986.
57. Elhassan B, Ozbaydar M, Massimini D, Higgins L, Warner JJP. Arthroscopic capsular release for refractory shoulder stiffness: a critical analysis of effectiveness in specific etiologies. *J Shoulder Elbow Surg.* 2010;19(4):580-587. doi:10.1016/j.jse.2009.08.004.

12

Injuries to the Biceps-Labral Complex

Nicholas A. Trasolini, MD and Seth Gamradt, MD

Pathophysiology

Anatomy of the Superior Glenoid Labrum

- The glenoid labrum is an elevated rim of fibrous tissue that increases the concavity and depth of the labrum, improving static stability of the glenohumeral joint.[1] The labrum also serves as a site of attachment for capsuloligamentous structures that provide dynamic glenohumeral stability.[2,3]
  - Specific locations along the labrum are often described like the face of a clock, with the superior portion extending from the 10 o'clock position posteriorly to the 2 o'clock position anteriorly.
  - The blood supply of the glenoid labrum comes from branches of the suprascapular, circumflex scapular, and posterior humeral circumflex arteries. The majority of the vascularity is limited to the peripheral labrum, with minimal blood supply to the free edge, particularly in superior and anterosuperior portions of the tissue.[4]
- The labrum contains free nerve endings in its periphery and adjacent connective tissue, but does not have mechanoreceptors, supporting a role in pain sensation but not proprioception.[5,6]
- The superior labrum has a more meniscal shape and more elastic capsular attachments that allow for greater mobility when compared to the inferior labrum.[4]
- The tendon of the long head of the biceps (LHB) brachii muscle inserts into the supraglenoid tubercle as an attachment to the superior labrum. This often results in a synovial recess between the glenoid rim and superior labrum.[4]
- Significant anatomic variations exist in the anterior-superior quadrant of the glenoid. Two common anomalies include the following:

Namdari S, Zmistowski B, Omid R, eds.
The Foundations of Shoulder and Elbow Surgery (pp 223-239).

- A "Buford complex" is defined as a thickened "cord-like" middle glenohumeral ligament that attaches to the superior labrum in the area of the biceps insertion associated with absent labral tissue in the anterosuperior region of the glenoid.[7] *Recommended reading for historical context and understanding variant anatomy*
- The prevalence of a sublabral foramen has been reported to be between 12% and 18.5%, and the Buford complex between 1.5% and 6.5%.[7,8]

Anatomy of the Proximal Biceps Tendon

- The LHB originates at the supraglenoid tubercle (5 mm medial to the superior rim of the glenoid at 12 o'clock[9]) and inserts at the biceps tuberosity on the proximal radius. In some normal variants, the tendon originates from the superior labrum directly.
- The blood supply of the long head of the biceps tendon (LHBT) has 3 sources: branches of the brachial artery crossing the musculotendinous junction, branches of the thoracoacromial artery crossing the osteotendinous junction, and (rarely) branches of the anterior circumflex humeral artery travelling in a mesotendon.[10]
  - A hypovascular watershed area exists between 1.2 and 3 cm from the biceps' origin.[10]
- The LHBT has sensory and sympathetic neural elements associated with pain sensation, with increased density at the origin.[11]
- There are 4 types of biceps origin from the scapula[9]:
  1. Labral attachment only to the posterior labrum (22%)
  2. Attachment mostly to the posterior labrum, but with a small contribution to the anterior labrum (33%)
  3. Equal contributions to anterior and posterior labrum (37%)
  4. Attachment mostly to the anterior labrum, with a small contribution to the posterior labrum (8%)
- Three zones of injury for the proximal biceps have been described: inside; junction; and bicipital tunnel.[12]
  - Inside: the superior labrum and biceps anchor, also referred to as the origin
  - Junction: the intra-articular biceps tendon and the biceps pulley
    - The biceps pulley is defined as a stabilizing fibrous sling composed of contributions from the superior glenohumeral ligament (SGHL), coracohumeral ligament (CHL), supraspinatus, and subscapularis.[13,14] It is located at the rotator interval prior to the biceps entering the bony bicipital groove.
  - Bicipital tunnel: the extra-articular tendon
    - There are 3 described zones for the extra-articular proximal biceps tendon[15]:
      - Zone 1: The bony bicipital groove, which starts at the articular margin and extends distally to the distal aspect of the subscapularis. The transverse humeral ligament helps contain the biceps in this area.
      - Zone 2: between the distal margin of the subscapularis and the proximal margin of the pectoralis major tendon
      - Zone 3: the subpectoralis region

Pathomechanics and Classification

Part I: Superior labral injuries

- Superior labrum anterior and posterior (SLAP) tear: an injury involving the superior aspect of the glenoid labrum, in which the labrum detachment or injury begins posteriorly and extends anteriorly, stopping at or above the midglenoid notch.[16]
- The original description of superior labral injuries in throwing athletes by Andrews et al, who described 3 biomechanical contributions[17]: *Recommended reading for historical context*
  1. Direct attachment of the biceps tendon to the superior labrum
  2. Forceful contraction of the biceps during deceleration phase of throwing[18]
  3. Elevation of the superior labrum during biceps muscle stimulation
- Other mechanisms of injury include inferior traction on the arm and fall onto an outstretched arm positioned in slight forward flexion and abduction.[19]
- There are 4 common pathomechanical theories for how SLAP tears occur[20]:
  1. Eccentric contraction of the biceps brachii, such as during the deceleration phase of throwing.[17]
  2. "Peel back": When the shoulder is placed in a position of abduction and maximal external rotation in the late-cocking phases of throwing or overhead sports, the rotation produces a twist at the base of the biceps, transmitting torsional force to the anchor. There can also be direct contact of the rotator cuff to the labrum ("internal impingement") in abduction/external rotation, particularly in patients with a glenohumeral internal rotation deficit and posterior capsular tightness.[21]
  3. "Weed pulling": Changing the vector of the biceps during different phases of throwing can loosen the anchor, similar to how pulling a weed straight from the ground is not as effective as toggling from side to side as one pulls.[22]
  4. Kinetic chain: This theory, popularized by Kibler, posits that a combination of factors put the shoulder at risk for a SLAP tear.[23-25]
     - A contracted posteroinferior capsule (glenohumeral internal rotation deficit) shifts the contact point superiorly, increasing labral shear.[26]
     - Labral shear force is at a maximum during late-cocking, the same time as "peel back" occurs.
     - Energy transfer from the trunk is simultaneously at a peak during this phase of throwing, exacerbating the other 2 effects.
- SLAP injuries were originally classified by Snyder and colleagues[16] *Recommended reading for historical context* with 4 types, but subsequent modifications were made by Maffet et al, Morgan et al, and others[16,27,28]:
  - Intrasubstance degeneration or fraying of the superior labrum without biceps anchor detachment
  - Detachment of the superior labrum from the glenoid with labral-biceps anchor instability
    - Anterior
    - Posterior
    - Combined
  - Bucket-handle tear of superior labrum with intact biceps anchor
  - Bucket-handle tears of the superior labrum are similar to those of type 3, but with the tear also extending into the biceps tendon.
  - An anterior-inferior Bankart lesion continues superiorly to include separation of the biceps tendon.

- An unstable anterior or posterior labrum flap tear is present in conjunction with a biceps tendon separation superiorly.
- The superior labrum-biceps tendon separation extends anteriorly beneath the middle glenohumeral ligament.
- A superior labral avulsion with posterior glenohumeral extension, which may be associated with a posterior shoulder dislocation or repetitive stress on the posterior labrum (eg, bench press)[29,30]
- A near complete detachment of the labrum due to anterior and posterior extension of the superior labral injury[29]
- A superior labral tear with extension into the rotator interval[29]
    - The Snyder classification has modest intraobserver and interobserver reliability, particularly with type III and IV lesions.[31,32]
    - Avulsion fractures of the supraglenoid tubercle have also been described as a SLAP variant.[33]

- There are pathologic biomechanical consequences of a SLAP tear:
    - Complete lesions of the superior portion of the labrum that destabilize the insertion of the biceps have been shown to cause increases in anteroposterior and superoinferior glenohumeral translation, as well as external rotation range of motion (ROM).[34,35]
        - However, type II SLAP tears do not significantly alter the path of glenohumeral articulation during shoulder motion.[36]
- Age-related histopathologic changes in the superior and anterosuperior regions of the labrum have been discovered in cadavers without known shoulder disease.[37]
- SLAP injuries are frequently associated with other intra-articular lesions, including Bankart tears or rotator cuff tears.[38]

Part II: proximal biceps injuries

- The LHBT originates both from the supraglenoid tubercle and the superior labrum; the strongest mechanical attachment is the bony attachment to the supraglenoid tubercle; the superior labral attachment acts as a secondary restraint.[39]
- The role of the LHBT in shoulder mechanics remains controversial.
    - In a cadaveric model, loading of the biceps shifted the humeral head to a more centered position on the glenoid, especially at the extremes of internal and external rotation.[40]
    - However, in vivo and cadaveric studies after biceps tenodesis have shown minimal effects on glenohumeral articulation and translation during functional shoulder movements.[41,42]
    - Yamaguchi and colleagues used electromyography to evaluate biceps activity during active shoulder motion when elbow motion was inhibited by bracing. This study of 44 shoulders found insignificant biceps activity, even in patients with known rotator cuff injuries.[43] These results were corroborated by Levy et al, using a similar study design.[44]
- Biceps lesions can be classified as inside, junction, or bicipital tunnel lesions.[12]
    - Inside lesions are associated with superior labral disruption (Part I).
    - Junction lesions occur in the intra-articular portion of the tendon or the biceps pulley.
        - Intra-articular lesions of the LHBT range from inflammation to complete tears. Tears commonly occur in the vascular watershed region 2.5 cm from the origin.[12,45]
        - Injuries to the biceps pulley occur with a fall onto an internally rotated arm. Bennett describes 5 such lesions[46]:
            1. Tears of the subscapularis without involvement of the medial head of the CHL
            2. Tears of the medial head of the CHL without subscapularis involvement
            3. Tears of both the subscapularis and the medial head of the CHL

4. Tears of the supraspinatus and the lateral head of the CHL
5. Tears of the subscapularis, medial and lateral head of the CHL, and including the leading edge of the supraspinatus tendon

- Habermeyer and colleagues focused on the SGHL rather than the CHL and classified pulley lesions into 4 types[47]:
  1. SGHL lesion leading to instability of the LHB during internal rotation
  2. SGHL lesion with a partial articular-side supraspinatus tendon tear
  3. SGHL lesion with a partial articular-side subscapularis tendon tear. In this case, the medially subluxated LHB leads to a deep surface tear of the subscapularis tendon.
  4. SGHL lesion with partial articular-side supraspinatus and subscapularis tendon tears

- Bicipital tunnel lesions are often missed during diagnostic arthroscopy.[48] Arthroscopy visualizes only 32% of the tendon, and a large percentage of proximal tears propagate distally out of the zone of visualization.[49]

Presentation and Diagnosis

Subjective Presentation

- Patients may present with vague anterior or deep shoulder pain, with limitations in lifting or throwing objects. There may be a history of an acute traumatic painful injury, such as during throwing, traction injuries, or falls.

Physical Examination

- Studies have shown limited specificity of physical examination for these lesions.[50-52]
- SLAP tears[53,54]
  - Inspection: No obvious deformities are visible.
  - Palpation: There is no directly palpable point of tenderness, but the biceps should be palpated to assess for concomitant LHB tendinitis or degeneration.
  - Motion: There is no direct limitation to motion, but there may be pain in the apprehension position (90-degree elevation, 90-degree abduction, 90-degree external rotation) or a clicking sensation during motion.
  - Provocative tests
    - Dynamic labral shear test[54]: The arm is placed in 90-degrees of elevation and abducted to the scapular plane with the elbow bent to 90 degrees. The examiner applies an anterior force to the shoulder as the arm is elevated from 60 degrees to 120 degrees and back to 60 degrees. A positive test is posterior superior shoulder pain with or without a click (sensitivity 72%, specificity 98%[54]).
    - Active compression (O'Brien's) test[55]: *Recommended reading for understanding development of diagnostic tests* With the arm at 90-degrees forward elevation, 10-degrees adduction, and internally rotated with the thumb pointing down, the examiner places downward pressure on the elbow while the patient resists. This is then repeated with the arm in external rotation (thumb facing lateral). A positive test is pain during the internally rotated position that improves in the second position (sensitivity 61%, specificity 82%[54]).
    - Anterior slide test[56]: The arm is placed at the side with the thumb pointing posteriorly. The examiner applies load in an anterosuperior direction from the elbow to the

shoulder. A positive test is pain or a painful click on the joint line (sensitivity 48% to 78.4%, specificity 82% to 91.5%[54,56]).

- Crank test: In the upright position, the arm is elevated to 160 degrees in the scapular plane. The examiner then applies load to the glenohumeral joint, while internally and externally rotating. A positive test is pain or a painful click.[57]
- Throwing test: The shoulder is abducted to 90 degrees with the elbow flexed to 90 degrees, and maximal external rotation (mimicking the late-cocking position). The patient steps forward to mimic throwing with the transition to the early acceleration phase while the examiner provides resistance. A positive test is pain with the maneuver.[51,58]

- LHBT tears[53]
  - Inspection: Complete tears may manifest as a "Popeye" deformity with a distal bulge in the biceps muscle compared to the contralateral side.
    - A Ludington test may assist in inspection: The patient places both hands on top of the head and then flexes the biceps to accentuate the deformity.[59]
  - Palpation: Focal tenderness can be elicited in the anterior shoulder along the biceps tendon. The preferred positions for palpation are either 10-degrees of internal rotation with the arm at the side (biceps at the anterior joint line), or with the arm externally rotated 30 degrees with elbow flexion or supination used to help localize the moving tendon.
  - Motion: Forward elevation may cause anterior shoulder pain, but isolated LHBT lesions should not limit shoulder motion directly.
  - Provocative tests
    - Yergason test[60] (also known as the supination sign): the patient fully pronates the forearm with the elbow flexed to 90 degrees. The examiner then resists supination of the forearm by the patient. A positive test is anterior shoulder pain (sensitivity 43%, specificity 79%[61]).
    - Speed test: The arm is flexed 90 degrees with the elbow fully extended and the palm up. The patient resists downward force by the examiner. A positive test is pain in the anterior shoulder. This test results in the most LBH muscle activation when compared to Yergason and O'Brien tests[62] (sensitivity 32% to 90%, specificity 14% to 75%[61,63,64]).
    - Upper cut test[54]: With the involved shoulder in a neutral position, the elbow flexed to 90 degrees, the forearm supinated, and the patient making a fist, the patient rapidly brings the arm toward the chin against resistance. A positive test is a painful pop over the anterior shoulder (sensitivity 73%, specificity 78%).
- Combined examination
  - There is significant overlap between the clinical syndrome associated with SLAP and LHBT injuries, so there are no reliable provocative tests to differentiate the two.
  - The "3-pack" test, a combination of the O'Brien test, throwing test, and palpation of the bicipital groove[51]
    - The "3-pack" test is designed to find lesions in all 3 LHBT zones. The O'Brien test is used to identify inside lesions, the throwing test is used to identify junction lesions, and the bicipital groove palpation is used to identify extra-articular bicipital tunnel lesions.
  - One study of 54 patients with heterogeneous labral tears found that combined physical examination tests outperformed magnetic resonance imaging (MRI) for diagnosis.[65]

Imaging

- Imaging modalities for SLAP injuries include MRI, MR arthrography, and computed tomography arthrography. An example of an MRI showing a SLAP tear is seen in Figure 12-1.

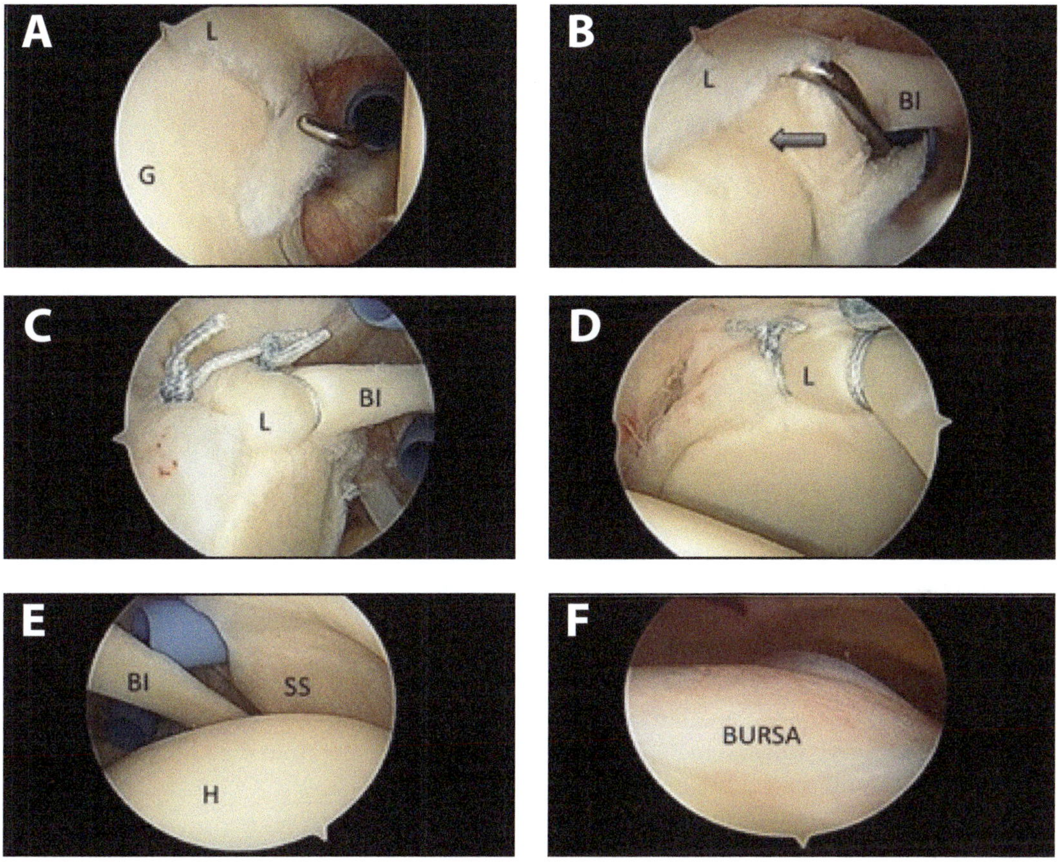

Figure 12-1. (A through F) MRI T2 coronal images with sequential cuts demonstrating a SLAP tear. The SS and IS are labeled for frame of reference. The blue arrow highlights the torn labrum. The white arrow highlights a paralabral cyst. The red arrow highlights proximity to the suprascapular nerve. Abbreviations: BI, biceps; G, glenoid; H, humerus; IS, infraspinatus; L, labrum; SS, supraspinatus.

- The accuracy of MRI for diagnosis is limited. Extensive literature has resulted in a wide range of reported diagnostic accuracy.
  - In a study of 144 cases and 100 controls, noncontrast MRI had a sensitivity of only 38% for type II SLAP tears but the specificity was 94%.[66]
  - In contrast, a study of 73 cases found a sensitivity of 86% and a specificity of only 13% for noncontrast MRI of SLAP tears.[67]
  - SLAP tears can also be frequently identified with noncontrast MRI in asymptomatic individuals, and thus may be a normal finding in patients 45 to 60 years old.[68]
- The addition of intra-articular contrast can assist in diagnosis.
  - In a study of 83 cases and 17 controls, community and musculoskeletal-trained radiologists both had improved sensitivity and specificity with the addition of intra-articular contrast.[69]
  - A cadaveric study of 43 shoulders found that MR arthrography and computed tomography arthrography could correctly identify a sublabral recess in 79% and 84%, respectively. The anterior-posterior extent of the recess was better assessed with MR.[70]
  - Clinically, MR arthrography has been shown to have a sensitivity of 90% but a specificity of only 50%.[71]

- LHBT pathology is also better visualized with intra-articular contrast.[72] Biceps pathologic findings include the following:
  - Increased tendon diameter consistent with an inflammatory process
  - Increased signal uptake on T2, indicating a spectrum of disease from tenosynovitis to partial tearing
  - Partial or complete tendon tears, as evidenced by loss of continuity of tendon fibers on MR
  - Tendon subluxation
- Some authors advocate for use of ultrasound in detection of biceps tendon injuries as well.[73] This has the advantage of being noninvasive and can be performed in the office. Positive findings are fluid around the biceps or a discontinuity in the tendon.

Arthroscopic Findings

- The arthroscopic diagnosis of a SLAP injury is made by discovery of a frayed or detached superior labrum.
- The arthroscopic diagnosis of LHBT injury is made by inspection of the tendon for synovitis, fraying, or tearing. It is important to pull the tendon into the joint, as only a portion is immediately visible.[73] Even with this maneuver, injuries to the distal portion of the tendon can be missed.[49]
- The sulcus score can be useful to differentiate a normal sulcus from a type II SLAP tear. It is calculated by comparing the depth of the sulcus to the length of the arthroscopic probe tip (2 mm) at various positions around the glenoid. Increased scores denote greater depth of probe penetration, which is more likely to be pathologic further from the 12 o'clock position.[74]

TREATMENT

Conservative

- In the majority of patients with SLAP and LHBT injuries, a trial of nonoperative treatment with rest, physical therapy, and graduated return to activities is warranted.
- Wilk and Hooks describe 4 phases for nonoperative treatment[75]:
  1. Phase 1: acute phase
     - Goals are to improve pain and inflammation, restore motion and muscle balance, promote dynamic stability, and correct postural adaptations.
     - Modalities: Anti-inflammatory medications, ice, laser, iontophoresis, active-assisted ROM, and stretching can all be used. In addition, improving scapular posture is important. Strengthening the rotator cuff musculature can also decrease the demands of the LHB for shoulder stability.
  2. Phase 2: intermediate phase
     - Goals are strengthening, flexibility, mobility, neuromuscular control and ROM of the elbow and shoulder joint complex.
     - Modalities: More aggressive isotronic exercises, Thrower's 10 program,[76] and neuromuscular drills. Improving periscapular muscle strength continues to be important in this phase. Isolated biceps strengthening is progressed and closed kinetic chain exercises remain a focus.
  3. Phase 3: advanced strengthening phase

        - Goals are to initiate aggressive strengthening exercises and functional drills, progress muscular endurance and power, and prepare for a return to sports activity.
        - Modalities include sustained holds, neuromuscular drills, eccentric exercises, and controlled sports activities.
    4. Phase 4: return to activity
- Some patients with LHBT injuries may benefit from corticosteroid injections,[77] but this is controversial because these medications have been shown to adversely affect tendons in vitro.[78]
- One study of 39 patients with SLAP tears found that nonoperative treatment was successful in 49% of patients. In that population, 71% returned to preoperative athletic levels.[79]

Surgical

- SLAP injuries
    - SLAP surgeries are becoming increasingly common, particularly in men 20 to 29 years old and 40 to 49 years old.[80]
    - Relative surgical indications include the following[81]:
        - Failure of nonoperative treatment
        - Younger patients
        - Active athletes (particularly overhead sports)
        - Type II SLAP tear
        - Physical examination and imaging support the diagnosis without another known cause for the symptoms.
    - Debridement vs repair
        - Most authors recommend debridement for type I and type III SLAP tears and repair for type II tears. Type IV tears have varied involvement of the biceps tendon and can be treated with either debridement or repair, with a concurrent biceps debridement, tenotomy, or tenodesis.[19]
    - Surgical technique
        - Initial diagnostic arthroscopy is crucial to determine whether concurrent pathology is present and to determine the stability of the biceps anchor.
        - If debridement is chosen, the use of an arthroscopic shaver is helpful for removal of frayed labral and biceps tissue. Care must be taken not to cause iatrogenic instability to the biceps-labral complex (BLC).
        - The current standard in arthroscopic repair of the superior labrum is with suture anchors using knotless anchors or standard repair techniques using arthroscopic knot tying.[19] Figure 12-2 shows a case example of this technique. Knotless anchors are theorized to cause less irritation of the articular side of the rotator cuff.
        - Accessory portals such as Neviaser's and Wilmington may be useful for anchor placement.[81]
        - In a meta-analysis, Kibler and Sciascia reported that most authors use between 2 and 4 suture anchors, with one at the 12 o'clock position and others either anterior or posterior.[82]
        - Biomechanical studies have validated current repair techniques.

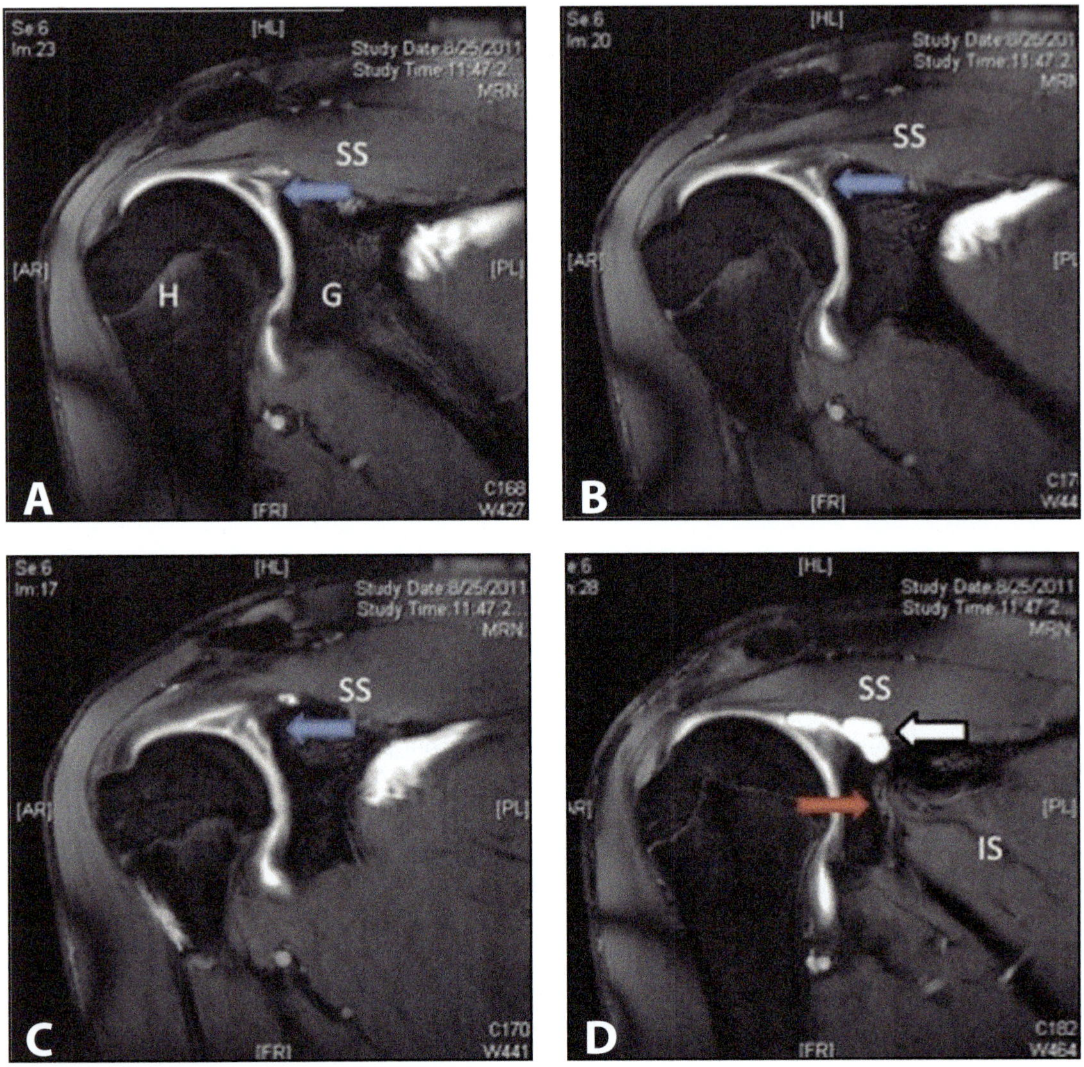

Figure 12-2. (A and B) Arthroscopic images demonstrating a type II SLAP tear. One can see the tear by elevating the torn portion of the labrum with a probe. The gray arrow highlights the torn portion. (C and D) This repair was performed with a 2-anchor technique. Abbreviations: BI, biceps; G, glenoid; H, humerus; IS, infraspinatus; L, labrum; SS, supraspinatus.

- Yoo et al found that for type II-B SLAP tears, one anchor posterior to the biceps with a simple suture was sufficient to withstand clinical loads and was superior to a horizontal mattress suture.[83]
- Panossian and colleagues showed that repair with 2 suture anchors, 1 anterior and 1 posterior to the biceps, restored glenohumeral stability to preinjury values.[35] However, some residual anterior capsular laxity can be present even after repair.[84]

- Biceps tenodesis is an alternative to repair for type II SLAP injuries and may have a role as a salvage procedure when a repair fails.[85]
- Combined tenodesis with repair is also an option, but resulted in worse outcomes in one small retrospective series.[86]

- LHB injuries

- Surgical treatment options for biceps lesions include debridement, tenotomy, and tenodesis. Biceps tenotomy and tenodesis have been studied extensively, without a clear consensus.[87]
- The most conservative surgical option is debridement, but the utility is limited to mild fraying without biceps instability. Overly aggressive debridement can result in spontaneous rupture of the tendon postoperatively.
- Biceps tenotomy involves cutting the biceps tendon from its origin.
  - This has been shown to have satisfactory clinical results, with improved pain and functional scores postoperatively. However, it frequently results in a cosmetic "Popeye" deformity and, less frequently, uncomfortable muscle cramping or soreness after activity.[88]
  - Advocates for tenotomy report fewer rehabilitation restrictions with shorter surgical time and complexity.
  - This procedure may be favored in older, less active patients and in patients who do not have concerns about cosmetic deformity.[72]
- Biceps tenodesis is becoming increasingly common.[89] This procedure involves releasing the biceps tendon from its insertion, and securing it to a more distal attachment.
  - Several open and arthroscopic techniques have been described, including tenodesis to the intact rotator cuff, to the conjoint tendon or the transverse humeral ligament, to the bicipital groove (ie, suprapectoral), or distally to the subpectoral aspect of the humerus.[87,90,91]
    - Suprapectoral tenodesis has the benefit of being possible through an all-arthroscopic technique, whereas subpectoral tenodesis is performed open. However, suprapectoral techniques often leave tendon within the bicipital groove, which evokes a theoretical concern of persistent irritation in that area.[92]
    - In a cadaveric study, arthroscopic suprapectoral tenodesis resulted in overtensioning the musculotendinous unit and lower failure strength compared to an open subpectoral technique.[93]
    - Clinical studies from separate groups have found no significant difference in patient satisfaction scores or functional outcomes between the 2 techniques with a minimum follow up of 18 to 24 months.[92,94]
  - Advocates for tenodesis report less cosmetic deformity and muscle cramping, but this remains controversial.
  - This procedure is favored in younger, more active patients; overhead athletes; and patients with concerns about cosmetic deformity.[72]
  - Reported complications include persistent groove pain, peripheral nerve injury, proximal humerus fracture through a suture anchor stress riser, complex regional pain, and infection.[95]

Postoperative Rehabilitation

- SLAP repairs
  - Postoperative rehabilitation after SLAP repair starts with immobilization, followed by early protected motion.[20]
    - It is important to protect against arm positions that promote the "peel back" phenomenon (external rotation and abduction).[21]
  - Early deltoid isometrics as well as hand and wrist movement are encouraged.
  - Return to motion typically proceeds from gentle passive motion to active assisted ROM then active ROM.

- Initial strengthening exercises are restricted to positions below 90 degrees of flexion.
- Gradual and protected return to sport, particularly overhead athletic activities, can typically begin after 3 months of therapy if ROM is restored to functional levels without significant discomfort.
- Postoperative neuromuscular control during throwing can be altered after SLAP repair. Studies have shown altered thoracic rotation, lead knee flexion, horizontal abduction, and external rotation in the late-cocking phase.[96,97]

- Biceps tenodesis
  - Postoperative rehabilitation after biceps tenodesis involves an initial period of sling immobilization for 3 to 4 weeks, followed by mobilization with a goal of full motion at 6 weeks. Elbow flexion and supination is restricted for 6 weeks to allow the tenodesis to heal.[72]

Outcomes

- SLAP repair
  - Outcomes of SLAP repairs with current techniques have been studied extensively. There is a consensus in retrospective studies that repair is effective, with excellent results in approximately 84% of patients in an aggregate analysis.
    - However, return to sports in overhead athletes is not guaranteed, and return to previous level of play occurs in only 64% of patients.[98,99]
    - In a cohort of elite overhead athletes, the return to preinjury levels was only 57%.[100]
    - Similarly, a large cohort of active military patients had a 37% failure rate and 28% revision rate for SLAP repairs.[101]
  - A recent randomized, controlled trial compared biceps tenodesis, repair, and sham surgery for type II SLAP tears and did not find a significant difference between procedures.[102]
  - Patients who have a poor outcome from initial SLAP repair often require reoperation because of failed conservative care.[103]
    - Risk factors for revision include the following[104]:
      - Older than 40 years old
      - Female sex
      - Obesity
      - Smoking
      - Concurrent biceps pathology
- Biceps tenotomy and tenodesis
  - There is a large body of literature looking at the outcomes of biceps tenotomy and tenodesis. Despite this, there is a paucity of level I data.
  - A recent systematic review by Slenker et al summarized the literature findings.[105]
    - Biceps tenotomy and tenodesis both have good clinical results (77% excellent outcomes for tenotomy and 74% for tenodesis). Both procedures also reliably improve patient-reported and functional outcome scores when compared to the preoperative condition.
    - Biceps tenotomy has a higher rate of "Popeye" deformity (43% vs 8%).

Conclusion

- Injuries to the BLC cause pain and loss of function.
- There is a spectrum of disease, including tenosynovitis, tendon tears, tendon instability, and labral tearing.
- Diagnosis on physical examination and imaging can be challenging and definitive diagnosis of BLC injuries can be made only arthroscopically.
- Initial management with nonoperative treatment is effective in many patients.
- When surgical interventions are indicated, options include labral repair, debridement, biceps tenotomy, and biceps tenodesis.
- Outcomes of surgical interventions depend on patient selection and postoperative functional demand.

References

1. Perry J. Anatomy and biomechanics of the shoulder in throwing, swimming, gymnastics, and tennis. *Clin Sports Med.* 1983;2(2):247-270.
2. Peat M. Functional anatomy of the shoulder complex. *Phys Ther.* 1986;66(12):1855-1865.
3. Warner JJP, Caborn DNM, Berger R, Fu FH, Seel M. Dynamic capsuloligamentous anatomy of the glenohumeral joint. *J Shoulder Elbow Surg.* 1993;2(3):115-133. doi:10.1016/S1058-2746(09)80048-7.
4. Cooper DE, Arnoczky SP, O'Brien SJ, Warren RF, DiCarlo E, Allen AA. Anatomy, histology, and vascularity of the glenoid labrum. An anatomical study. *J Bone Joint Surg Am.* 1992;74(1):46-52.
5. Vangsness CT Jr, Ennis M, Taylor JG, Atkinson R. Neural anatomy of the glenohumeral ligaments, labrum, and subacromial bursa. *Arthroscopy.* 1995;11(2):180-184. doi:10.1016/0749-8063(95)90064-0.
6. Veeger HEJ, van der Helm FCT. Shoulder function: The perfect compromise between mobility and stability. *J Biomech.* 2007;40(10):2119-2129. doi:10.1016/j.jbiomech.2006.10.016.
7. Williams MM, Snyder SJ, Buford D. The buford complex—The "cord-like" middle glenohumeral ligament and absent anterosuperior labrum complex: a normal anatomic capsulolabral variant. *Arthroscopy.* 1994;10(3):241-247. doi:10.1016/S0749-8063(05)80105-7.
8. Ilahi OA, Labbe MR, Cosculluela P. Variants of the anterosuperior glenoid labrum and associated pathology. *Arthroscopy.* 2002;18(8):882-886. doi:10.1053/jars.2002.36119.
9. Vangsness CT Jr, Jorgenson SS, Watson T, Johnson DL. The origin of the long head of the biceps from the scapula and glenoid labrum. An anatomical study of 100 shoulders. *J Bone Joint Surg.* 1994;76(6):951-954.
10. Cheng NM, Pan WR, Vally F, Le Roux CM, Richardson MD. The arterial supply of the long head of biceps tendon: Anatomical study with implications for tendon rupture. *Clin Anat.* 2010;23(6):683-692. doi:10.1002/ca.20992.
11. Alpantaki K, McLaughlin D, Karagogeos D, Hadjipavlou A, Kontakis G. Sympathetic and sensory neural elements in the tendon of the long head of the biceps. *J Bone Joint Surg Am.* 2005;87(7):1580-1583. doi:10.2106/JBJS.D.02840.
12. Taylor SA, O'Brien SJ. Clinically relevant anatomy and biomechanics of the proximal biceps. *Clin Sports Med.* 2016;35(1):1-18. doi:10.1016/j.csm.2015.08.005.
13. Werner A, Mueller T, Boehm D, Gohlke F. The stabilizing sling for the long head of the biceps tendon in the rotator cuff interval. A histoanatomic study. *Am J Sports Med.* 2000;28(1):28-31. doi:10.1177/03635465000280011701.
14. Martetschläger F, Tauber M, Habermeyer P. Injuries to the biceps pulley. *Clin Sports Med.* 2016;35(1):19-27. doi:10.1016/j.csm.2015.08.003.
15. Taylor SA, Fabricant PD, Bansal M, et al. The anatomy and histology of the bicipital tunnel of the shoulder. *J Shoulder Elbow Surg.* 2015;24(4):511-519. doi:10.1016/j.jse.2014.09.026.
16. Snyder SJ, Karzel RP, Del Pizzo W, Ferkel RD, Friedman MJ. SLAP lesions of the shoulder. *Arthroscopy.* 1990;6(4):274-279. doi:10.1016/j.arthro.2010.06.004.
17. Andrews JR, Carson WG Jr, McLeod WD. Glenoid labrum tears related to the long head of the biceps. *Am J Sports Med.* 1985;13(5):337-341. doi:10.1177/036354658501300508.
18. Jobe FW, Moynes DR, Tibone JE, Perry J. An EMG analysis of the shoulder in pitching. A second report. *Am J Sports Med.* 1984;12(3):218-220. doi:10.1177/036354658401200310.
19. Mileski RA, Snyder SJ. Superior labral lesions in the shoulder: pathoanatomy and surgical management. *J Am Acad Orthop Surg.* 1998;6(2):121-131.

20. Wilk K, Reinold MM, Dugas JR, Arrigo CA, Moser MW, Andrews JR. Current concepts in the recognition and treatment of superior labral (SLAP) lesions. *J Ortho Sports Phys Ther.* 2005;35(5):273-291.
21. Burkhart SS, Morgan CD. The peel-back mechanism: its role in producing and extending posterior type II SLAP lesions and its effect on SLAP repair rehabilitation. *Arthroscopy.* 1998;14(6):637-640. doi:10.1016/S0749-8063(98)70065-9.
22. Dugas JR, Andrews JR. Thrower's shoulder: two perspectives. In: McGinty JB, ed. *Operative Arthroscopy.* 3rd ed. Philadelphia, PA: Lippincott Williams & Wilkins; 2003:585.
23. Kibler WB. The role of the scapula in athletic shoulder function. *Am J Sports Med.* 1998;26(2):325-337. doi:10.1177/03635465980260022801.
24. Kibler WB, Wilkes T, Sciascia A. Mechanics and pathomechanics in the overhead athlete. *Clin Sports Med.* 2013;32(4):637-651. doi:10.1016/j.csm.2013.07.003.
25. BurkhartSS, MorganCD, KiblerWB. The disabled throwing shoulder: spectrum of pathology Part I: pathoanatomy and Biomechanics. *Arthroscopy.* 2003;19(4):404-420. doi:10.1053/jars.2003.50128.
26. Grossman MG1, Tibone JE, McGarry MH, Schneider DJ, Veneziani S, Lee TQ. A cadaveric model of the throwing shoulder: a possible etiology of superior labrum anterior-to-posterior lesions. *J Bone Joint Surg Am.* 2005;87(4):824-831. doi:10.2106/JBJS.D.01972.
27. Maffet MW, Gartsman GM, Moseley B. Superior labrum-biceps tendon complex lesions of the shoulder. *Am J Sports Med.* 1995;23(1):93-98. doi:10.1177/036354659502300116.
28. Morgan CD, Burkhart SS, Palmeri M, Gillespie M. Type II slap lesions: three subtypes and their relationships to superior instability and rotator cuff tears. *Arthroscopy.* 1998;14(6):553-565. doi:10.1016/S0749-8063(98)70049-0.
29. Mohana-Borges AVR, Chung CB, Resnick D. Superior labral anteroposterior tear: classification and diagnosis on MRI and MR arthrography. *AJR Am J Roentgenol.* 2003;181(6):1449-1462. doi:10.2214/ajr.181.6.1811449.
30. Seroyer S, Tejwani SG, Bradley JP. Arthroscopic capsulolabral reconstruction of the type VIII superior labrum anterior posterior lesion: mean 2-year follow-up on 13 shoulders. *Am J Sports Med.* 2007;35(9):1477-1483. doi:10.1177/0363546507302546.
31. Gobezie R, Zurakowski D, Lavery K, Millett PJ, Cole BJ, Wamer JJP. Analysis of interobserver and intraobserver variability in the diagnosis and treatment of SLAP tears using the Snyder classification. *Am J Sports Med.* 2008;36(7):1373-1379. doi:10.1177/0363546508314795.
32. Jia X, Yokota A, McCarty EC, et al. Reproducibility and reliability of the Snyder classification of superior labral anterior posterior lesions among shoulder surgeons. *Am J Sports Med.* 2011;39(5):986-991. doi:10.1177/0363546510392332.
33. Iannotti JP, Wang ED. Avulsion fracture of the supraglenoid tubercle: a variation of the SLAP lesion. *J Shoulder Elbow Surg.* 1992;1(1):26-30. doi:10.1016/S1058-2746(09)80012-8.
34. Pagnani MJ, Deng XH, Warren RF, Torzilli PA, Altchek DW. Effect of lesions of the superior portion of the glenoid labrum on glenohumeral translation. *J Bone Joint Surg Am.* 1995;77(7):1003-1010. doi:10.2106/00004623-199507000-00005.
35. Panossian VR, Mihata T, Tibone JE, Fitzpatrick MJ, McGarry MH, Lee TQ. Biomechanical analysis of isolated type II SLAP lesions and repair. *J Shoulder Elbow Surg.* 2005;14(5):529-534. doi:10.1016/j.jse.2004.11.002.
36. Youm T, Tibone JE, Elattrache NS, McGarry MH, Lee TQ. Simulated type II superior labral anterior posterior lesions do not alter the path of glenohumeral articulation: a cadaveric biomechanical study. *Am J Sports Med.* 2008;36(4):767-774. doi:10.1177/0363546507312169.
37. Pfahler M, Haraida S, Schulz C, et al. Age-related changes of the glenoid labrum in normal shoulders. *J Shoulder Elbow Surg.* 2003;12(1):40-52. doi:10.1067/mse.2003.3.
38. Kim TK, Queale WS, Cosgarea AJ, McFarland EG. Clinical features of the different types of SLAP lesions. *J Bone Joint Surg Am.* 2003;85(1):1421-1427.
39. Healey JH, Barton S, Noble P, Kohl HW, Ilahi OA. Biomechanical evaluation of the origin of the long head of the biceps tendon. *Arthroscopy.* 2001;17(4):378-382. doi:10.1053/jars.2001.21244.
40. Youm T, ElAttrache NS, Tibone JE, McGarry MH, Lee TQ. The effect of the long head of the biceps on glenohumeral kinematics. *J Shoulder Elbow Surg.* 2009;18(1):122-129. doi:10.1016/j.jse.2008.06.003.
41. Giphart JE, Elser F, Dewing CB, Torry MR, Millett PJ. The long head of the biceps tendon has minimal effect on in vivo glenohumeral kinematics: a biplane fluoroscopy study. *Am J Sports Med.* 2012;40(1):202-212. doi:10.1177/0363546511423629.
42. Strauss EJ, Salata MJ, Sershon RA, et al. Role of the superior labrum after biceps tenodesis in glenohumeral stability. *J Shoulder Elbow Surg.* 2014;23(4):485-491. doi:10.1016/j.jse.2013.07.036.
43. Yamaguchi K, Riew KD, Galatz LM, Syme JA, Neviaser RJ. Biceps activity during shoulder motion: an electromyographic analysis. *Clin Orthop Relat Res.* 1997;(336):122-129.
44. Levy AS, Kelly BT, Lintner SA, Osbahr DC, Speer KP. Function of the long head of the biceps at the shoulder: electromyographic analysis. *J Shoulder Elbow Surg.* 10(3):250-255. doi:10.1067/mse.2001.113087.
45. Boileau P, Ahrens PM, Hatzidakis AM. Entrapment of the long head of the biceps tendon: The hourglass biceps—A cause of pain and locking of the shoulder. *J Shoulder Elbow Surg.* 2004;13(3):249-257. doi:10.1016/j.jse.2004.01.001.

46. Bennett WF. Arthroscopic repair of anterosuperior (supraspinatus/subscapularis) rotator cuff tears: a prospective cohort with 2- to 4-year follow-up. Classification of biceps subluxation/instability. *Arthroscopy.* 2003;19(1):21-33. doi:10.1053/jars.2003.50023.
47. Habermeyer P, Magosch P, Pritsch M, Scheibel MT, Lichtenberg S. Anterosuperior impingement of the shoulder as a result of pulley lesions: a prospective arthroscopic study. *J Shoulder Elbow Surg.* 2004;13(1):5-12. doi:10.1016/j.jse.2003.09.013.
48. Taylor SA, Khair MM, Gulotta LV, et al. Diagnostic glenohumeral arthroscopy fails to fully evaluate the biceps-labral complex. *Arthroscopy.* 2015;31(2):215-224. doi:10.1016/j.arthro.2014.10.017.
49. Gilmer BB, DeMers AM, Guerrero D, Reid JB, Lubowitz JH, Guttmann D. Arthroscopic versus open comparison of long head of biceps tendon visualization and pathology in patients requiring tenodesis. *Arthroscopy.* 2015;31(1):29-34. doi:10.1016/j.arthro.2014.07.025.
50. Cook C, Beaty S, Kissenberth MJ, Siffri P, Pill SG, Hawkins RJ. Diagnostic accuracy of five orthopedic clinical tests for diagnosis of superior labrum anterior posterior (SLAP) lesions. *J Shoulder Elbow Surg.* 2012;21(1):13-22. doi:10.1016/j.jse.2011.07.012.
51. Taylor SA, Newman AM, Dawson C, et al. The "3-pack" examination is critical for comprehensive evaluation of the biceps-labrum complex and the bicipital tunnel: a prospective study. *Arthroscopy.* 2017;33(1):28-38. doi:10.1016/j.arthro.2016.05.015.
52. Meserve BB, Cleland JA, Boucher TR. A meta-analysis examining clinical test utility for assessing superior labral anterior posterior lesions. *Am J Sports Med.* 2009;37(11):2252-2258. doi:10.1177/0363546508325153.
53. McFarland EG, Borade A. Examination of the biceps tendon. *Clin Sports Med.* 2016;35(1):29-45. doi:10.1016/j.csm.2015.08.004.
54. Kibler WB, Sciascia AD, Hester P, Dome D, Jacobs C. Clinical utility of traditional and new tests in the Diagnosis of biceps tendon injuries and superior labrum anterior and posterior lesions in the shoulder. *Am J Sports Med.* 2009;37(9):1840-1847. doi:10.1177/0363546509332505.
55. O'Brien SJ, Pagnani MJ, Fealy S, McGlynn SR, Wilson JB. The active compression test: a new and effective test for diagnosing labral tears and acromioclavicular joint abnormality. *Am J Sports Med.* 1998;26(5):610-613. doi:10.1177/03635465980260050201.
56. Kibler WB. Specificity and sensitivity of the anterior slide test in throwing athletes with superior glenoid labral tears. *Arthroscopy.* 1995;11(3):296-300.
57. Guanche CA, Jones DC. Clinical testing for tears of the glenoid labrum. *Arthroscopy.* 2003;19(5):517-523. doi:10.1053/jars.2003.50104.
58. Taylor SA, McCarthy MM, Newman AM, O'Brien SJ. Arthroscopy of the subdeltoid space and biceps transfer. In: Craig, EV. *Master Techniques in Orthopaedic Surgery: The Shoulder.* 3rd ed. Baltimore, MD: Lippincott Williams & Wilkins; 2012.
59. Ludington NA. Rupture of the long head of the biceps flexor cubiti muscle. *Ann Surg.* 1923;77(3):358-363.
60. Yergason R. Supination sign. *J Bone Joint Surg Am.* 1931;13(1):160.
61. Holtby R, Razmjou H. Accuracy of the Speed's and Yergason's tests in detecting biceps pathology and SLAP lesions: comparison with arthroscopic findings. *Arthroscopy.* 2004;20(3):231-236. doi:10.1016/j.arthro.2004.01.008.
62. Wood VJC, Sabick MB, Pfeiffer RP, Kuhlman SM, Christensen JH, Curtin MJ. Glenohumeral muscle activation during provocative tests designed to diagnose superior labrum anterior-posterior lesions. *Am J Sports Med.* 2011;39(12):2670-2678. doi:10.1177/0363546511419822.
63. Gill HS, El Rassi G, Bahk MS, Castillo RC, McFarland EG. Physical examination for partial tears of the biceps tendon. *Am J Sports Med.* 2007;35(8):1334-1340. doi:10.1177/0363546507300058.
64. Bennett WF. Specificity of the Speed's test: arthroscopic technique for evaluating the biceps tendon at the level of the bicipital groove. *Arthroscopy.* 1998;14(8):789-796.
65. Liu SH, Henry MH, Nuccion S, et al. Diagnosis of glenoid labral tears. *Am J Sports Med.* 1996;24(2):149-154. doi:10.1177/036354659602400205.
66. Connolly KP, Schwartzberg RS, Reuss B, Crumbie D Jr, Homan BM. Sensitivity and specificity of noncontrast magnetic resonance imaging reports in the diagnosis of type-II superior labral anterior-posterior lesions in the community setting. *J Bone Joint Surg Am.* 2013;95(4):308-313. doi:10.1016/S0021-9355(13)70579-4.
67. Phillips JC, Cook C, Beaty S, Kissenberth MJ, Siffri P, Hawkins RJ. Validity of noncontrast magnetic resonance imaging in diagnosing superior labrum anterior-posterior tears. *J Shoulder Elbow Surg.* 2013;22(1):3-8. doi:10.1016/j.jse.2012.03.013.
68. Schwartzberg R, Reuss BL, Burkhart BG, Butterfield M, Wu JY, McLean KW. High prevalence of superior labral tears diagnosed by MRI in middle-aged patients with asymptomatic shoulders. *Orthop J Sport Med.* 2016;4(1):232596711562321. doi:10.1177/2325967115623212.
69. Reuss BL, Schwartzberg R, Zlatkin MB, Cooperman A, Dixon JR. Magnetic resonance imaging accuracy for the diagnosis of superior labrum anterior-posterior lesions in the community setting: Eighty-three arthroscopically confirmed cases. *J Shoulder Elbow Surg.* 2006;15(5):580-585. doi:10.1016/j.jse.2005.10.011.
70. Waldt S, Metz S, Burkart A, et al. Variants of the superior labrum and labro-bicipital complex: a comparative study of shoulder specimens using MR arthrography, multi-slice CT arthrography and anatomical dissection. *Eur Radiol.* 2006;16(2):451-458. doi:10.1007/s00330-005-2864-0.

71. Amin MF, Youssef AO. The diagnostic value of magnetic resonance arthrography of the shoulder in detection and grading of SLAP lesions: comparison with arthroscopic findings. *Eur J Radiol.* 2012;81(9):2343-2347. doi:10.1016/j.ejrad.2011.07.006.
72. Mellano CR, Shin JJ, Yanke AB, Verma NN. Disorders of the long head of the biceps tendon. *Instr Course Lect.* 2015;64:567-576.
73. Sethi N, Wright R, Yamaguchi K. Disorders of the long head of the biceps tendon. *J Shoulder Elbow Surg.* 1999;8(6):644-654. doi:10.1016/B978-1-4160-3857-3.50008-9.
74. Mihata T, McGarry MH, Tibone JE, Abe M, Lee TQ. Type II SLAP lesions: a new scoring system—The sulcus score. *J Shoulder Elbow Surg.* 2005;14(1 suppl):19-23. doi:10.1016/j.jse.2004.10.004.
75. Wilk KE, Hooks TR. The painful long head of the biceps brachii: nonoperative treatment approaches. *Clin Sports Med.* 2016;35(1):75-92. doi:10.1016/j.csm.2015.08.012.
76. Wilk KE, Andrews JR, Arrigo CA. *Preventive and Rehabilitative Exercises for the Shoulder and Elbow.* 6th ed. Birmingham, AL: American Sports Medicine Institute; 2001.
77. Schickendantz M, King D. Nonoperative management (including ultrasound-guided injections) of proximal biceps disorders. *Clin Sports Med.* 2016;35(1):57-73. doi:10.1016/j.csm.2015.08.006.
78. Dean BJF, Franklin SL, Murphy RJ, Javaid MK, Carr AJ. Glucocorticoids induce specific ion-channel-mediated toxicity in human rotator cuff tendon: a mechanism underpinning the ultimately deleterious effect of steroid injection in tendinopathy? *Br J Sports Med.* 2014;48(22):1620-1626. doi:10.1136/bjsports-2013-093178.
79. Edwards SL, Lee JA, Bell JE, et al. Nonoperative treatment of superior labrum anterior posterior tears. *Am J Sports Med.* 2010;38(7):1456-1461. doi:10.1177/0363546510370937.
80. Zhang AL, Kreulen C, Ngo SS, Hame SL, Wang JC, Gamradt SC. Demographic trends in arthroscopic SLAP repair in the United States. *Am J Sports Med.* 2012;40(5):1144-1147. doi:10.1177/0363546512436944.
81. Werner BC, Holzgrefe RE, Brockmeier SF. Arthroscopic surgical techniques for the management of proximal biceps injuries. *Clin Sports Med.* 2016;35(1):113-135. doi:10.1016/j.csm.2015.08.001.
82. Kibler WB, Sciascia A. Current practice for the surgical treatment of SLAP lesions: a systematic review. *Arthroscopy.* 2016;32(4):669-683. doi:10.1016/j.arthro.2015.08.041.
83. Yoo JC, Ahn JH, Lee SH, et al. A biomechanical comparison of repair techniques in posterior type II superior labral anterior and posterior (SLAP) lesions. *J Shoulder Elbow Surg.* 2008;17(1):144-149. doi:10.1016/j.jse.2007.03.025.
84. Mihata T, McGarry MH, Tibone JE, Fitzpatrick MJ, Kinoshita M, Lee TQ. Biomechanical assessment of type II superior labral anterior-posterior (SLAP) lesions associated with anterior shoulder capsular laxity as seen in throwers. *Am J Sports Med.* 2008;36(8):1604-1610. doi:10.1177/0363546508315198.
85. Boileau P, Parratte S, Chuinard C, Roussanne Y, Shia D, Bicknell R. Arthroscopic treatment of isolated type II slap lesions: biceps tenodesis as an alternative to reinsertion. *Am J Sports Med.* 2009;37(5):929-936. doi:10.1177/0363546508330127.
86. Chalmers PN, Monson B, Frank RM, et al. Combined SLAP repair and biceps tenodesis for superior labral anterior-posterior tears. *Knee Surgery Sports Traumatol Arthrosc.* 2016;24(12):3870-3876. doi:10.1007/s00167-015-3774-6.
87. Frank RM, Cotter EJ, Strauss EJ, Jazrawi LM, Romeo AA. Management of biceps tendon pathology. *J Am Acad Orthop Surg.* 2018;26(4):e77-e89. doi:10.5435/JAAOS-D-17-00085.
88. Kelly AM, Drakos MC, Fealy S, Taylor SA, O'Brien SJ. Arthroscopic release of the long head of the biceps tendon. *Am J Sports Med.* 2005;33(2):208-213. doi:10.1177/0363546504269555.
89. Erickson BJ, Jain A, Cvetanovich GL, et al. Biceps tenodesis: an evolution of treatment. *Am J Orthop (Belle Mead NJ).* 2017;46(4):E219-E223.
90. Romeo AA, Mazzocca AD, Tauro JC. Arthroscopic biceps tenodesis. *Arthroscopy.* 2004;20(2):206-213. doi:10.1016/j.arthro.2003.11.033.
91. Mazzocca AD, Rios CG, Romeo AA, Arciero RA. Subpectoral biceps tenodesis with interference screw fixation. *Arthroscopy.* 2005;21(7):1-7. doi:10.1016/j.arthro.2005.04.002.
92. Gombera MM, Kahlenberg CA, Nair R, Saltzman MD, Terry MA. All-arthroscopic suprapectoral versus open subpectoral tenodesis of the long head of the biceps brachii. *Am J Sports Med.* 2015;43(5):1077-1083. doi:10.1177/0363546515570024.
93. Werner BC, Lyons ML, Evans CL, et al. Arthroscopic suprapectoral and open subpectoral biceps tenodesis: a comparison of restoration of length-tension and mechanical strength between techniques. *Arthroscopy.* 2015;31(4):620-627. doi:10.1016/j.arthro.2014.10.012.
94. Werner BC, Evans CL, Holzgrefe RE, et al. Arthroscopic suprapectoral and open subpectoral biceps tenodesis: a comparison of minimum 2-year clinical outcomes. *Am J Sports Med.* 2014;42(11):2583-2590. doi:10.1177/0363546514547226.
95. Virk MS, Nicholson GP. Complications of proximal biceps tenotomy and tenodesis. *Clin Sports Med.* 2016;35(1):181-188. doi:10.1016/j.csm.2015.08.011.
96. Chalmers PN, Trombley R, Cip J, et al. Postoperative restoration of upper extremity motion and neuromuscular control during the overhand pitch: evaluation of tenodesis and repair for superior labral anterior-posterior tears. *Am J Sports Med.* 2014;42(12):2825-2836. doi:10.1177/0363546514551924.

97. Laughlin WA, Fleisig GS, Scillia AJ, Aune KT, Cain EL, Dugas JR. Deficiencies in pitching biomechanics in baseball players with a history of superior labrum anterior-posterior repair. *Am J Sports Med.* 2014;42(12):2837-2841. doi:10.1177/0363546514552183.
98. Gorantla K, Gill C, Wright RW. The outcome of type II SLAP repair: a systematic review. *Arthroscopy.* 2010;26(4):537-545. doi:10.1016/j.arthro.2009.08.017.
99. Sayde WM, Cohen SB, Ciccotti MG, Dodson CC. Return to play after type ii superior labral anterior-posterior lesion repairs in athletes: a systematic review. *Clin Orthop Relat Res.* 2012;470(6):1595-1600. doi:10.1007/s11999-012-2295-6.
100. Neri BR, Elattrache NS, Owsley KC, Mohr K, Yocum LA. Outcome of type II superior labral anterior posterior repairs in elite overhead athletes: effect of concomitant partial-thickness rotator cuff tears. *Am J Sports Med.* 2011;39(1):114-120. doi:10.1177/0363546510379971.
101. Provencher MT, McCormick F, Dewing C, McIntire S, Solomon D. A prospective analysis of 179 type 2 superior labrum anterior and posterior repairs: outcomes and factors associated with success and failure. *Am J Sports Med.* 2013;41(4):880-886. doi:10.1177/0363546513477363.
102. Schrøder CP, Skare Ø, Reikerås O, Mowinckel P, Brox JI. Sham surgery versus labral repair or biceps tenodesis for type II SLAP lesions of the shoulder: a three-armed randomised clinical trial. *Br J Sports Med.* 2017;51(24):1759-1766. doi:10.1136/bjsports-2016-097098.
103. Katz LM, Hsu S, Miller SL, et al. Poor outcomes after SLAP repair: descriptive analysis and prognosis. *Arthroscopy.* 2009;25(8):849-855. doi:10.1016/j.arthro.2009.02.022.
104. Taylor SA, Degen RM, White AE, et al. Risk factors for revision surgery after superior labral anterior-posterior repair: a national perspective. *Am J Sports Med.* 2017;45(7):1640-1644. doi:10.1177/0363546517691950.
105. Slenker NR, Lawson K, Ciccotti MG, Dodson CC, Cohen SB. Biceps tenotomy versus tenodesis: clinical outcomes. *Arthroscopy.* 2012;28(4):576-582. doi:10.1016/j.arthro.2011.10.017.

13

Shoulder Fractures

Christopher McDowell, DO and Luke Austin, MD

Sternoclavicular Injuries

- Epidemiology
  - Sternoclavicular (SC) injuries are rare: 3% of shoulder girdle injuries[1]
  - Eighty percent of SC joint dislocations are directly related to high-energy trauma: 47% motor vehicle accidents and 31% sports-related injury[2]
- Mechanism of injury (MOI)[3,4]
  - Direct: An anteromedial force applied to the junction of the medial clavicle creates a posterior dislocation.
  - Indirect: Force applied through aspects of the shoulder creates a dislocation of the SC joint in the opposite direction of the force, given the nature of the clavicle as a fulcrum.
- Radiographs and imaging
  - Anteroposterior chest radiograph
    - Asymmetry of the clavicle. The medial head of the clavicle may appear larger (anterior dislocation) or smaller (posterior dislocation) than the contralateral side.
  - Hobbs view[4]
    - The patient leans over the plate to obtain a 90-degree cephalocaudal lateral view. The beam is angled from behind the neck.
  - Serendipity view
    - X-ray is obtained with a 40-degree cephalic tilt in an anterior to posterior direction aimed at the manubrium. Anterior dislocation will show the medial clavicle above the interclavicular line, and posterior dislocation will show the medial clavicle below the interclavicular line.

Namdari S, Zmistowski B, Omid R, eds.
The Foundations of Shoulder and Elbow Surgery (pp 241-259).

- Computed tomography (CT)
  - CT is the best study for evaluation of subtle fracture lines, minor subluxation, and dislocations of the SC joint.
- Classification
  - Anatomic classification is based on the direction of the medial clavicle in relation to the sternum (eg, anterior vs posterior).
  - Sprain or subluxations[5]
    - Mild: stable joint with no compromise of ligaments
    - Moderate: subluxation in either direction with partial ligamentous disruptions
    - Severe: unstable joint with no intact ligaments
- Treatment
  - Acute (less than 10 days)
    - Anterior: Closed reduction using a direct posterior force on the medial clavicle with general anesthesia or conscious sedation. Application of figure-of-eight sling, clavicle strap or sling, and swathe for 4 to 6 weeks.[6]
    - Posterior: Prior to reduction, a general or vascular surgeon should be made aware and available if any of the posterior neurovascular structures are damaged during the reduction process. Closed or open reduction under general anesthesia is obtained using a towel clip attached to the medial clavicle applying a direct anterior force on the clavicle.[7]
  - Chronic (greater than 10 days)
    - Closed reduction was more likely to be successful if performed within 10 days.[5]
    - Chronic dislocations are managed nonoperatively as long as there are no signs of disruption to the mediastinal structures in a posterior dislocation.[4]
    - Chronic anterior dislocations have poor cosmesis, but function is not compromised.[4]

Acromioclavicular Injuries

- Epidemiology
  - Common in contact athletes and account for 40% to 50% of athletic shoulder injuries.[8]
  - Most common in second decade of life.[9]
  - Male-to-female ratio of 5:1[9]
- MOI
  - Failure of the acromioclavicular (AC) ligaments followed by the failure of the coracoclavicular (CC) ligaments and the deltotrapezial fascia.[9]
    - AC joint stability is a combination of the capsule, static, and dynamic structures.[10]
    - The capsule is the primary restraint of the distal clavicle in the anterior and posterior direction.
    - Static
      - AC ligaments (anterior, posterior, superior, inferior), CC ligaments (trapezoid and conoid), and coracoacromial ligaments
        - AC ligaments provide primary posterior and superior stability.
        - CC ligaments provide vertical stability.
    - Dynamic

    - Deltoid and trapezius
  - Direct: fall onto superolateral shoulder with arm adducted, generating an inferior and medial force through the acromion[11]
- Radiographs and imaging
  - Shoulder trauma series
    - AP shoulder, scapular-Y, and axillary views should be taken in the upright patient. The arm should not be supported to allow for gravity to pull on the injured side (eg, gravity stress).
  - Zanca view[12]
    - The Zanca view is the most accurate view when evaluating for AC injuries. X-ray is obtained in an anterior to posterior direction with 10 to 15 degrees of cephalic tilt. It should be obtained with comparison views to the contralateral limb to evaluate CC distance and native anatomy.
  - Stress view[12]
    - The stress view was historically used to help differentiate between type II and III injuries. It is no longer routinely used. Classically it was obtained with 10 to 15 pounds (4.5 to 6.8 kg) in the injured hand; an AP chest to include both shoulders was obtained to compare the amount of displacement of the injured AC joint to the contralateral side.
  - Cross-body adduction view
    - The cross-body adduction view is performed with the shoulder in adduction and the x-ray beam angled parallel to the body of the scapula.
    - It is positive when the distal clavicle rides over the top of the acromion, indicating higher-grade injury.
- Classification[9]
  - Rockwood classification for AC injuries
    - Type I: sprain of the AC ligament with normal radiographs
    - Type II: AC ligament tear, CC ligaments intact, distal clavicle unstable horizontally
    - Type III: AC and CC ligaments torn with displacement of the AC joint, distal clavicle unstable vertically and horizontally
    - Type IV: posterior displacement of the distal clavicle through the trapezius
    - Type V: displacement of the AC joint greater than 100%, deltoid and trapezius muscles detached
    - Type VI: dislocation of the AC joint with the clavicle displaced inferior to the acromion or coracoid
- Treatment
  - Nonoperative
    - Period of immobilization with sling or shoulder immobilizer should be prescribed
    - Resume a rehabilitation program once the pain has resolved, focusing on passive and active range of motion followed by strengthening.
    - Avoid contact sports for 2 to 3 months to allow for ligamentous healing.[13]
    - Nonoperative methods are indicated for types I to II and type III in the nonlaborer or recreational athlete.[14-16] *Recommended reading for classic description of acromioclavicular injuries*
    - The success of nonoperative management is improved with a supervised rehabilitation program.[17]
  - Operative
    - Types III and V[14]

        - These types are rarely treated surgically. Evidence shows more significant improvement in cosmesis than function.[15]
        - Operative methods are in high demand by overhead athletes or laborers.[16,18,19]
        - Persistent symptoms may warrant a delayed reconstruction.[17]
    - Type IV
        - Nonreducible dislocations indicate an entrapped distal clavicle into the trapezial fascia, requiring an open reduction and ligament reconstruction with fascial repair.
        - There are multiple surgical techniques. All have adequate outcomes if able to achieve a reduced AC joint that is stable in horizontal and vertical planes.[11,17,20-22]
    - Type VI
        - Type VI is a rare injury.
        - Nonreducible dislocations should be reduced with open reduction and ligament reconstruction.

Clavicle Fractures

- Epidemiology
    - Four percent of all fractures[23]
    - Forty-four percent are fractures of the shoulder girdle.[24]
    - Middle third fractures 80% of the time[24]
    - Distal clavicle 10% to 20%[25]
- MOI
    - Direct: Most occur as a fall onto the shoulder. The next most common mechanism is from direct impact (10%).[26]
- Radiographs and imaging
    - Standard upright views of the shoulder
        - If concerns for fracture, compare to the contralateral side
    - Clavicle trauma series
        - Four-view trauma series[27] (Figure 13-1)
            - Anterior-posterior view
            - Anterior-posterior with 20-degree cephalad tilt
            - Orthogonal views 45 degrees caudad and 45 degrees cephalad
        - Four-view radiographic series improves the interobserver reliability of initial displacement and surgeon's decision to treat.
    - CT
        - CT is useful to help delineate proximal-third fractures from SC joint dislocation and can identify intra-articular involvement.
    - Classification
        - Allman classification[28] as modified by Neer[29] and Craig[30]
            - Group I: middle-third fracture
            - Group II: distal-third fractures
                - Type I: minimally displaced, fracture distal to the intact CC ligaments
                - Type II: displaced with fracture medial to the CC ligaments
                    - IIA: conoid and trapezoid remain intact and attached to the distal segment.

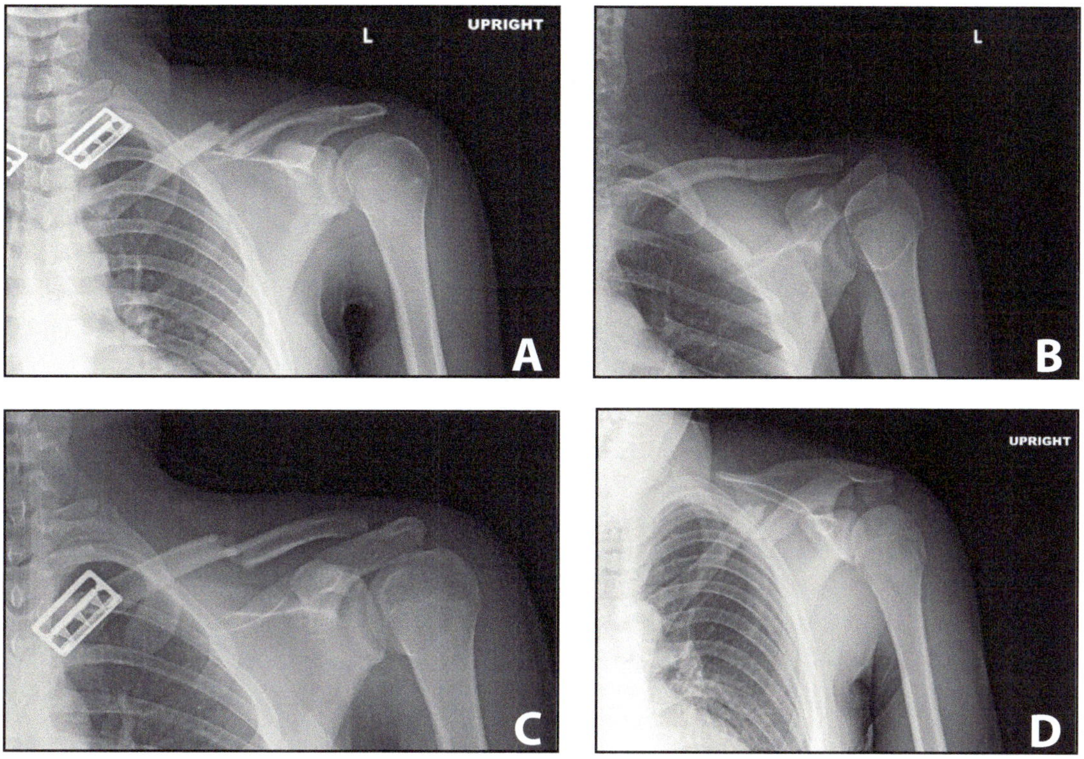

Figure 13-1. (A) Upright anteroposterior view of a left-displaced midshaft clavicle fracture. (B) Upright anteroposterior view with 20-degree cephalic tilt of a left-displaced midshaft fracture. (C) Upright orthogonal view with 45-degree cephalad tilt. (D) Upright orthogonal view with 45-degree caudal tilt.

        - IIB: conoid torn, trapezoid remains intact and attached to the distal segment
      - Type III: fracture of the articular surface of the AC joint
      - Type IV: physeal separation
      - Type V: comminuted
    - Group III: Proximal-third fractures
      - Type I: minimally displaced
      - Type II: displaced
      - Type III: intra-articular
      - Type IV: physeal separation
      - Type V: comminuted
  - Nonoperative
    - Nonoperative procedures are recommended for most minimally displaced fractures.
    - Use of a sling for comfort is recommended. The figure-of-eight bandage is no longer recommended.[31]
    - The period of immobilization is typically 4 to 6 weeks.[32,33]
    - Functional outcomes of a united midshaft clavicle fracture are good in nonoperative and operative patients.[32,34] *Recommended reading for level-one evidence of clavicle fracture management*
    - Pediatric clavicle fractures[35]
      - No significant differences in the functional outcome and range of motion when compared to operative fixation regardless of initial fracture pattern and displacement

- Operative
  - Group I (midshaft)
    - Accepted indications include the following[34,36]:
      - Displaced fractures
        - Greater than 2 cm of shortening or 100% displacement in any plane
      - Open fracture or threatened skin
      - Neurovascular compromise
      - Floating shoulder (double disruption of the superior shoulder suspensory complex [SSSC]; eg, fractures of the glenoid neck and clavicle)
    - Open reduction and internal fixation (ORIF) or intramedullary fixation
      - No difference in long-term function or nonunion in fractures amenable to intramedullary fixation[37,38]
    - Decreased time to radiographic union and higher patient satisfaction at 6 weeks and 3 months with surgical intervention for displaced fractures[32,34]
    - For displaced midshaft clavicle fractures, the nonunion rate is 2% with plate fixation compared to 17% when treated nonoperatively.[39]
    - Surgical fixation provides improved outcome in patients with risk factors of nonunion, including smoking, comminution, and displacement.[39]
  - Group II (lateral)
    - ORIF have shown to be a favorable treatment option with several described techniques.[40-42]
      - Indicated in type II (A and B nonunion rate up 33%) and type V[41]
      - Stabilization can be achieved with hook plate, ligament reconstruction, interfragmentary fixation, or K-wire.
  - Group III (medial)
    - ORIF with plate, suture, or interosseous wires[43]
      - Surgical management is rarely required, but indicated if mediastinal structures are currently at risk or may become at risk because of increased displacement.[36]

Scapula Fractures

- Fractures are rare and associated with high energy. The scapula can be subdivided further into specific anatomic landmarks.
  - Each bony prominence of the scapula has specific operative indications to maintain function of the shoulder.
- Epidemiology
  - Scapula fractures are rare and associated with high energy.
  - Ninety percent of patients have a concomitant injury:
    - Ipsilateral arm injury; 50%[44,45]
    - Thoracic injury; 80%[46]
    - Head injury; 48%[45]
    - Spinal fracture; 26%[45]
  - Patient mean age is 35 to 42 years old.[44]
  - Delayed diagnosis in 12.5% of cases is due to a high level of concomitant injuries.[47]

- MOI
  - Force vector directed from a lateral to medial direction pointed toward the thorax and neck, leading to a high rate of associated injuries.[44]
  - High-energy trauma: The scapula is well protected by surrounding musculature and has the ability to recoil and absorb energy prior to fracture.
- Radiographs and imaging
  - Standard trauma series
    - Because of the high-energy nature of the injury, the following are recommended: AP chest, lateral cervical spine, and AP pelvis to rule out concomitant injuries[48]
  - Shoulder trauma series
    - AP shoulder, scapular-Y, and axillary views are recommended.[49]
  - Anteroposterior view of shoulder (Grashey View)
    - The glenopolar angle measures the rotational malalignment of the glenoid about an AP axis perpendicular to the scapular plane.[50]
    - The angle formed by a line connecting the superior most point of the glenoid with the inferior most point of the glenoid intersecting with a line connecting the superior most point of the glenoid with the inferior most point of the scapular body. Normal is considered between 30 and 45 degrees.[50]
  - Stryker notch view
    - This is used when there is concern for a coracoid fracture.
    - The patient is supine with cassette behind the shoulder. The beam has a 10-degree cephalic tilt aiming toward the coracoid.
  - CT
    - Because of the complexity of injury and surrounding bony landmarks, CT scan is an effective modality to further delineate fracture patterns and associated injuries. Three-dimensional reconstructions are valuable in determining injury pattern.[51]

Scapular Body Fractures

- Treatment options
  - Nonoperative
    - Nondisplaced scapula fracture
      - The vast majority are nondisplaced or minimally displaced because of the strong nature of the surrounding ligaments.[52]
      - Sling use for 2 to 3 weeks with early passive range of motion exercise starting within 2 weeks are recommended.
    - Allow for management of associated injuries
  - Operative
    - Severe scapular malunion can lead to loss of motion, endurance, and dysfunction.[53]
    - Surgical indications[54]
      - Medial displacement of lateral border greater than 25 mm
      - Angular deformity greater than 45 degrees
      - Twenty-five percent glenoid involvement
      - Glenopolar angle less than 22 degrees
      - Floating shoulder: double disruption of shoulder suspensory complex (see as follows)

- ORIF[54] (Figure 13-2)
  - The Judet approach allows exposure to the scapula body, glenoid neck, posterior and inferior glenoid fragments, and the acromial process.
    - The posterior approach uses the internervous plane between the infraspinatus (suprascapular nerve) and teres minor (axillary nerve).

Glenoid Fractures

- Epidemiology
  - Thirty-eight percent of all scapula fractures[55]
- MOI
  - Direct: high energy of humeral head driving into the glenoid fossa[56,57]
  - The anterior and posterior rim fractures secondary to dislocation 8% of the time.[58]
  - Classification
    - Ideberg classification of intra-articular glenoid fractures[56,57]
      - Type I
        - IA: anterior glenoid rim fracture
        - IB: posterior glenoid rim fracture
      - Type II
        - IIA: transverse fracture through the glenoid fossa with inferior exit
        - IIB: oblique fracture through the glenoid fossa with inferior exit
      - Type III
        - Oblique fracture through the glenoid with superior exit
      - Type IV
        - Transverse fracture exiting through the medial border of the scapula, involving scapula neck and body
      - Type V
        - Combination of Types II, III, and IV
      - Type VI
        - Comminuted glenoid
  - Treatment options
    - Nonoperative
      - Non–displaced intra-articular glenoid fractures[59]
      - Sling for comfort, early passive range of motion within 2 weeks[57]
      - X-rays until radiographic union has occurred
    - Operative
      - Surgical indications
        - Greater than 4 mm articular step-off or fracture gap[59]
        - Twenty percent to 30% of articular surface involvement[56,57,59,60]
        - Glenohumeral instability[56,57,59,60]
      - ORIF
        - The Judet approach allows exposure to the scapula body, glenoid neck, posterior and inferior glenoid fragments, and the acromial process.
        - Anterior glenoid fragments and coracoid process are approached through the deltopectoral approach.[60]
        - Periarticular scapular-specific plates and 2.7 mm reconstruction plates are used for their ability to conform to the scapular surface.[60]

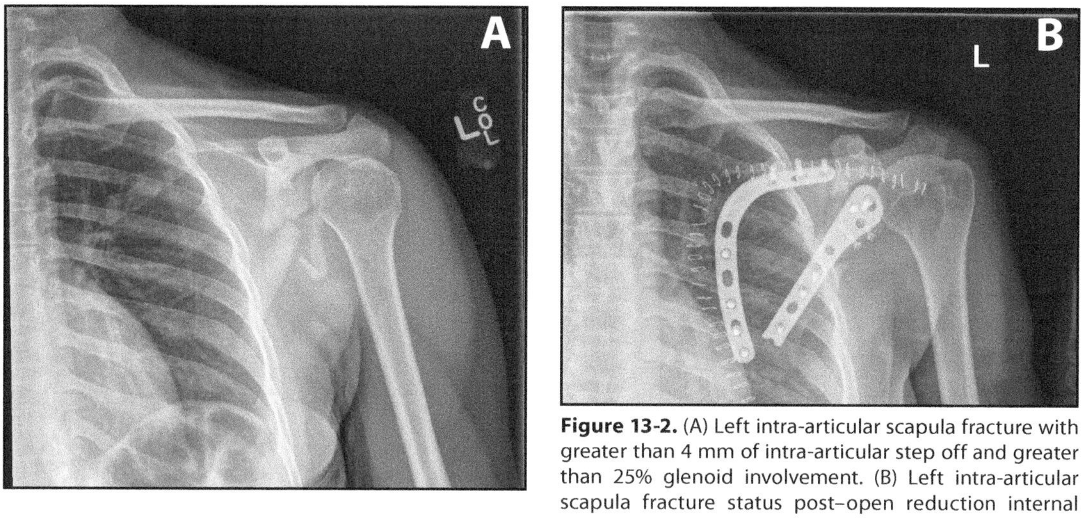

Figure 13-2. (A) Left intra-articular scapula fracture with greater than 4 mm of intra-articular step off and greater than 25% glenoid involvement. (B) Left intra-articular scapula fracture status post–open reduction internal fixation with periarticular scapular plates.

Acromial Fractures

- Epidemiology
  - Nine percent of scapula fractures[61]
- MOI
  - Direct: lateral force to shoulder[62]
  - Indirect: avulsion fractures from deltoid or AC ligament stress[61,63]
- Classification
  - Kuhn classification of acromial fractures[61]
    - Type I
      - Minimally displaced
      - IA: avulsion fractures associated with no direct trauma
      - IIB: direct trauma to the acromion
    - Type II
      - Displaced but subacromial space intact
    - Type III
      - Displaced and associated narrowing of the subacromial space
- Treatment options
  - Nonoperative
    - Minimally or nondisplaced fractures of the acromion[53]
    - Sling for comfort, begin passive range of motion when pain free[61]
    - X-rays until radiographic union
  - Operative indications have not been widely discussed. Proposed indications include the following[53]:
    - Painful nonunion
    - Concomitant operative ipsilateral scapular fracture
    - More than 1 cm displacement
    - Two disruptions in the SSSC

        - Kuhn type III fractures
    - ORIF using a neutralization plate with lag screw technique or tension band technique has been successfully described.[62,64,65]

Coracoid Fractures

- Epidemiology
    - Three percent to 13% of all scapula fractures[66]
    - Often associated with AC dislocation (up to 58% incidence), superior scapular margin (36%), clavicular fracture (20%), or acromial fracture (19.4%)[67]
- MOI
    - Most commonly through the base of the coracoid[68]
- Classification
    - Ogawa classification of coracoid fractures[67]
        - Type I
            - Proximal to the CC ligament
        - Type II
            - Distal to the CC ligament
- Treatment options
    - Nonoperative
        - Indicated in minimal or nondisplaced coracoid fractures and Ogawa type II fractures[67,68]
        - Sling for comfort, early range of motion when pain free[52]
    - Operative
        - Operative indications[67,69]
            - Painful nonunion
            - Concomitant operative ipsilateral scapular fracture
            - More than 1 cm displacement
            - Two disruptions in the SSSC
        - ORIF
            - Fixation with two 2.7-mm or 3.5-mm screws for base fractures. A plate may be added for additional stability.[65,69]

Floating Shoulder

- Epidemiology
    - Floating shoulder is rare, comprising 0.1% of all fractures.[70]
- MOI
    - High-energy trauma, often associated with injury to the chest, lung, or head.[70]
- Radiographs and imaging[70]
    - Standard trauma series
        - Standard trauma radiographs are necessary because of high-energy pattern; AP chest, lateral C-spine, and AP pelvis are recommended.[53]
    - Shoulder trauma series
        - AP shoulder, scapular-Y, axillary views

- Note the amount of displacement in key ligamentous structures and associated fractures.
- CT
  - It was previously believed that CT was not helpful in determining the amount of displacement of scapular neck displacement. However, with the development and advancement of 3-dimensional reconstructions, reformatted images are recommended for preoperative planning.[51]
- Classification
  - Double disruptions of the SSSC
    - SSSC was originally described by Goss as a bone and soft-tissue ring at the end of a superior and inferior bone strut.[52]
      - Superior strut: middle third of the clavicle
      - Inferior strut: lateral scapular body
  - Parts of the SSSC
    - Glenoid process
    - Coracoid
    - CC ligaments
    - Distal clavicle
    - AC joint
    - Acromion
    - Coracoacromial ligament[71] *Recommended reading for providing an understanding in decision making of superior shoulder suspensory complex injuries*
  - Unstable vs stable injuries
    - Double disruption of shoulder suspensory complex may indicate an unstable shoulder and require surgical repair.
    - Disruption of the AC and CC ligaments[71]
    - Combination of scapular neck fracture and ipsilateral clavicle fracture is the most common unstable pattern.[70,72]
- Treatment options
  - The literature has not supported repair of all floating shoulders.[73]
  - Nonoperative
    - Indication: minimally displaced fractures both in the scapular body and clavicle[49,70]
    - Intact AC and CC ligaments[71]
  - Operative
    - Indication: double disruption of SSSC leading to unstable shoulders in active individuals
    - Preoperative planning is important to determine which bony and ligamentous structures are leading to the shoulder instability.
    - ORIF, repair, and reconstruction should be tailored to each patient's specific injury.

Scapulothoracic Dissociation

- Epidemiology[74]
  - Rare, life-threatening injury

  - Mortality: 10% of cases
  - Flail extremity: 52% of cases
  - Early above-elbow amputation: 21% of cases
- MOI
  - Direct force over shoulder with traction applied to the upper extremity[52]
  - High-energy distraction force[75]
  - Forty-four percent to 50% of patients are involved in motorcycle crashes.
  - Thirty-five percent are involved in automobile crashes.[74]
- Radiographs and imaging
  - Anteroposterior chest view
    - Increased soft-tissue density around the scapula indicates a hematoma from a muscular or vascular insult. Disruption of bony landmarks at the AC joint, clavicle, or SC joint.
    - A scapular index greater than 1.29 is consistent with scapulothoracic dissociation.[76,77]
      - The ratio of the distance from the thoracic spinous process to the medial border of the scapula on the injured side to normal side
  - Computed tomography angiography (CTA)
    - CTA is necessary to identify any vascular insult.
  - Magnetic resonance imaging and CT myelography
    - Identify any neurological insult, with CT myelography being the modality of choice for identifying psuedomeningocele.[78]
- Classification
  - May be combination of a laterally displaced scapula with separation of the ipsilateral AC joint, distracted clavicle fracture, SC joint disruption, disruption of the brachial plexus and subclavian vessels, and intact overlying skin[79-81]
  - Zelle classification of scapulothoracic dissociation[76]
    - Type I
      - Musculoskeletal injury alone
    - Type II
      - IIA: musculoskeletal injury with vascular disruption
      - IIB: musculoskeletal injury with neurologic impairment
    - Type III
      - Musculoskeletal injury with neurologic and vascular injury
    - Type IV
      - Musculoskeletal injury with complete brachial plexus avulsion
- Treatment options
  - Perform Advanced Trauma Life Support (ATLS) and maintain a high level of suspicion; usually associated with polytrauma and distracting injuries[75]
  - No established treatment algorithm; ongoing discussion with orthopedics, vascular and general surgery. Treatment is generally dictated by vascular injury in hopes to stop any ischemic insult.[75]
  - Stabilization of associated bone or joint injures is required.
  - Angiography and vascular repair performed as necessary
  - Delayed nerve transfer up to 6 months after injury has become a recent option compared to arthrodesis or above-elbow amputation.[82]
  - Electromyography at 3 to 4 weeks and repeat every 6 weeks for signs of neurologic recovery[83]

Proximal Humerus Fracture

- Epidemiology
  - Female-to-male ratio of 2:1
  - Fragility fracture
    - Increased incidence in the older population
  - Third most common fracture in patients older than 65 years old.[84,85]
  - The majority are nondisplaced.
- MOI
  - In older patients: fall from standing height onto an outstretched upper extremity
  - In younger patients: high-energy trauma (eg, motor vehicle accidents)
- Radiographs and imaging
  - Shoulder trauma series
    - AP, scapular-Y, and axillary view are recommended
  - CT
    - In the setting of 3-part or 4-part fractures, CT is helpful to evaluate for tuberosity, humeral bone stock, and for head splitting of greater than 50% articular involvement.[86]
- Classification
  - Neer classification for proximal humerus[87] *Recommended reading for establishing classification and management of proximal humerus fractures*
    - Four parts: greater tuberosity; lesser tuberosity; humeral shaft; and humeral head
    - A part is defined as displacement greater than 1 cm or greater than 45 degrees of angulation.
      - May have proximal fractures that are considered 1-part by Neer classification (eg, nondisplaced)
- Treatment options
  - Nonoperative treatment
    - Minimally displaced or nondisplaced fractures[88]
    - Patients who are medically unfit for surgery[88]
    - Nonoperative treatment of all proximal humerus fractures showed 98% radiographic union in a systematic review by Iyengar.[89]
      - Subsequent forward flexion was significantly affected, with the increasing amount of parts in nonoperative treatment with 151 degrees in 1-part compared to 127 degrees in a 4-part fracture.[89]
    - Short-term sling immobilization and early physical therapy[90] are recommended.
    - Frequent radiographs are required to follow for radiographic union.
  - Operative
    - Two-part
      - ORIF with locking-plate technology
        - Locking-screw technology has allowed for a more secure fixation in comminuted and osteoporotic bone.[86]
        - Surgical fixation is recommended if there is significant displacement, block to motion, and involvement of the anatomic neck.[86]
        - ORIF is recommended for greater tuberosity fracture greater than 5 mm displacement to reduce potential for subacromial impingement.[91]

- For displaced lesser tuberosity fracture, operative fixation restores function and range of motion.[92]
- Closed reduction and percutaneous pinning
  - Inferior to ORIF in stability[93]
  - Can be a reliable surgical option in patients with minimal comminution and a stable calcar
  - Must be able to achieve an adequate closed reduction
  - Pins must be placed in multiplanar fashion to achieve stability.[93]
- Intramedullary nail fixation (Figure 13-3)
  - Implant design updates have allowed for a resurgence in intramedullary nail fixation for specific fracture patterns.
  - Common indications: 2-part surgical neck fractures or concomitant humeral shaft fracture [94,95]
  - Allows for compression at fracture site

- Three-part and 4-part
  - ORIF
    - Three-part and 4-part fractures in active patients younger than 65 years[86]
  - Intramedullary nailing for select 3-part fractures[86]
    - ORIF with locking plates in valgus impacted 4-part fractures often require bone grafting.[96]
  - Hemiarthoplasty (Figure 13-4)
    - Anatomically reduced tuberosities and the presence of a functioning rotator cuff are required for success with hemiarthroplasty.
    - Technically challenging; tuberosity alignment, humeral height, and version are all variables that must be corrected.[97]
    - Performed in patients younger than 65 years old when ORIF is not a viable option
    - High rate of failure and need to convert to a reverse total shoulder arthroplasty[86,98]
  - Reverse total shoulder arthroplasty (Figure 13-5)
    - Surgical options for patients with acute 3- or 4-part fractures in those older than 65 years old with nonreconstructable tuberosities[86]
    - Associated with low complication rate and minor impairment when compared to the contralateral side[99]
    - Improved forward flexion and functional outcomes when compared to a hemiarthroplasty in older patients[100]
    - May also be used to salvage a failed nonoperative treatment, ORIF, or hemiarthoplasty[86]

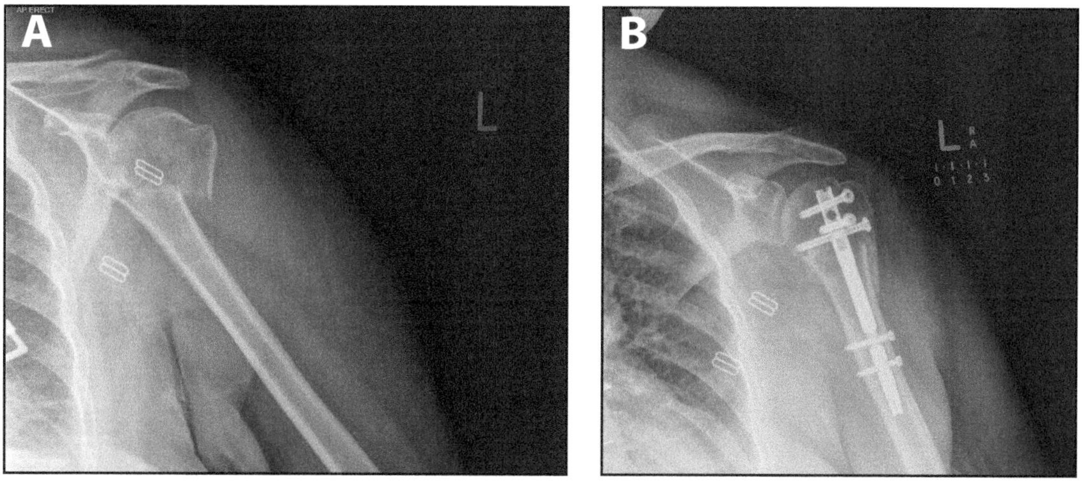

Figure 13-3. (A) Left 2-part surgical neck proximal humerus fracture. (B) Left 2-part surgical neck proximal humerus fracture status postintramedullary nailing.

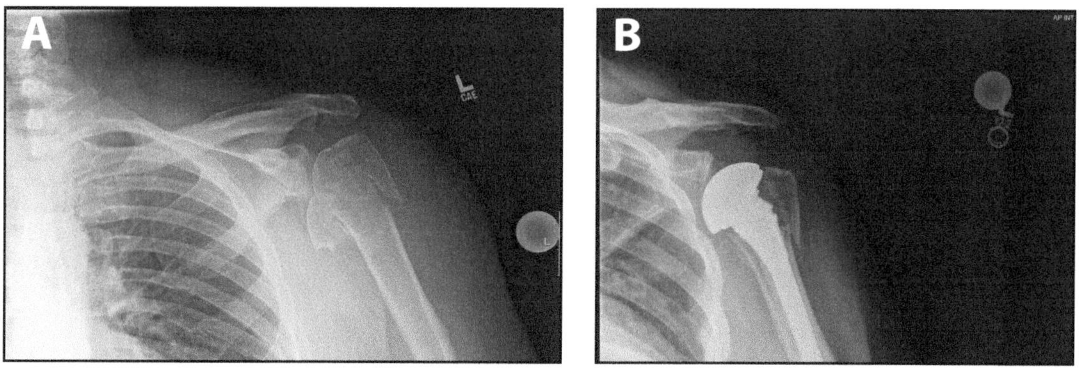

Figure 13-4. (A) Left 4-part proximal humerus fracture. (B) Left 4-part proximal humerus fracture status posthemiarthroplasty.

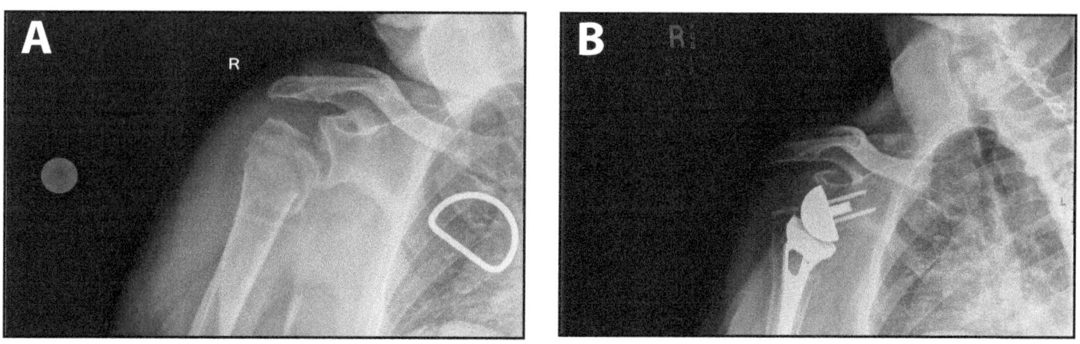

Figure 13-5. (A) Right 4-part proximal humerus fracture. (B) Right 4-part proximal humerus fracture status post–reverse total shoulder arthroplasty.

References

1. Cave EF. Shoulder girdle injuries. In: Cave EF, ed. *Fractures and Other Injuries*. Chicago, IL: Year Book Publishers; 1958:258-259.
2. Nettles JL, Linscheid RL. Sternoclavicular dislocations. *J Trauma*. 1968;8(2):158-164. doi:10.1097/00005373-196803000-00004.
3. Wirth MA, Rockwood CA. Disorders of the sternoclavicular joint. In: Rockwood CA Jr, Matsen FA III, Wirth MA, Lippitt SB, eds. *The Shoulder*. 4th ed. Philadelphia, PA: Saunders Elsevier; 2009:527-556.
4. Wirth MA, Rockwood CA. Acute and chronic traumatic injuries of the sternoclavicular joint. *J Am Acad Orthop Surg*. 1996;4(5):268-278. doi:10.5435/00124635-199609000-00005.
5. Groh GI, Wirth MA. Management of traumatic sternoclavicular joint injuries. *J Am Acad Orthop Surg*. 2011;19(1):1-7. doi:10.5435/00124635-201101000-00001.
6. Féry A, Sommelet J. Sternoclavicular dislocations. Observations on the treatment and result of 49 cases [in French]. *Int Orthop*. 1988;12(3):187-195. doi:10.1007/bf00547162.
7. Groh GI, Wirth MA, Rockwood CA Jr. Treatment of traumatic posterior sternoclavicular joint dislocations. *J Shoulder Elbow Surg*. 2011;20(1):107-113. doi:10.1016/j.jse.2010.03.009.
8. Kaplan LD, Flanigan DC, Norwig J, Jost P, Bradley J. Prevalence and variance of shoulder injuries in elite collegiate football players. *Am J Sports Med*. 2005;33(8):1142-1146. doi:10.1177/0363546505274718.
9. Rockwood CJ, Williams G, Young D. Disorders of the acromioclavicular joint. In: Rockwood CJ, Matsen FA III, eds. *The Shoulder*. 2nd ed. Philadelphia, PA: Saunders Elsevier; 1998:483-553.
10. Fukuda K, Craig E, An KN, Cofield RH, Chao EY. Biomechanical study of the ligamentous system of the acromioclavicular joint. *J Bone Joint Surg Am*. 1986;68(3):434-440.
11. Rios CG, Arciero RA, Mazzocca AD. Anatomy of the clavicle and coracoid process for reconstruction of the coracoclavicular ligaments. *Am J Sports Med*. 2007;35(5):811-817. doi:10.1177/0363546506297536.
12. Mazzocca AD, Arciero RA, Bicos J. Evaluation and treatment of acromioclavicular joint injuries. *Am J Sports Med*. 2007;35(2):316-329. doi:10.1177/0363546506298022.
13. Simovitch R, Sanders B, Ozbaydar M, Lavery K, Warner JJ. Acromioclavicular joint injuries: diagnosis and management. *J Am Acad Orthop Surg*. 2009;17(4):207-219. doi:10.5435/00124635-200904000-00002.
14. Wojtys EM, Nelson G. Conservative treatment of Grade III acromioclavicular dislocations. *Clin Orthop Relat Res*. 1991(268):112-119.
15. Smith TO, Chester R, Pearse EO, Hing CB. Operative versus non-operative management following Rockwood grade III acromioclavicular separation: a meta-analysis of the current evidence base. *J Orthop Traumatol*. 2011;12(1):19-27. doi:10.1007/s10195-011-0127-1.
16. Gstettner C, Tauber M, Hitzl W, Resch H. Rockwood type III acromioclavicular dislocation: surgical versus conservative treatment. *J Shoulder Elbow Surg*. 2008;17(2):220-225. doi:10.1016/j.jse.2007.07.017.
17. Beitzel K, Cote MP, Apostolakos J, et al. Current concepts in the treatment of acromioclavicular joint dislocations. *Arthroscopy*. 2013;29(2):387-397. doi:10.1016/j.arthro.2012.11.023.
18. Korsten K, Gunning AC, Leenen LP. Operative or conservative treatment in patients with Rockwood type III acromioclavicular dislocation: a systematic review and update of current literature. *Int Orthop*. 2013;38(4):831-838. doi:10.1007/s00264-013-2143-7.
19. Bradley JP, Elkousy H. Decision making: operative versus nonoperative treatment of acromioclavicular joint injuries. *Clin Sports Med*. 2003;22(2):277-290.
20. Mazzocca AD, Santangelo SA, Johnson ST, Rios CG, Dumonski ML, Arciero RA. A biomechanical evaluation of an anatomical coracoclavicular ligament reconstruction. *Am J Sports Med*. 2006;34(2):236-246. doi:10.1177/0363546505281795.
21. Jari R, Costic RS, Rodosky MW, Debski RE. Biomechanical function of surgical procedures for acromioclavicular joint dislocations. *Arthroscopy*. 2004;20(3):237-245. doi:10.1016/j.arthro.2004.01.011.
22. Nuber GW, Bowen MK. Acromioclavicular joint injuries and distal clavicle fractures. *J Am Acad Orthop Surg*. 1997;5(1):11-18. doi:10.5435/00124635-199701000-00002.
23. Lenza M, Buchbinder R, Johnston RV, Belloti JC, Faloppa F. Surgical versus conservative interventions for treating fractures of the middle third of the clavicle. *Cochrane Database Syst Rev*. 2013;6(6):CD009363. doi:10.1002/14651858.CD009363.pub2.
24. Nowak J, Mallmin H, Larsson S. The etiology and epidemiology of clavicular fractures. A prospective study during a two-year period in Uppsala, Sweden. *Injury*. 2000;31(5):353-358. doi:10.1016/s0020-1383(99)00312-5.
25. Robinson CM, Cairns DA. Primary nonoperative treatment of displaced lateral fractures of the clavicle. *J Bone Joint Surg Am*. 2004;86(4):778-782. doi:10.2106/00004623-200404000-00016.
26. Stanley D, Trowbridge EA, Norris SH. The mechanism of clavicular fracture. A clinical and biomechanical analysis. *J Bone Joint Surg Br*. 1988;70(3):461-464.

27. Austin LS, O'Brien MJ, Zmistowski B, et al. Additional x-ray views increase decision to treat clavicular fracture surgically. *J Shoulder Elbow Surg.* 2012;21(10):1263-1268. doi:10.1016/j.jse.2011.08.050.
28. Allman FL Jr. Fractures and ligamentous injuries of the clavicle and its articulation. *J Bone Joint Surg Am.* 1967;49(4):774-784.
29. Neer CS II. Fractures of the distal third of the clavicle. *Clin Orthop Relat Res.* 1968;58:43-50.
30. Craig EV. Fractures of the clavicle. In: Rockwood CA Jr, Matsen FA 3rd, eds. *The Shoulder.* Philadelphia, PA: Saunders Elsevier; 1990:367-412.
31. Andersen K, Jensen PO, Lauritzen J. Treatment of clavicular fractures. Figure-of-eight versus a simple sling. *Acta Orthop Scand.* 1987;58(1):71-74. doi:10.3109/17453678709146346.
32. Ahrens PM, Garlick NI, Barber J, Tims EM, Clavicle Trial Collaborative Group. The Clavicle Trial: a multicenter randomized controlled trial comparing operative with nonoperative treatment of displaced midshaft clavicle fractures. *J Bone Joint Surg Am.* 2017;99(16):1345-1354. doi:10.2106/JBJS.16.01112.
33. Banerjee R, Waterman B, Padalecki J, Robertson W. Management of distal clavicle fractures. *J Am Acad Orthop Surg.* 2011;19(7):392-401. doi:10.5435/00124635-201107000-00002.
34. Canadian Orthopaedic Trauma Society. Nonoperative treatment compared with plate fixation of displaced midshaft clavicle fractures. A multicenter, randomized clinical trial. *J Bone Joint Surg Am.* 2007;89(1):1-10. doi:10.2106/JBJS.F.00020.
35. Hagstrom LS, Ferrick M, Galpin R. Outcomes of operative versus nonoperative treatment of displaced pediatric clavicle fractures. *Orthopedics.* 2015;38(2):e135-e138. doi:10.3928/01477447-20150204-62.
36. van der Meijden OA, Gaskill TR, Millett PJ. Treatment of clavicle fractures: current concepts review. *J Shoulder Elbow Surg.* 2012;21(3):423-429. doi:10.1016/j.jse.2011.08.053.
37. Houwert RM, Smeeing DP, Ali UA, Hietbrink F, Kruyt MC, van der Meijden OA. Plate fixation or intramedullary fixation for midshaft clavicle fractures: a systematic review and meta-analysis of randomized controlled trials and observational studies. *J Shoulder Elbow Surg.* 2016;25(7):1195-1203. doi:10.1016/j.jse.2016.01.018.
38. Fuglesang HFS, Flugsrud GB, Randsborg PH, Oord P, Benth JŠ, Utvåg SE. Plate fixation versus intramedullary nailing of completely displaced midshaft fractures of the clavicle: a prospective randomised controlled trial. *Bone Joint J.* 2017;99-B(8):1095-1101. doi:10.1302/0301-620X.99B8.BJJ-2016-1318.R1.
39. Woltz S, Krijnen P, Schipper IB. Plate fixation versus nonoperative treatment for displaced midshaft clavicular fractures: a meta-analysis of randomized controlled trials. *J Bone Joint Surg Am.* 2017;99(12):1051-1057. doi:10.2106/JBJS.16.01068.
40. Han L, Hu Y, Quan R, Fang W, Jin B, Huang L. Treatment of Neer IIb distal clavicle fractures using anatomical locked plate fixation with coracoclavicular ligament augmentation. *J Hand Surg Am.* 2017;42(12):1036.e1-1036.e6. doi:10.1016/j.jhsa.2017.08.005.
41. Oh JH, Kim SH, Lee JH, Shin SH, Gong HS. Treatment of clavicle fracture: a systematic review of treatment modalities in 425 fractures. *Arch Orthop Trauma Surg.* 2011;131(4):525-533. doi:10.1007/s00402-010-1196-y.
42. Kirsch JM, Blum L, Hake ME. distal clavicle fractures: open reduction and internal fixation with a hook plate. *J Orthop Trauma.* 2018;32(suppl 1):S2-S3. doi:10.1097/BOT.0000000000001214.
43. Sidhu VS, Hermans D, Duckworth DG. The operative outcomes of displaced medial-end clavicle fractures. *J Shoulder Elbow Surg.* 2015;24(11):1728-1734. doi:10.1016/j.jse.2015.04.011.
44. Veysi VT, Mittal R, Agarwal S, Dosani A, Giannoudis PV. Multiple trauma and scapula fractures: so what? *J Trauma.* 2003;55(6):1145-1457. doi:10.1097/01.TA.0000044499.76736.9D.
45. Tadros AM, Lunsjo K, Czechowski J, Abu-Zidan FM. Multiple-region scapular fractures had more severe chest injury than single-region fractures: a prospective study of 107 blunt trauma patients. *J Trauma.* 2007;63(4):889-893. doi:10.1097/01.ta.0000235876.32569.db.
46. Weening B, Walton C, Cole PA, Alanezi K, Hanson BP, Bhandari M. Lower mortality in patients with scapular fractures. *J Trauma.* 2005;59(6):1477-1481. doi:10.1097/01.ta.0000199191.14780.75.
47. Tadros AM, Lunsjo K, Czechowski J, Abu-Zidan FM. Causes of delayed diagnosis of scapular fractures. *Injury.* 2008;39(3):314-318. doi:10.1016/j.injury.2007.10.014.
48. Baldwin KD, Ohman-Strickland P, Mehta S, Hume E. Scapula fractures: a marker for concomitant injury? A retrospective review of data in the National Trauma Database. *J Trauma.* 2008;65(2):430-435. doi:10.1097/TA.0b013e31817fd928.
49. Schroder LK, Gauger EM, Gilbertson JA, Cole PA. Functional outcomes after operative management of extra-articular glenoid neck and scapular body fractures. *J Bone Joint Surg Am.* 2016;98(19):1623-1630. doi:10.2106/JBJS.15.01224.
50. Romero J, Schai P, Imhoff AB. Scapular neck fracture—the influence of permanent malalignment of the glenoid neck on clinical outcome. *Arch Orthop Trauma Surg.* 2001;121(6):313-316. doi:10.1007/s004020000224.
51. Armitage BM, Wijdicks CA, Tarkin IS, et al. Mapping of scapular fractures with three-dimensional computed tomography. *J Bone Joint Surg Am.* 2009;91(9):2222-2228. doi:10.2106/JBJS.H.00881.

52. Goss TP. Scapular fractures and dislocations: diagnosis and treatment. *J Am Acad Orthop Surg.* 1995;3(1):22-33. doi:10.5435/00124635-199501000-00004.
53. Cole PA, Gauger EM, Schroder LK. Management of scapular fractures. *J Am Acad Orthop Surg.* 2012;20(3):130-141. doi:10.5435/JAAOS-20-03-130.
54. Jones CB, Cornelius JP, Sietsema DL, Ringler JR, Endres TJ. Modified Judet approach and minifragment fixation of scapular body and glenoid neck fractures. *J Orthop Trauma.* 2009;23(8):558-564. doi:10.1097/BOT.0b013e3181a18216.
55. Jaeger M, Lambert S, Südkamp NP, et al. The AO Foundation and Orthopaedic Trauma Association (AO/OTA) scapula fracture classification system: focus on glenoid fossa involvement. *J Shoulder Elbow Surg.* 2013;22(4):512-520. doi:10.1016/j.jse.2012.08.003.
56. Ideberg R. Fractures of the scapula involving the glenoid fossa. In: Bateman JE, Welsh RP, eds. *Surgery of the Shoulder.* Philadelphia, PA: BC Decker; 1984:63.
57. Goss TP. Fractures of the glenoid cavity. *J Bone Joint Surg Am.* 1992;74(2):299-305.
58. Hovelius L. Anterior dislocation of the shoulder in teen-agers and young adults. Five year prognosis. *J Bone Joint Surg Am.* 1987;69(3):393-399.
59. Anavian J, Khanna G, Plocher EK, Wijdicks CA, Cole PA. Progressive displacement of scapula fractures. *J Trauma.* 2010;69(1):156-161. doi:10.1097/TA.0b013e3181b40393.
60. Mayo KA, Benirschke SK, Mast JW. Displaced fractures of the glenoid fossa. Results of open reduction and internal fixation. *Clin Orthop Relat Res.* 1998;(347):122-130.
61. Kuhn JE, Blasier RB, Carpenter JE. Fractures of the acromion process: a proposed classification system. *J Orthop Trauma.* 1994;8(1):6-13. doi:10.1097/00005131-199402000-00002.
62. Hill BW, Anavian J, Jacobson AR, Cole PA. Surgical management of isolated acromion fractures: technical tricks and clinical experience. *J Orthop Trauma.* 2014;28(5):e107-e113. doi:10.1097/BOT.0000000000000040.
63. Warner JJ, Port J. Stress fracture of the acromion. *J Shoulder Elbow Surg.* 1994;3(4):262-265. doi:10.1016/S1058-2746(09)80045-1.
64. Ogawa K, Naniwa T. Fractures of the acromion and the lateral scapular spine. *J Shoulder Elbow Surg.* 1997;6(6):544-548. doi:10.1016/s1058-2746(97)90087-2.
65. Anavian J, Wijdicks CA, Schroder LK, Vang S, Cole PA. Surgery for scapula process fractures: good outcome in 26 patients. *Acta Orthop.* 2009;80(3):344-350. doi:10.3109/17453670903025394.
66. McGinnis M, Denton JR. Fractures of the scapula: a retrospective study of 40 fractured scapulae. *J Trauma.* 1989;29(11):1488-1493.
67. Ogawa K, Yoshida A, Takahashi M, et al. Fractures of the coracoid process. *J Bone Joint Surg Br.* 1997;79(1):17-19. doi:10.1302/0301-620x.79b1.6912.
68. Butters KP. Fractures and dislocations of the scapula. In: Rockwood CA Jr, Green DP, Bucholz RW, Heckman JD, eds. *Fractures in Adults.* 4th ed. Philadelphia, PA: Lippincott-Raven; 1996:1163-1164.
69. Hill BW, Jacobson AR, Anavian J, Cole PA. Surgical management of coracoid fractures: technical tricks and clinical experience. *J Orthop Trauma.* 2014;28(5):e114-e122. doi:10.1097/01.bot.0000435632.71393.bb.
70. DeFranco MJ, Patterson BM. The floating shoulder. *J Am Acad Orthop Surg.* 2006;14(8):499-509. doi:10.5435/00124635-200608000-00007.
71. Williams GR Jr, Naranja J, Klimkiewicz J, Karduna A, Iannotti JP, Ramsey M. The floating shoulder: a biomechanical basis for classification and management. *J Bone Joint Surg Am.* 2001;83(8):1182-1187. doi:10.2106/00004623-200108000-00007.
72. Edwards SG, Whittle AP, Wood GW II. Nonoperative treatment of ipsilateral fractures of the scapula and clavicle. *J Bone Joint Surg Am.* 2000;82(6):774-780. doi:10.2106/00004623-200006000-00003.
73. Egol KA, Connor PM, Karunakar MA, Sims SH, Bosse MJ, Kellam JF. The floating shoulder: clinical and functional results. *J Bone Joint Surg Am.* 2001;83(8):1188-1194. doi:10.2106/00004623-200108000-00008.
74. Damschen DD, Cogbill TH, Siegel MJ. Scapulothoracic dissociation caused by blunt trauma. *J Trauma.* 1997;42(3):537-540.doi:10.1097/00005373-199703000-00024.
75. Choo AM, Schottel PC, Burgess AR. Scapulothoracic dissociation: evaluation and management. *J Am Acad Orthop Surg.* 2017;25(5):339-347. doi:10.5435/JAAOS-D-15-00509.
76. Zelle BA, Pape HC, Gerich TG, Garapati R, Ceylan B, Krettek C. Functional outcome following scapulothoracic dissociation. *J Bone Joint Surg Am.* 2004;86(1):2-8. doi:10.2106/00004623-200401000-00002.
77. Kelbel JM, Jardon OM, Huurman WW. Scapulothoracic dissociation: a case report. *Clin Orthop Relat Res.* 1986;(209):210-214.
78. Giuffre JL, Kakar S, Bishop AT, Spinner RJ, Shin AY. Current concepts of the treatment of adult brachial plexus injuries. *J Hand Surg Am.* 2010;35(4):678-688. doi:10.1016/j.jhsa.2010.01.021.
79. Oreck SL, Burgess A, Levine AM. Traumatic lateral displacement of the scapula: a radiographic sign of neurovascular disruption. *J Bone Joint Surg Am.* 1984;66(5):758-763.

80. Ebraheim NA, Pearlstein SR, Savolaine ER, Gordon SL, Jackson WT, Corray T. Scapulothoracic dissociation (closed avulsion of the scapula, subclavian artery, and brachial plexus): a newly recognized variant, a new classification, and a review of the literature and treatment options. *J Orthop Trauma.* 1987;1(1):18-23. doi:10.1097/00005131-198701010-00003.
81. Rubenstein JD, Ebraheim NA, Kellam JF. Traumatic scapulothoracic dissociation. *Radiology.* 1985;157(2):297-298. doi:10.1148/radiology.157.2.4048434.
82. Masmejean EH, Asfazadourian H, Alnot JY. Brachial plexus injuries in scapulothoracic dissociation. *J Hand Surg Br.* 2000;25(4):336-340. doi:10.1054/jhsb.2000.0393.
83. O'Shea K, Feinberg JH, Wolfe SW. Imaging and electrodiagnostic work-up of acute adult brachial plexus injuries. *J Hand Surg Eur Vol.* 2011;36(9):747-759. doi:10.1177/1753193411422313.
84. Baron JA, Karagas M, Barrett J, et al. Basic epidemiology of fractures of the upper and lower limb among Americans over 65 years of age. *Epidemiology.* 1996;7(6):612-618. doi:10.1097/00001648-199611000-00008.
85. Gupta AK, Harris JD, Erickson BJ, et al. Surgical management of complex proximal humerus fractures—a systematic review of 92 studies including 4500 patients. *J Orthop Trauma.* 2015;29(1):54-59. doi:10.1097/BOT.0000000000000229.
86. Kancherla VK, Singh A, Anakwenze OA. Management of acute proximal humeral fractures. *J Am Acad Orthop Surg.* 2017;25(1):42-52. doi:10.5435/JAAOS-D-15-00240.
87. Neer CS II. Displaced proximal humeral fractures. I. Classification and evaluation. *J Bone Joint Surg Am.* 1970;52(6):1077-1089.
88. Acevedo DC, Vanbeek C, Lazarus MD, Williams GR, Abboud JA. Reverse shoulder arthroplasty for proximal humeral fractures: update on indications, technique, and results. *J Shoulder Elbow Surg.* 2014;23(2):279-289. doi:10.1016/j.jse.2013.10.003.
89. Iyengar JJ, Devcic Z, Sproul RC, Feeley BT. Nonoperative treatment of proximal humerus fractures: a systematic review. *J Orthop Trauma.* 2011;25(10):612-617. doi:10.1097/BOT.0b013e3182008df8.
90. Hanson B, Neidenbach P, de Boer P, Stengel D. Functional outcomes after nonoperative management of fractures of the proximal humerus. *J Shoulder Elbow Surg.* 2009;18(4):612-621. doi:10.1016/j.jse.2009.03.024.
91. Platzer P, Kutscha-Lissberg F, Lehr S, Vecsei V, Gaebler C. The influence of displacement on shoulder function in patients with minimally displaced fractures of the greater tuberosity. *Injury.* 2005;36(10):1185-1189. doi:10.1016/j.injury.2005.02.018.
92. Robinson CM, Teoh KH, Baker A, Bell L. Fractures of the lesser tuberosity of the humerus. *J Bone Joint Surg Am.* 2009;91(3):512-520. doi:10.2106/JBJS.H.00409.
93. Magovern B, Ramsey ML. Percutaneous fixation of proximal humerus fractures. *Orthop Clin North Am.* 2008;39(4):405-416. doi:10.1016/j.ocl.2008.05.005.
94. Gradl G, Dietze A, Kääb M, Hopfenmüller W, Mittlmeier T. Is locking nailing of humeral head fractures superior to locking plate fixation? *Clin Orthop Relat Res.* 2009;467(11):2986-2993. doi:10.1007/s11999-009-0916-5.
95. Aaron D, Shatsky J, Paredes JC, Jiang C, Parsons BO, Flatow EL. Proximal humeral fractures: Internal fixation. *Instr Course Lect.* 2013;62:143-154.
96. Kim SH, Lee YH, Chung SW, et al. Outcomes for four-part proximal humerus fractures treated with a locking compression plate and an autologous iliac bone impaction graft. *Injury.* 2012;43(10):1724-1731. doi:10.1016/j.injury.2012.06.029.
97. Boileau P, Krishnan SG, Tinsi L, Walch G, Coste JS, Molé D. Tuberosity malposition and migration: reasons for poor outcomes after hemiarthroplasty for displaced fractures of the proximal humerus. *J Shoulder Elbow Surg.* 2002;11(5):401-412. doi:10.1067/mse.2002.124527.
98. Reppetto I, Alessio-Mazzola M, Cerruti, Sanguineti, Formica M, Felli L. Surgical management of complex proximal humeral fractures: pinning, locked plate and arthroplasty: clinical results and functional outcome on retrospective series of patients. *Musculoskelet Surg.* 2017;101(1):153-158. doi:10.1007/s12306-017-0451-6.
99. Schliemann B, Theisen C, Kösters C, Raschke MJ, Weimann A. Reverse total shoulder arthroplasty for type I fracture sequelae after internal fixation of proximal humerus fractures. *Arch Orthop Trauma Surg.* 2017;137(12):1677-1683. doi:10.1007/s00402-017-2789-5.
100. Mata-Fink A, Meinke M, Jones C, Kim B, Bell JE. Reverse shoulder arthroplasty for treatment of proximal humeral fractures in older adults: a systematic review. *J Shoulder Elbow Surg.* 2013;22(12):1737-1748. doi:10.1016/j.jse.2013.08.021.

14

Shoulder Arthritis
Glenohumeral Arthritis

Wayne W. Chan, MD, PhD; Surena Namdari, MD, MSc; and Gerald R. Williams Jr, MD

- Arthritis is a general term used to describe a wide range of pathologic conditions that result in loss of cartilage at the joint surfaces.
- The shoulder (ie, glenohumeral [GH] joint) is the third most commonly affected large joint, after the hip and knee.
- Etiologies of GH arthritis
  - Broadly categorized as osteoarthritis (OA), inflammatory arthritis, and other arthritides
  - Exact cause remains unclear
- OA can be divided into primary and secondary types.
  - Primary OA is without an identifiable etiology.
  - Secondary OA include post-traumatic (ie, instability or intra-articular fracture) and post-surgical (ie, capsulorrhaphy) arthritis.
- Inflammatory arthritides are systemic diseases.
  - Rheumatoid arthritis (RA) represents the most common form.
  - Arthritis from inflammatory bowel disease, ankylosing spondylitis (AS), and psoriatic arthritis are also in the family of inflammatory arthritides.
- Other arthritides encompasses a wide range of diagnoses.
  - Crystal deposition diseases (gout and pseudogout) can involve the shoulder.
  - Arthritis can be associated with acromegaly, GH dysplasia, neuropathic arthropathy, and septic arthropathy.
  - Atraumatic osteonecrosis or avascular necrosis (AVN) can result in humeral head subchondral bone collapse and may be secondary to systemic corticosteroid use, alcoholism, Gaucher disease, sickle cell disease, and irradiation.
  - Rotator cuff tear arthropathy (RCTA) is a unique form of arthritis with well-known pathoanatomy but poorly understood etiology.

Namdari S, Zmistowski B, Omid R, eds.
The Foundations of Shoulder and Elbow Surgery (pp 261-283).

Diagnosis

- The majority of patients with GH arthritis can be diagnosed based on history, physical examination, and plain radiographs.
- Differential diagnoses
  - Cervical spine disease
  - Cardiac or pulmonary etiologies
  - Diaphragmatic irritation
  - Charcot arthropathy
  - Tumors
  - Acute trauma
- Specific clinical features are dependent on the type of arthritis.
  - The predominant symptom is shoulder pain that has worsened over time.
  - Initially, the pain occurs with use of the joint and is relieved by rest.
  - With disease progression, the pain and discomfort can be brought on by minimal activity and may even occur at rest and at nighttime.
  - Associated symptoms usually include stiffness, weakness, grinding, and clicking with movement and functional limitation of the affected arm.
  - Inflammatory arthritis: morning stiffness that improves throughout the day and swelling around the shoulder
- Physical examination
  - Decreased motion (active and passive) and crepitus
  - Generalized atrophy of the shoulder girdle muscles secondary to disuse
  - Other physical findings are more specific to the disease process.
- Imaging for shoulder arthritis
  - AP view in the scapular plane both in internal and ER and an axillary view[1]
  - The major indication for using computed tomography (CT) is to quantitate posterior glenoid erosion and version for operative planning.
    - Imaging can also assist in evaluating glenoid bone stock, central erosion, and rotator cuff muscle quality.[2]
  - Magnetic resonance imaging (MRI)
    - MRI is the preferred imaging modality in the setting of inflammatory arthritis.
    - MRI is helpful in quantifying rotator cuff tear size, retraction, muscle atrophy, and fatty degeneration,[3] which may be helpful in preoperative planning.

Specific Arthritides Affecting the Shoulder

Osteoarthritis

- Most common of all arthritis, OA is irreversible and progressive, characterized by focal loss of articular cartilage with hypertrophic reaction in the subchondral bone.
- Patients may present as early as 40 to 50 years old with shoulder pain and stiffness. More than 50% of patients are unable to sleep on the affected side and cannot perform common functional tasks.
- Etiologies: 2 major hypotheses[4,5]

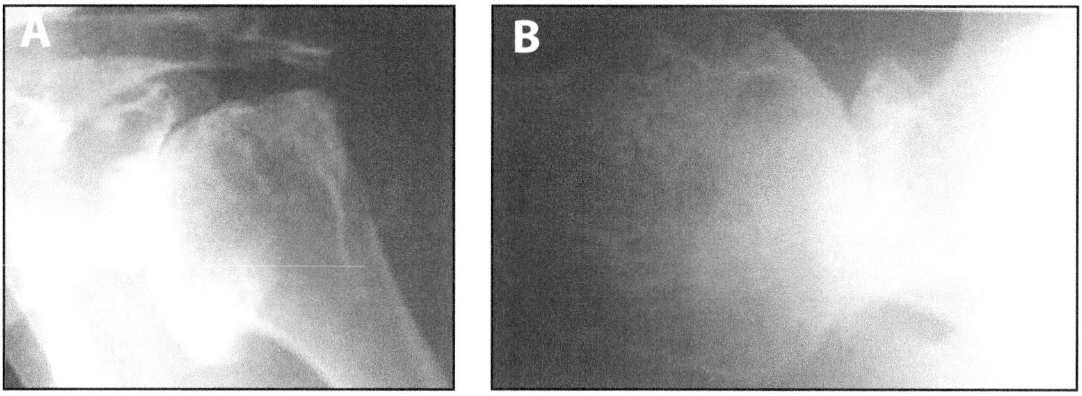

Figure 14-1. Radiographs of a patient with GH OA. (A) The AP view shows joint-space narrowing, subchondral sclerosis, and osteophytes on the inferior aspect of the humeral head and neck. (B) The axillary view is better for evaluating GH joint-space narrowing.

  - Physical forces cause failure of articular cartilage.
  - Failure of the regulation between degradation and repair of articular cartilage
  - Common pathway is eventual cartilage breakdown
  - Factors associated with the development of OA include the following:
    - Aging; trauma; and genetic factors
  - Although the shoulder is not considered a weight-bearing joint, the muscles around the shoulder can generate significant forces across the joint.
- Physical examination
  - A symmetric restriction both of active and passive motions is seen.
  - A greater loss of external rotation (ER) compared with internal rotation secondary to anterior soft-tissue contractures (capsule and subscapularis tendon) is seen.
    - Loss of ER is a more sensitive test of intra-articular disease than loss of elevation.
    - Anterior tightness can translate the humeral head posteriorly, leading to posterior glenoid wear in up to 45% of patients.
    - Chronic posterior subluxation can lead to attenuated posterior capsule
  - The rotator cuff is typically intact, with incidence of full-thickness tears around 5%
  - A slight prominence of the coracoid process and loss of normal shoulder contour is caused by a posteriorly subluxated humeral head in the setting of posterior glenoid wear.
  - Localized posterior joint line tenderness is also common.[6]
- Radiographic features
  - Asymmetrical joint-space narrowing, subchondral sclerosis, subchondral cyst formation, and osteophyte formation[7] (Figure 14-1)
  - Osteophyte formation is commonly seen on the inferior aspect of the humeral head and neck, but can also be present circumferentially. May envelope and tension adjacent capsule, contributing to loss of ER.
  - Axillary view is preferred for evaluating GH joint-space narrowing and can often show humeral head flattening that is not always appreciated on the anteroposterior (AP) view.
  - The axillary view can also give a rough estimate of posterior glenoid wear, humeral head subluxation, and glenoid version.
- Glenoid morphology

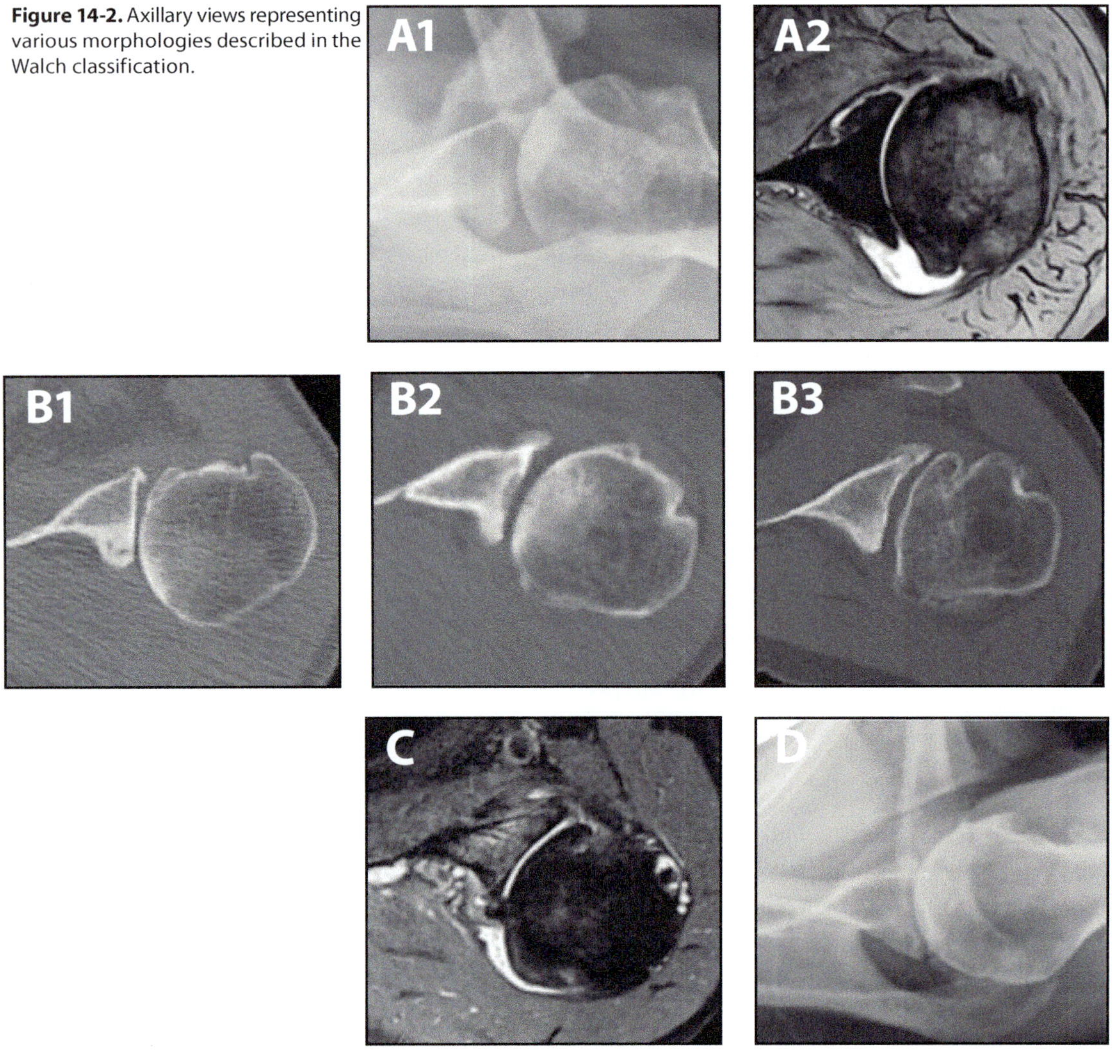

Figure 14-2. Axillary views representing various morphologies described in the Walch classification.

- Walch classification[8] *Recommended reading for updated classification of glenoid morphology* of glenoid morphology with OA (Figure 14-2)
  - Type A: The humeral head is centered, resulting from symmetric loads across the glenoid.
    - A1: minor erosion
    - A2: Major erosion marked by central erosion, leading to a centered glenoid cupula. A line connecting the anterior and posterior rims of the glenoid transects the humeral head.
  - Type B: The humeral head is subluxated posteriorly, with asymmetric distributed loads.
    - B1: shows narrowing of the posterior joint space, subchondral sclerosis, and osteophytes
    - B2: demonstrates a posterior cupula that gives an unusual biconcave aspect of the glenoid
    - B3: demonstrates severe glenoid wear, leading to loss of biconcavity
  - Type C: Defined by a glenoid retroversion of more than 25 degrees, regardless of the erosion.

        - Retroversion is dysplastic in origin, and the humeral head is well centered or slightly subluxated posteriorly
    - Type D: Defined by glenoid anteversion or anterior humeral head subluxation.

Rotator Cuff Tear Arthropathy

- RCTA is severe GH joint destruction that occurs in association with a chronic, massive rotator cuff defect.
- Clinical features of RCTA have been described in the literature since the 19th century; however, its pathogenesis remains elusive.
- Two main theories have been proposed.
    - In 1981, McCarty and colleagues[9] introduced the term *Milwaukee shoulder* to describe 4 patients with GH degenerative joint disease and rotator cuff defects whose joint fluid contained active collagenase, neutral proteinase, and hydroxyapatite crystals.
    - In 1983 Neer and colleagues[10] put forth the concept that mechanical and nutritional factors lead to RCTA. *Recommended reading for historical context*
- Characteristics
    - Rotator cuff insufficiency
    - Degenerative changes of the GH joint
    - Superior migration of the humeral head
    - Recurrent (often hemorrhagic) effusions
- Limited active elevation of the shoulder is the most significant physical examination finding
    - Loss of motion is related to the rotator cuff deficiency
    - GH incongruity that results from the high-riding humeral head
    - Marked atrophy of the supraspinatus and infraspinatus muscles, and patients may also have recurrent swelling (ie, Codman's "fluid sign")
    - In the setting of an incompetent coracoacromial arch as a static humeral head restraint, patients will have superior escape of the humeral head and "pseudoparalysis" of the arm
- Radiographic features
    - Osteopenia, proximal humeral head migration, narrowing or obliteration of the acromiohumeral space, acromial erosions, and superior glenoid bone loss (Figure 14-3)
    - Humeral head collapse, osteophytes, cyst formation, and subchondral sclerosis may also be seen.
    - Axillary view is useful for evaluating glenoid erosion and medial migration.
    - Anterior subluxation on the axillary view suggests anterosuperior escape.
- Although hemiarthroplasty with an anatomic, slightly oversized, or hooded humeral component was a historic treatment option for RCTA, the reverse shoulder arthroplasty has emerged as the procedure of choice with reasonable outcomes at long-term follow-up.[11,12]

Dislocation Arthropathy

- Dislocation arthropathy is GH arthritis occurring in the setting of a history of dislocation or after surgery for instability.
- Samilson and Prieto classification[13]
    - Mild arthrosis: evidence on the AP radiograph of an inferior humeral or glenoid osteophyte, or both, measuring less than 3 mm

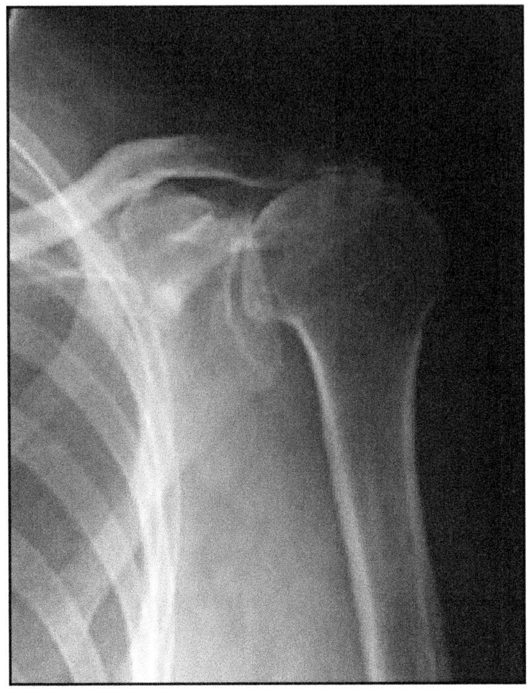

Figure 14-3. Radiograph of a patient with cuff tear arthropathy, showing osteopenia, proximal humeral head migration, narrowing of the acromiohumeral space, acromion erosions, and superior glenoid bone loss.

  - Moderate arthrosis: evidence on the AP radiograph of an inferior humeral or glenoid osteophyte, or both, measuring 3 to 7 mm, with slight GH joint irregularity
  - Severe arthrosis: evidence on the AP radiograph of an inferior humeral or glenoid osteophyte, or both, measuring greater than 7 mm, with GH narrowing and sclerosis
- GH dislocation requiring reduction is associated with a 10-fold to 20-fold increase in the risk of subsequent development of severe arthrosis.[14]
- The most common cause of arthritis in patients younger than 50 years old undergoing total shoulder arthroplasty (TSA) is capsulorrhaphy.[15]
  - Often results from excessive tightening of the soft tissues
  - When performed for anterior instability, there is a loss of ER.
  - Humeral head shifts posteriorly (eccentric load on the glenoid) posterior glenoid wear
- Hovelius conducted a 10-year[16] and 25-year[17] prospective study in patients following traumatic dislocation.
  - There was a 26% incidence of moderate to severe arthropathy at 25 years, compared to 9% after 10 years.
  - Advanced arthritis can occur even after a single GH dislocation without surgery.
  - Surgically stabilized shoulders did not differ from solitary dislocations in development of arthropathy (21% vs 17%), but had a lower incidence of arthropathy compared to shoulders that stabilized over time (21% vs 43%).
  - Factors affecting development of arthritis[17]
    - Older than 25 years old at first dislocation associated with less arthropathy
    - Recurrent dislocation
    - Injury sustained during high-energy sports
    - Person with alcoholism

Osteonecrosis

- Death of bone tissue
- Can be classified as traumatic or atraumatic
- Bone death (both osteocytes and marrow contents) can have numerous causes.
  - Steroid ingestion is the predominant identifiable risk factor (short-term use as well as intra-articular injections).
  - Excessive intake of alcohol
  - Gaucher disease, trauma, sickle cell disease, and many more
- Humeral head blood supply
  - The posterior humeral circumflex artery provides about two-thirds of the blood supply.[18] *Recommended reading for study design and clinical importance*
- At the time of collapse, the overlying subchondral bone and cartilage remain intact.
  - Radiographically termed the *crescent sign*, it corresponds to the area of maximum joint reaction force.
  - Further loading results in complete segmental failure with incongruity of the subchondral bone.
- Ficat and Arlet system modified by Cruess[19]
  - Stage 1: subtle changes within the humeral head
  - Stage 2: Focal sclerosis without collapse. The AP view in ER will typically show this (as will MRI).
  - Stage 3: Collapse or crescent sign. There is no displacement of the articular surface greater than 1 to 2 mm.
  - Stage 4: displaced cartilaginous flap with humeral head softening and collapse
  - Stage 5: wear of the cartilage and bone both of the humerus and glenoid
- Treatment
  - Stage 1 disease (silent) is inoperable but there is some debate about core decompression.
  - Stage 2 disease is treated with core decompression ± bone grafting if the patient fails conservative treatment.
  - Stage 3 (subchondral fracture) and stage 4 (collapse) are treated with hemiarthroplasty.
  - Stage 5 (glenoid involvement) is treated with TSA.
  - In patients with atraumatic osteonecrosis, hemiarthroplasty and TSA can provide lasting pain relief and improved function.[20]

Rheumatoid Arthritis

- RA is a chronic, progressive inflammatory disease that affects multiple organ systems, including the musculoskeletal system.
- Etiology is thought to be an antigen-driven mechanism that results in activation of immune pathways, causing tissue destruction, especially in and around synovial joints.
- Incidence of RA has been reported to be between 20 and 40 per 100,000 white adults, with a prevalence rate of 0.5% to 2%.[21,22]
- There is a 2-fold to 4-fold higher frequency in women.[23-25]

- Clinical features
  - Morning joint stiffness and polyarticular arthritis
  - Shoulders are asymptomatic early in the inflammatory disease process, with only 4% of rheumatoid patients initially presenting with shoulder symptoms.[26]
  - Progression of the disease leads to as many as 91% of patients reporting shoulder symptoms.[27]
  - When the GH joint is involved, it is often bilateral and is usually associated with deformities of the hand and elbow.[28]
- Physical examination
  - Examination typically reveals boggy synovitis, generalized atrophy, and decreased active and passive ranges of motion.
  - In contrast to OA, the loss of active motion in RA is often greater than the loss of passive motion.
  - Higher prevalence of dysfunctional or torn rotator cuff tendons may also result in weakness and atrophy.
- Radiographic features of a rheumatoid shoulder parallel those of any joint affected by RA.[29]
  - Regional osteopenia, symmetrical joint-space narrowing, and juxta-articular erosions may be seen.
  - Erosions are best seen at the synovial reflection on the superior aspect of the humeral head.
  - Osteophytes are not a prominent feature, but may be present.
  - Central glenoid erosion may also be present on the AP view, seen as medialization of the glenoid joint surface.
  - In rotator cuff insufficiency, the AP view will help determine superior migration of the humerus, which contributes to superior glenoid erosion.
  - An axillary view is the best way to estimate joint-space narrowing as well as medial erosion of the glenoid surface with respect to the coracoid process (Figure 14-4A).
  - The extent of humeral head deformity associated with juxta-articular erosions is best evaluated with the axillary view and can be verified on MRI (Figure 14-4B).
- Neer identified 3 clinical types of RA involving the GH joint.
  1. Dry type is characterized by loss of joint space, formation of subchondral cysts, sclerosis, and marginal osteophytes (not unlike OA).
  2. Wet type results from proliferation of exuberant granulation tissue at the articular margins. Marginal erosions, sometimes quite large, are characteristic of this pattern.
  3. Wet resorptive type is the most destructive, characterized by centralization.
     - It evolves in response to a rapid and severe articular cartilage and bone loss.
     - Medial migration with the loss of bone mass results in a loss of the normal physical contour of the shoulder.
- Surgical management depends on the stage of disease
  - Patients with early disease may benefit from joint debridement, bursectomy, and synovectomy.
  - If glenoid bone stock is adequate and the humeral head can be centered on the glenoid by a functional cuff, TSA provides pain relief superior to hemiarthroplasty.[30,31]
  - In advanced disease, reverse total shoulder arthroscopy is often indicated because of significant bone loss or proximal humeral migration associated with rotator cuff dysfunction.[32,33]

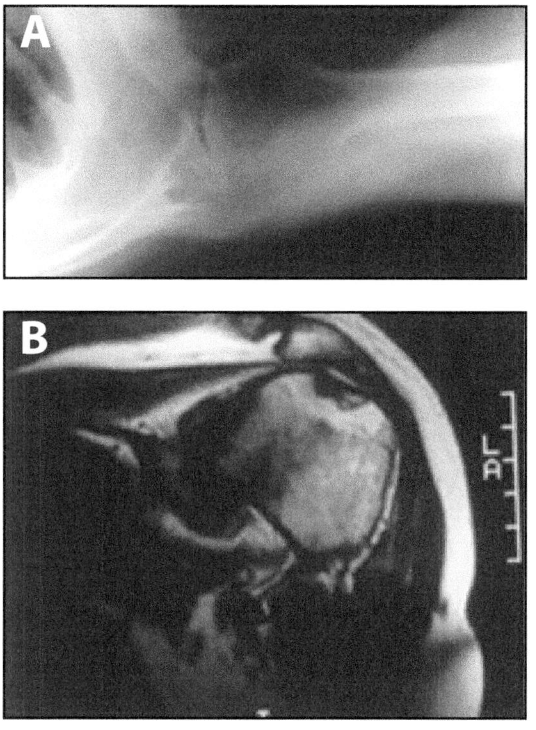

Figure 14-4. Axillary radiographs of a patient with RA of the shoulder. (A) There are marginal erosions of the humeral head and medialization of the glenoid joint surface beyond the base of the coracoid process. (B) MRI confirms the severe joint destruction with juxta-articular erosions, in addition to thinning of the superior cuff.

Rapidly Destructive Articular Disease

- Rapidly destructive articular disease (RDAD) is an unusual form of arthropathy recognized most often in the hip, and has been suspected to cause a similar condition in the shoulder.
- It is often seen in older women.
- Osteoporosis-induced subchondral insufficiency fracture may play a significant role in the pathogenesis of the disorder.

Dialysis Arthropathy

- As many as 50% to 69% of patients undergoing dialysis for end-stage renal disease develop dialysis arthropathy.
- Up to one-third of the time it involves the shoulder.
- ESRD and dialysis both contribute to the pathophysiology.
- Etiologies include amyloid depositions, oxalosis, nonbacterial infections (hepatitis C), apatite crystal deposition, and iron or aluminum overload.

Spondyloarthropathy

- Involvement of the shoulder typically occurs somewhat early in the disease process.
- Entities such as psoriatic arthritis, enteropathic arthritis, and AS are known to involve the shoulder.
- In AS, the frequent involvement of the hips and shoulder (50%) follows spinal involvement. Sometimes the first symptoms are in the shoulder, and bilateral involvement is common.

Figure 14-5. Plain radiograph of a patient with neuropathic shoulder. There is notable subchondral sclerosis, destruction of articular cartilage, and substantial deformity of the humeral head.

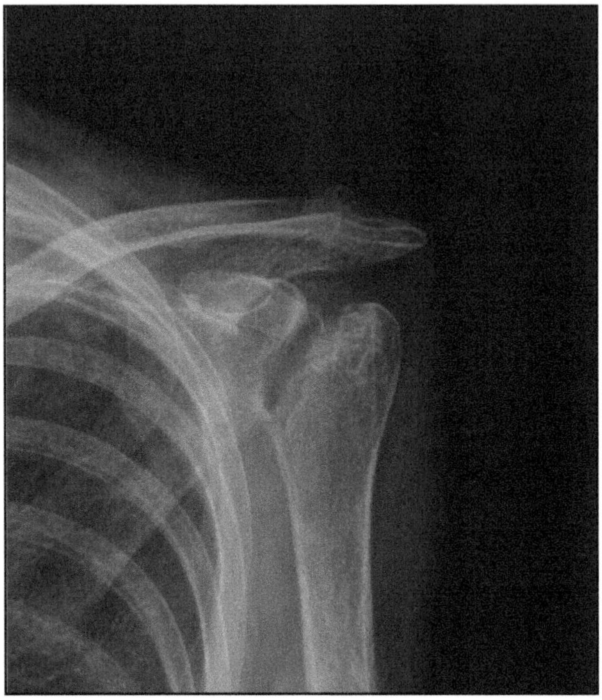

- The hatchet sign is a characteristic destructive abnormality and involves the superior lateral aspect of the humeral head. A rotator cuff tear often accompanies this lesion.
- Psoriatic arthritis involves the shoulder in 30% to 50% of patients.
- Reiter disease can cause acute shoulder pain in 8% of patients.
- Enteric arthritis parallels the activity of the inflammatory bowel disease. Shoulder involvement occurs in 5% to 10% of patients and is usually associated with sacroiliitis and spondylitis.

Neuropathic Arthropathy

- Syringomyelia is the most common cause of neuropathic arthropathy of the shoulder and occurs in 20% to 40% of patients with the disease (Figure 14-5).
- The shoulder is more commonly affected than the elbow.
- Other causes include diabetes mellitus, syphilis, and peripheral neuropathies.

Hemophilia Arthropathy

- GH arthropathy has been observed as a sequela to hemophilia.
- Shoulder involvement is more common in adults than in juveniles and proceeds slowly over the years, manifesting as erosions and thinning of the glenoid.

Endocrine/Metabolic Arthropathy

- Arthropathy associated with hemochromatosis can affect the shoulder.
- Ochronosis arthropathy affecting the spine and hips precedes shoulder involvement by many years.
- Acromegaly can result in peripheral joint arthropathy.
- Hyperparathyroidism can cause GH arthropathy.

Nonoperative Management of Shoulder Arthritis

- Physical therapy geared toward gentle stretching can help with shoulder stiffness. Aggressive strengthening can often exacerbate symptoms and should be avoided.
- For patients with an inflammatory component, an initial period of rest may be beneficial; however, extended rest can worsen symptoms and exacerbate stiffness.
- Cold treatment can be good for inflammatory flare-ups. The analgesic effects of cold have been attributed to depression of excitability of nerve fibers, decreasing pain.
- Dry heat may enhance joint motion and increases tissue elasticity, which can be beneficial in chronic arthritis.
- Occupational therapy can assist patients in addressing functional limitations (ability to dress and perform personal hygiene).
- Intra-articular corticosteroid injections can be effective in providing temporary pain relief. Corticosteroids can have negative effects on articular cartilage and should be used cautiously.
- Viscosupplementation of the GH joint remains controversial and is not currently approved by the Food and Drug Administration.

Surgical Management

- When nonoperative management strategies have been exhausted, there are several surgical options available to patients with GH arthritis.
  1. Arthroscopic joint debridement,[34-37] with or without capsular release
  2. Humeral hemiarthroplasty,[38-40] with or without glenoid reaming
  3. TSA[41-44]
  4. Reverse TSA[32,45-49] *Boileau et al[46] is recommended reading for historical context and adoption of new technology; Frankle et al[47] is recommended reading for historical context and adaptation of technology*
  5. Arthrodesis (limited role in the treatment of GH OA)

Debridement and Capsular Release

- Indicated in high-demand, young patients (typically less than 50 years old) with mild to moderate GH arthritis
- Effective procedure for pain relief and restoration of motion
- A nonconcentric or incongruent joint is a relative contraindication to debridement because the results have been poor.[37,50]
- Although the debridement can be done by open technique, most are performed arthroscopically.
- Arthroscopy can be both diagnostic and therapeutic for early-stage arthritis, especially in cases in which there are small focal lesions that are not easily seen by imaging studies.
- Though mechanical causes of pain and stiffness (loose bodies, unstable chondral flaps, capsular contracture, biceps tendon pathology, etc) can be treated arthroscopically, diffuse loss of articular cartilage cannot be restored. Because of this, results of arthroscopy in the setting of arthritis can be unpredictable.
- Outcomes

- Weinstein and colleagues[37] noted good to excellent outcomes in 80% of patients undergoing arthroscopic debridement for early GH OA.
  - The average age of the group was 46 years old, and all patients reported at least some improvement in pain.
  - At final follow-up (12 to 63 months), only 2 patients had reported a return of pain to preoperative levels. There was a trend toward increasing severity of articular cartilage damage and unfavorable results.
- Cameron and colleagues[34] reported on arthroscopic debridement of grade 4 GH articular lesions.
  - The procedure provided pain relief for at least 28 months in their patients.
  - Chondral lesions greater than 2 cm^2 were predictive of ultimate failure of the debridement.
- Skelley et al[51] examined 33 patients, with a mean age of 55 years old and grade II to IV chondral changes.
  - Pain and preoperative pain scores returned to baseline at 3.8 months, with 61% of the patients reporting dissatisfaction with the outcome.
  - Subsequently, 42% of the patients underwent a TSA at an average of 8.8 months.
  - Remaining patients had similar preoperative and postoperative American Shoulder and Elbow Surgeons (ASES) and visual analog scale scores.
- Mitchell and colleagues[52] described a more durable outcome.
  - At 5 years, 77% of patients with 49 shoulders avoided TSA.
  - The procedure includes chondroplasty, capsular release synovectomy, humeral osteoplasty, axillary nerve neurolysis, subacromial decompression, loose body removal, microfracture, and biceps tenodesis.

Hemiarthroplasty

- Hemiarthroplasty can be a reasonable option for arthritis that preserves glenoid bone stock.
- Although total shoulder arthroscopy is the procedure of choice for GH arthritis, there are several scenarios in which hemiarthroplasty is indicated.
  - A young patient with isolated humeral head arthrosis (ie, uninvolved glenoid) and an intact rotator cuff (such as in osteonecrosis or post-traumatic arthropathy)
  - Arthritis in the setting of an irreparable rotator cuff tear, proximal humeral head migration, and preserved preoperative active overhead elevation. Typically, this can be seen with RCTA, OA, or RA.
    - Prosthetic glenoid component under these conditions can prematurely loosen; therefore, hemiarthroplasty, or more commonly reverse TSA, is a better choice.
  - Inadequate glenoid bone stock to accept a prosthesis
- Outcomes
  - Levine and colleagues[53] followed 30 patients longitudinally who were treated with hemiarthroplasty for GH OA with an average follow-up of 17 years.
    - At final follow-up forward elevation improved from 104 degrees to 142 degrees and ER with the arm at 90-degrees abduction increased from 21 degrees to 61 degrees.
    - Only 25% of patients were satisfied at final follow-up.
    - Patients with concentric glenoid and primary OA fared better than those with eccentric wear and secondary OS.
  - Sperling and colleagues[44] prospectively followed 62 patients who underwent uncemented humeral hemiarthroplasty with a mean follow-up of 15 years.

        - Patients showed significant improvement in pain relief, active abduction, and ER.
        - Humeral periprosthetic lucency was present in 34% patients, and glenoid erosion was present in 72% of patients.
        - Outcomes were reported as excellent (10%), satisfactory (30%), and unsatisfactory; unsatisfactory results were related to motion restriction.
        - Implant survival was 82% at 10 years and 75% at 15 years.
- Hemiarthroplasty with glenoid reaming (ie, ream-and-run arthroplasty)
    - In patients who demand a high level of physical activity, a ream-and-run arthroplasty eliminates the concern for glenoid component failure (Figure 14-6).
    - Careful patient selection is required, as is a high level of technical expertise and dedication from the patient to consistent postoperative rehabilitation.
    - Described by Weldon and colleagues,[54] *Recommended reading for historical context and developing new techniques* it restores a concentric glenoid surface and stimulates fibrocartilage ingrowth.
        - A capsular release is performed while preserving the labrum.
        - Residual cartilage is curetted from the surface of the glenoid.
        - In patients with a notable biconcavity, a burr is used to smooth down the ridge prior to reaming the glenoid concentrically.
        - The goal of reaming is to achieve a concentric glenoid articulation while prioritizing preserving glenoid bone stock over normalizing glenoid version.
    - Results
        - Saltzman and colleagues[55] evaluated the ream-and-run procedure in patients younger than 55 years old and found significant functional and pain improvement.
        - Modest results were also achieved in the treatment of patients with a biconcave glenoid, with 75% survivorship with a mean follow-up of 3.7 years.[56]
        - Younger patients and early postoperative stiffness were associated with worse outcomes.[56]
- Interpositional arthroplasty
    - Alternative to prosthetic resurfacing of the glenoid, using either the lateral meniscus allograft or Achilles tendon allograft
    - Ball and colleagues first described the use of lateral meniscus for interpositional tissue.[57]
    - Krishnan and colleagues[38] reported on 36 shoulders in which they concluded that biological resurfacing of the glenoid can provide pain relief similar to total shoulder arthroscopy.
        - Achilles tendon allograft was their graft of choice for this procedure.
    - Nicholson and colleagues[58] concluded that glenoid resurfacing with lateral meniscus allograft was not perfect but did provide significant pain relief, increased range of motion, and patient satisfaction in the short-term.
    - Namdari and colleagues[59] performed a systematic review using a variety of tissue sources.
        - There were modest improvements in outcomes scores and a reoperation rate of 26%.
        - They reported a complication rate of 13%, including infection, stiffness, and brachial neuritis.
    - Puskas et al investigated their own prospective cohort, using either capsular interposition, meniscal allograft, or human dermal allograft combined with either a resurfacing or stemmed hemiarthroplasty.[60]

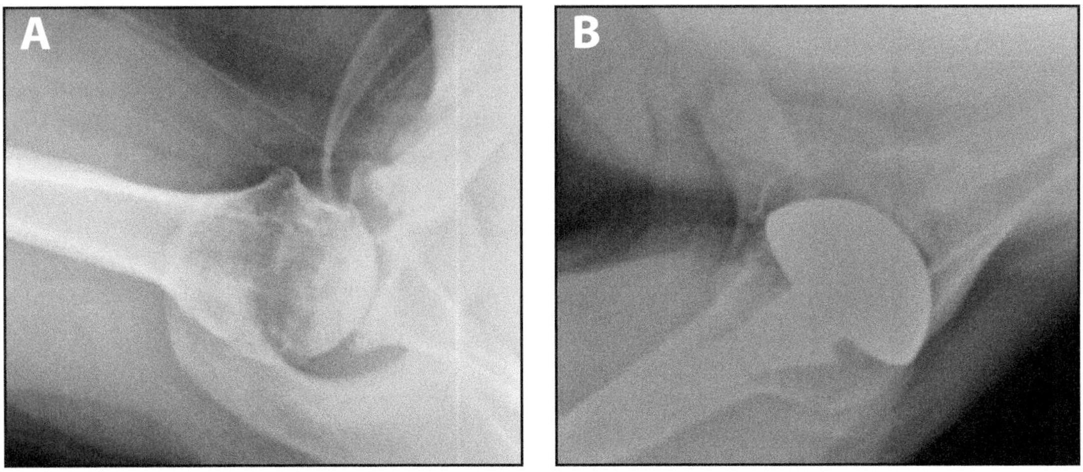

Figure 14-6. Hemiarthroplasty with concentric glenoid reaming (ream-and-run). (A) Preoperative axillary radiograph showing Walch B2 (biconcave) glenoid. (B) Postoperative axillary radiograph with no posterior subluxation.

    - Follow-up ranged from 16 months to 34 months, with 4 of the 6 patients undergoing capsular interposition, 3 out of the 5 receiving meniscal allograft, and 5 of the 6 patients implanted with human dermal allograft undergoing a revision surgery, with a combined 10 of the 17 patients undergoing conversion to either an anatomic or reverse TSA.
  - As recent studies demonstrate poor outcomes, this technique has fallen out of favor.

Total Shoulder Arthroplasty

- Indications
  - Indications include severe pain that has failed to respond to conservative measures (after 6 to 12 months) and a degree of dysfunction that is unacceptable to the patient.
- Though controversial, TSA is generally reserved for patients over 50 years old, whereas hemiarthroplasty is considered for patients younger than 50 years old.
  - Patients younger than 40 years old or physically active, and older patients with symptomatic GH arthritis and an intact rotator cuff present a significant problem. Prosthetic replacement places them at high risk for multiple revisions. Nonoperative treatment should be maximized and other surgical options such as debridement should be considered.
  - Risks of nonoperative treatment include worsening of concomitant conditions associated with the arthritis (stiffness and posterior subluxation).
    - Patients with OA and mild stiffness or posterior erosion should be counseled about the risk of progression glenoid bone loss, subluxation, and disease progression that could influence ability to perform anatomic arthroplasty in the future.
    - RA patients with an intact and functional cuff and good bone stock should be cautioned about the development of irreparable cuff deficiency and nonreconstructible bone loss with further nonoperative management.
- Preoperative imaging
  - The AP view is taken in internal and ER to assess bone quality, identification of inferior osteophytes, joint space loss, and diameter of the humeral canal.
  - Evaluation of the acromiohumeral distance can suggest the presence of significant rotator cuff deficiency if the distance measures less than 7 mm.

- The axillary radiograph is useful in identifying glenoid version as well as the posterior glenoid wear.
- CT scan is better for assessing glenoid bone stock and version.
  - Accurate determination of whether glenoid replacement is feasible, need for eccentric reaming, or if bone grafting or use of an augmented glenoid component may be necessary.
  - Measurement of glenoid version is performed by a CT scan.[2]
    - A line drawn down the transverse axis of the scapula and another line perpendicular to this defines neutral version.
    - A line connecting the anterior and posterior rims of the glenoid is drawn (not including osteophytes) and this angle is amount of retroversion (Figure 14-7).
  - Because posterior glenoid erosion and posterior subluxation are common with severe internal rotation contracture, CT scanning should be considered in all patients with ER of 30 degrees or less.
  - Posterior erosion in B-type glenoid increases with age, leading to an excess of glenoid retroversion and humeral subluxation.
    - The humeral head can be fixed in a posterior subluxated position, resulting in a longer, more demanding surgical procedure because extensive release of soft tissues and bony reconstruction may be required
    - Evaluation of the relationship between the humeral head and the glenoid is recommended because the asymmetric load distribution in the horizontal plane may expose the glenoid component to loosening as a result of the rocking horse effect of the humeral component at the glenoid component.

- Humeral head implants
  - Eighty-five percent of all humeral heads can be reconstructed within 2 mm of their natural dimensions with 8 head sizes.[61]
    - Maintaining the ratio of humeral head radius to humeral head thickness to a narrow range allows for maximization of humeral surface area available for contact.
  - As a general guideline, a head size within 4 mm of the original thickness and positioning it within the same range as the original head should be the goal of prosthetic reconstruction.
  - Third-generation modular systems have several advantages:
    - They allow for anatomic variation.
    - Platform systems allow head removal while maintaining the humeral stem.
    - There is less inventory.
  - Implant malpositioning of 8 mm in any direction results in a statistically significant decrease in passive GH motion, similar to that caused by using an excessively thick humeral head.[62]
    - Articular malpositioning of no more than 4 mm may produce only a small, clinically irrelevant alteration in humeral translation and range of motion.
- Glenoid implants
  - Normal glenoid version ranges from 2 degrees of anteversion to 9 degrees of retroversion.
  - Conforming radii of curvature yield more physiologic translations and exhibit lower loosening scores than conforming designs.[63,64]
    - The best scores are associated with implants with radial mismatches of greater than 5.5 mm.

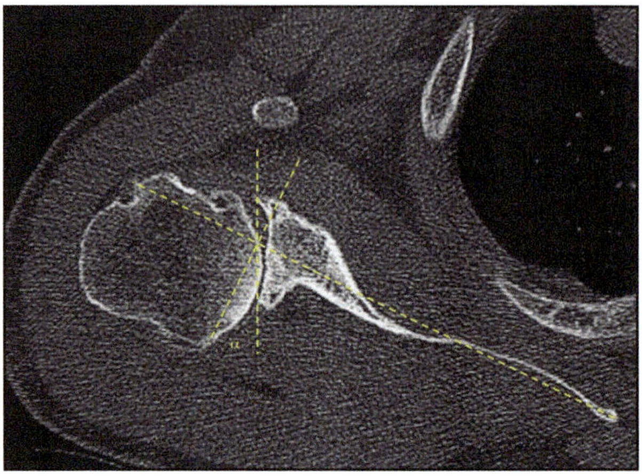

Figure 14-7. CT axillary cut of glenoid showing calculation of Friedman's line and glenoid retroversion.

- The radius of curvature of new prosthetic glenoids is 2 to 6 mm larger than that of the humeral head in an attempt to recreate physiologic translation and allow for the correct balance of stability and function.
- Clavert and colleagues used a cadaver model to show that glenoid retroversion of 15 degrees or more cannot be corrected with reaming.[65]
- Nowak et al used a computer model to simulate glenoid resurfacing.[66]
  - Glenoid retroversion of less than 12 degrees allowed for all implants; some implants were possible with retroversion of 12 degrees to 18 degrees.
  - Unable to implant either 46 mm or 52 mm glenoid components in any patient with retroversion greater than 18 degrees
  - Posterior penetration of the superior peg was the most common mode of compromise (with linear pegs).
- The prevalence of radiolucent line formation around the glenoid component is much higher than the humeral component and has been reported to occur in 30% to 96% of components. The rate of glenoid loosening is much lower (up to 12.5%) than the rate of lucent line formation but is the most common prosthesis-related cause for revision surgery.
- Finite element analysis studies have shown the following:
  - Curved-back glenoid components have better loosening performance than flat-back components.
- Intermediate reports using a metal-backed prosthesis are similar to all-polyethylene components, but they have increased rates of early failure[67] and are not commonly used.
- An all-polyethylene component distributes stress more physiologically to bone, and cemented all-polyethylene components remain the gold standard.

- Outcomes
  - Total shoulder arthroscopy in GH OA has been successful in relieving pain, increasing range of motion, and improving activities of daily living.
  - Pain relief and improved function occurs in approximately 90% of patients, with survivorship of more than 90% at 10 years and more than 80% at 20 years.[44]
  - In patients with RA, total shoulder arthroscopy offers better pain relief, range of motion, and patient satisfaction than a hemiarthroplasty.[68]
  - Sperling and colleagues[44] reported on shoulder arthroplasty for RA in 247 patients.

    - Follow-up averaged 11.6 years.
    - Results included significant long-term pain relief and better active abduction and ER both with hemiarthroplasty and TSA.
    - Among patients with an intact rotator cuff, improvement in pain and abduction were significantly greater, and the risk of revision was significantly lower for TSA.
  - Augmented glenoid components are available to address severe posterior glenoid wear.
    - Results at a 2-year minimum follow-up are comparable to a standard polyethylene implant.[69]
  - Recently 21 patients were followed for 2 years following augmented glenoid implantation.[70]
    - Significant improvements in ASES, Simple Shoulder Test, and range of motion
    - Radiographic improvement in glenoid version
    - Central peg ingrowth in all patients

Reverse Shoulder Arthroplasty

- The "reversed shoulder" is a ball-and-socket design in which the ball is on the glenoid side and the socket is on the humeral side (Figure 14-8).
- It has been available in the United States since 2004 and has been used in Europe for 2 decades.[48]
- Current designs use a medialized center of rotation to decrease torque on the glenoid anchoring points and to increase the deltoid lever arm.[71]
- Best indication is the patient with end-stage severe cuff arthropathy who is older and low demand with active elevation less than 90 degrees.
- The reverse total shoulder arthroscopy systems currently used have complete conformity of the articular surfaces (equal radii of curvature) and a high degree of constraint (high wall height), thereby enforcing ball-and-socket kinematics.
- Two basic designs
  - Medialized center of rotation (original Grammont design)
  - Lateralized center of rotation
- Design
  - Reverse of the ball and socket and components overcomes the absence of rotator cuff muscles.
  - The center of sphere (glenosphere) must be at or within the glenoid neck.
  - Medialization of the glenosphere results in forces acting on a fixed center of rotation, thus transforming torque generated by the deltoid into compressive forces at the prosthesis bone interface. This solved the formerly inevitable problem of loosening of the glenosphere.
  - Early attempts at a lateralized glenoid and deeper humeral socket led to early catastrophic failure.
  - Medialization of the glenoid limits range of motion and leads to scapular notching.
  - Lateralization of the glenosphere allows the prosthesis to overcome these range of motion limitations and scapular notching but increases shear forces at the prosthesis bone interface.
- Indications
  - A patient older than 70 years old with an irreparable rotator cuff tear associated with pseudoparalysis.
  - RCTA
  - Expanded indication for acute 3 or 4 part proximal humerus fractures in older patients

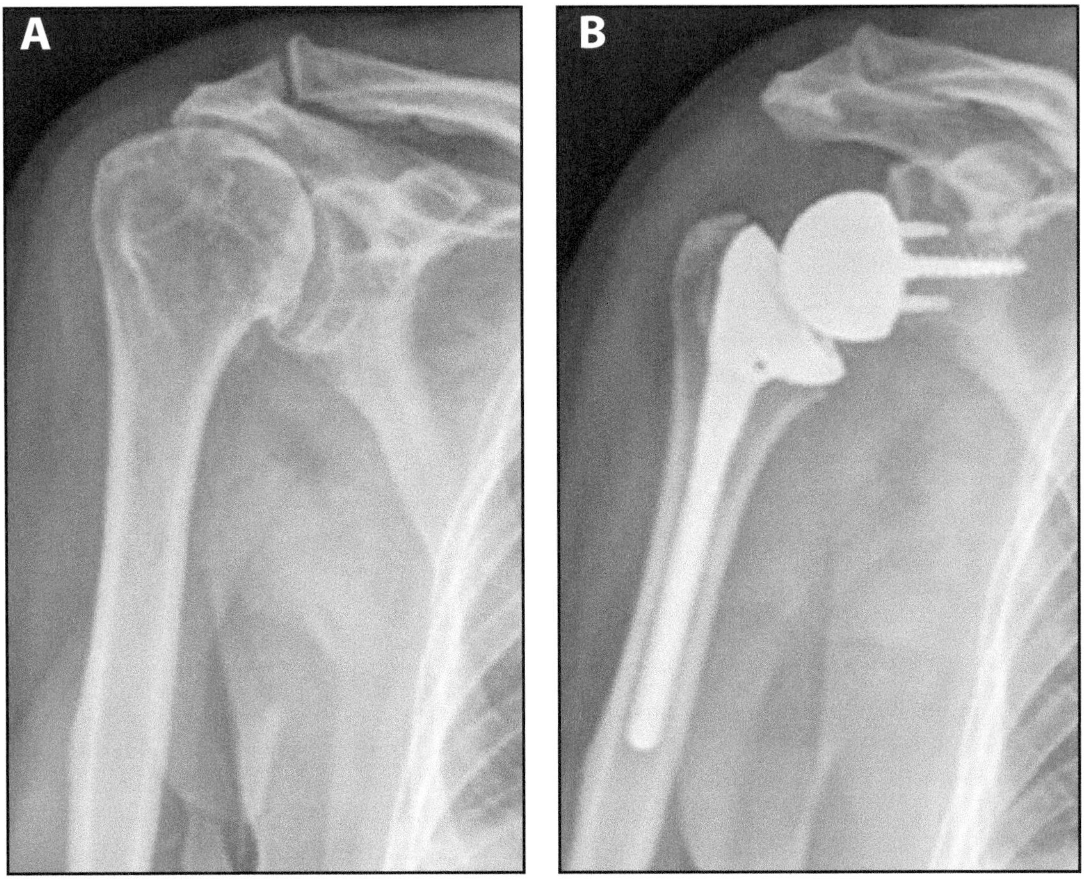

Figure 14-8. (A) Preoperative radiographs of cuff tear arthropathy and (B) postoperative radiographs of a reverse shoulder prosthesis.

- Results are less dependent on tuberosity healing (unlike hemiarthroplasty).
- Patients generally have faster recovery and do not need extended sling immobilization.

- Good option for revision shoulder surgery (failed anatomic total shoulder arthroscopy or proximal humerus open reduction and internal fixation)
- Preserved deltoid function
- Adequate glenoid bone stock

- Contraindications
  - Complete axillary nerve palsy
  - Young age
  - Poor glenoid bone stock
- Complications
  - Deep infection
    - Recent studies report infection rates in primary RTSA from 2.2% to 5.0%.[72,73]
  - Hematoma formation
  - Glenoid complications
    - Glenoid loosening occurs in 4.1% of cases.
    - Risk factors include young age (less than 70 years old), female sex, and superolateral approach.

  - Scapular notching
    - Notching of the bone of the inferior and posterior scapular neck has an incidence of 50% to 96%.
    - One study correlated the presence of notching to the presence of RCTA and Goutallier stage 3 to 4 of the infraspinatus.
    - Significance of notching is unclear.
      - Werner showed that notching stabilized in 50% of shoulders at 1 year and no correlation between notching and clinical results.[74]
      - Sirveaux et al showed poorer clinical results when significant notching occurred.[49]
      - Increased risk of glenoid component loosening
    - Placement of the baseplate as inferior as possible helps prevent notching.
      - Kelly showed that placement of the drill hole for the baseplate was 11.5 ± 1 mm above the inferior glenoid rim (12 mm rule).[75]
    - Inferior tilt of 10 to 15 degrees is recommended to limit notching and also provides a compressive force at the baseplate-bone interface.
    - Lateralized design minimizes impingement of polyethylene humeral cup on the scapular neck.
      - Results in a shorter deltoid lever arm and has the theoretical disadvantage of increased shear stresses at the glenoid component–bone interface.
  - Instability
    - Occurs in 3.4% of primary cases
    - Usually anterior and occurs with arm in extension and internal rotation
    - May be prevented by the following:
      - Use of the superolateral approach
      - Avoid retroversion of the humeral component
      - Establish optimal length of the humerus
      - Appropriate tensioning of the deltoid
  - Acromial fracture
    - Increasing the passive tension of the deltoid muscle can result in insufficiency fractures of the acromion.
    - Deltoid tension is difficult to assess intraoperatively. Undertensioning can lead to instability, and overtensioning can limit range of motion and may cause an acromial stress fracture.[76]
    - Incidence is around 3%, and patients have worse functional outcomes following acromial fractures.[77]
    - Generally treated nonoperatively
- Outcomes
  - Clinical outcome of reverse shoulder arthroplasty for RCTA is generally more favorable than when performed for other diagnoses (eg, failed prosthetic arthroplasty or fracture).
  - Several series have been published of short- to mid-term results showing overall improvement in pain, function, and active forward flexion from 105 degrees to 140 degrees.
  - Active ER is typically improved when a lateralized prosthesis is used to tension the remaining posterior rotator cuff.[78]
  - Al-Hadithy and others evaluated outcomes of reverse shoulder arthroplasty.[79]

        - Constant scores improved from 34 points to 71 points, and shoulder forward flexion improved from 55 degrees to 110 degrees over an average follow-up of 5 years.
        - Scapular notching was present in 68% of shoulders but no observed association with deterioration of constant score at 24 months and final follow-up.
    - Bacle and colleagues followed up on their initial mid-term outcome study looking at long-term outcomes (minimum 10-year follow-up).[80]
        - Overall prosthetic survival was excellent (93%).
        - Patients showed deteriorating functional outcomes, and high rates of scapular notching (73%) and complications (29%) long-term.
        - Despite the cautious optimism with reversed shoulder arthroplasty, complications and reoperation remain a concern.

Conclusion

- Multiple types of GH arthritis exist. The most common are OA, RA, and RCTA.
- Pathogenesis of all types of GH arthritis is poorly understood.
- Clinical presentation, prognosis, and recommended treatment are largely dependent on the arthritis type.
- When nonoperative measures fail, surgical management includes several options.
- Debridement and capsular releases may have a role for the active, high-demand, young patients with mild to moderate arthritis.
- Indications for hemiarthroplasty continue to be refined and in the future may become the procedure of choice for end-stage shoulder arthritis in younger, active patients.
- TSA is preferred in patients older than 50 years old with an intact and functional rotator cuff and adequate glenoid bone stock to accept a glenoid component.
- RTSA is most commonly used for the low-demand, older patient with GH arthritis in the setting of a massive, irreparable rotator cuff defect.

References

1. Green A, Norris TR. Imaging techniques for glenohumeral arthritis and glenohumeral arthroplasty. *Clin Orthop Relat Res.* 1994;(307):7-17.
2. Friedman RJ, Hawthorne KB, Genez BM. The use of computerized tomography in the measurement of glenoid version. *J Bone Joint Surg Am.* 1992;74(7):1032-1037.
3. Iannotti JP, Zlatkin MB, Esterhai JL, Kressel HY, Dalinka MK, Spindler KP. Magnetic resonance imaging of the shoulder. Sensitivity, specificity, and predictive value. *J Bone Joint Surg Am.* 1991;73(1):17-29.
4. Kumar V, Cotran RS, Robbins SL. Osteoarthritis. In: Kumar V, Robbins SL, Cotran RS, eds. Philadelphia, PA: Saunders Elsevier; 1992;693-696.
5. Howell DS, Treadwell BV, Trippel SB. Etiopathogensis of osteoarthritis. In: Moskowitz RW, Howell DS, Goldberg VM, Mankin HJ, eds. *Osteoarthritis: Diagnosis and Medical/Surgical Management.* 2nd ed. Philadelphia, PA: Saunders Elsevier; 1992:233-252.
6. Collins DN. Pathophysiology, Classification, and Pathoanatomy of Glenohumeral Arthritis and Related Disorders. In: Iannotti JP, Williams GR, eds. *Disorders of the Shoulder: Diagnosis and Management.* Philadelphia: Lippincott, Williams & Wilkins; 2007:563-632.
7. Neer CS II. Replacement arthroplasty for glenohumeral osteoarthritis. *J Bone Joint Surg Am.* 1974;56(1):1-13.
8. Bercik MJ, Kruse K II, Yalizis M, Gauci MO, Chaoui J, Walch G. A modification to the Walch classification of the glenoid in primary glenohumeral osteoarthritis using three-dimensional imaging. *J Shoulder Elbow Surg.* 2016;25(10):1601-1606. doi:10.1016/j.jse.2016.03.010.

9. McCarty DJ, Halverson PB, Carrera GF, Brewer BJ, Kozin F. "Milwaukee shoulder"—association of microspheroids containing hydroxyapatite crystals, active collagenase, and neutral protease with rotator cuff defects. I. Clinical aspects. *Arthritis Rheum.* 1981;24(3):464-473. doi:10.1002/art.1780240303.
10. Neer CS II, Craig EV, Fukuda H. Cuff-tear arthropathy. *J Bone Joint Surg Am.* 1983;65(9):1232-1244.
11. Favard L, Levigne C, Nerot C, Gerber C, De Wilde L, Mole D. Reverse prostheses in arthropathies with cuff tear: are survivorship and function maintained over time? *Clin Orthop Relat Res.* 2011;469(9):2469-2475. doi:10.1007/s11999-011-1833-y.
12. Ek ET, Neukom L, Catanzaro S, Gerber C. Reverse total shoulder arthroplasty for massive irreparable rotator cuff tears in patients younger than 65 years old: results after five to fifteen years. *J Shoulder Elbow Surg.* 2013;22(9):1199-1208. doi:10.1016/j.jse.2012.11.016.
13. Samilson RL, Prieto V. Dislocation arthropathy of the shoulder. *J Bone Joint Surg Am.* 1983;65(4):456-460.
14. Marx RG, McCarty EC, Montemurno TD, Altchek DW, Craig EV, Warren RF. Development of arthrosis following dislocation of the shoulder: a case-control study. *J Shoulder Elbow Surg.* 2002;11(1):1-5. doi:10.1067/mse.2002.119388.
15. Saltzman MD, Mercer DM, Warme WJ, Bertelsen AL, Matsen FA III. Comparison of patients undergoing primary shoulder arthroplasty before and after the age of fifty. *J Bone Joint Surg Am.* 2010;92(1):42-47. doi:10.2106/JBJS.I.00071.
16. Hovelius L, Augustini BG, Fredin H, Johansson O, Norlin R, Thorling J. Primary anterior dislocation of the shoulder in young patients. A ten-year prospective study. *J Bone Joint Surg Am.* 1996;78(11):1677-1684. doi:10.2106/00004623-199611000-00006.
17. Hovelius L, Saeboe M. Neer Award 2008: Arthropathy after primary anterior shoulder dislocation—223 shoulders prospectively followed up for twenty-five years. *J Shoulder Elbow Surg.* 2009;18(3):339-347. doi:10.1016/j.jse.2008.11.004.
18. Hettrich CM, Boraiah S, Dyke JP, Neviaser A, Helfet DL, Lorich DG. Quantitative assessment of the vascularity of the proximal part of the humerus. *J Bone Joint Surg Am.* 2010;92(4):943-948. doi:10.2106/JBJS.H.01144.
19. Cruess RL. Osteonecrosis of bone. Current concepts as to etiology and pathogenesis. *Clin Orthop Relat Res.* 1986;(208):30-39.
20. Schoch BS, Barlow JD, Schleck C, Cofield RH, Sperling JW. Shoulder arthroplasty for atraumatic osteonecrosis of the humeral head. *J Shoulder Elbow Surg.* 2016;25(2):238-245. doi:10.1016/j.jse.2015.07.019.
21. *Rheumatoid Arthritis.* Philadelphia, PA: WB Saunders; 1997.
22. Myasoedova E, Davis JM III, Crowson CS, Gabriel SE. Epidemiology of rheumatoid arthritis: rheumatoid arthritis and mortality. *Curr Rheumatol Rep.* 2010;12(5):379-385.
23. Silman AJ, Hochberg MC. *Epidemiology of the Rheumatic Diseases.* Oxford, England: Oxford University Press; 1993.
24. Chan KW, Felson DT, Yood RA, Walker AM. Incidence of rheumatoid arthritis in central Massachusetts. *Arthritis Rheum.* 1993;36(12):1691-1696. doi:10.1002/art.1780361207.
25. Hochberg MC. Adult and juvenile rheumatoid arthritis: current epidemiologic concepts. *Epidemiol Rev.* 1981;3:27-44. doi:10.1093/oxfordjournals.epirev.a036238.
26. Haskard DO, Grahame R. Management of chronic inflammatory arthropathy. In: Watsons M, ed. *Surgical Disorders of the Shoulder.* New York, NY: Churchill-Livingstone; 1991:203-215.
27. Petersson CJ. Painful shoulders in patients with rheumatoid arthritis. Prevalence, clinical and radiological features. *Scand J Rheumatol.* 1986;15(3):275-279. doi:10.3109/03009748609092592.
28. Bennett WF, Gerber C. Operative treatment of the rheumatoid shoulder. *Curr Opin Rheumatol.* 1994;6(2):177-182. doi:10.1097/00002281-199403000-00010.
29. Larson A, Dale K, Eek M. Radiographic evaluation of rheumatoid arthritis and related conditions by standard reference film. *Acta Radiol Diagn (Stockh).* 1977;18(4):481-491. doi:10.1177/028418517701800415.
30. Tan V, Leggin B, Williams GR Jr. Complications of shoulder arthroplasty. In: Iannotti JP, Williams GR, eds. *Disorders of the Shoulder: Diagnosis and Management.* Philadelphia, PA: Lippincott Williams & Wilkins; 2007:1608-1623.
31. Sperling JW, Cofield RH, Schleck CD, Harmsen WS. Total shoulder arthroplasty versus hemiarthroplasty for rheumatoid arthritis of the shoulder: results of 303 consecutive cases. *J Shoulder Elbow Surg.* 2007;16(6):683-690. doi:10.1016/j.jse.2007.02.135.
32. Rittmeister M, Kerschbaumer F. Grammont reverse total shoulder arthroplasty in patients with rheumatoid arthritis and nonreconstructible rotator cuff lesions. *J Shoulder Elbow Surg.* 2001;10(1):17-22. doi:10.1067/mse.2001.110515.
33. Holcomb JO, Hebert DJ, Mighell MA, et al. Reverse shoulder arthroplasty in patients with rheumatoid arthritis. *J Shoulder Elbow Surg.* 2010;19(7):1076-1084. doi:10.1016/j.jse.2009.11.049.
34. Cameron BD, Galatz LM, Ramsey ML, Williams GR, Iannotti JP. Non-prosthetic management of grade IV osteochondral lesions of the glenohumeral joint. *J Shoulder Elbow Surg.* 2002;11(1):25-32. doi:10.1067/mse.2002.120143.

35. Kerr BJ, McCarty EC. Outcome of arthroscopic débridement is worse for patients with glenohumeral arthritis of both sides of the joint. *Clin Orthop Relat Res.* 2008;466(3):634-638. doi:10.1007/s11999-007-0088-0.
36. Ogilvie-Harris DJ, Wiley AM. Arthroscopic surgery of the shoulder. A general appraisal. *J Bone Joint Surg Br.* 1986;68(2):201-207.
37. Weinstein DM, Bucchieri JS, Pollock RG, Flatow EL, Bigliani LU. Arthroscopic debridement of the shoulder for osteoarthritis. *Arthroscopy.* 2000;16(5):471-476. doi:10.1053/jars.2000.5042.
38. Krishnan SG, Nowinski RJ, Harrison D, Burkhead WZ. Humeral hemiarthroplasty with biologic resurfacing of the glenoid for glenohumeral arthritis. Two to fifteen-year outcomes. *J Bone Joint Surg Am.* 2007.89(4):727-734. doi:10.2106/JBJS.E.01291.
39. Lynch JR, Franta AK, Montgomery WH Jr, Lenters TR, Mounce D, Matsen FA III. Self-assessed outcome at two to four years after shoulder hemiarthroplasty with concentric glenoid reaming. *J Bone Joint Surg Am.* 2007;89(6):1284-1292. doi:10.2106/JBJS.E.00942.
40. Wirth MA, Tapscott RS, Southworth C, Rockwood CA Jr. Treatment of glenohumeral arthritis with a hemiarthroplasty: a minimum five-year follow-up outcome study. *J Bone Joint Surg Am.* 2006;88(5):964-973. doi:10.2106/JBJS.D.03030.
41. Antoniou J, Tsai A, Baker D, Schumacher R, Williams GR, Iannotti JP. Milwaukee shoulder: correlating possible etiologic variables. *Clin Orthop Relat Res.* 2003;(407):79-85. doi:10.1097/00003086-200302000-00015.
42. Austin LS, Williams GR Jr, Iannotti JP. Unconstrained prosthetic arthroplasty for glenohumeral arthritis with an intact or repairable rotator cuff: indications, technique, and results. In: Iannotti JP, Williams GR, eds. *Disorders of the Shoulder: Diagnosis and Management.* Philadelphia, PA: Lippincott Williams & Wilkins; 2007:697-726.
43. Orfaly RM, Rockwood CA Jr, Esenyel CZ, Wirth MA. Shoulder arthroplasty in cases with avascular necrosis of the humeral head. *J Shoulder Elbow Surg.* 2007;16(3 suppl):S27-S32. doi:10.1016/j.jse.2006.06.005.
44. Sperling JW, Cofield RH, Rowland CM. Minimum fifteen-year follow-up of Neer hemiarthroplasty and total shoulder arthroplasty in patients aged fifty years or younger. *J Shoulder Elbow Surg.* 2004;13(6):604-613. doi:10.1016/S1058274604001296.
45. Safran O, Seebauer L, Iannotti JP. Cuff deficiency: unconstrained and constrained shoulder arthroplasty. In: Iannotti JP, Williams GR, eds. *Disorders of the Shoulder: Diagnosis and Management.* Philadelphia, PA: Lippincott Williams & Wilkins; 2007:727-751.
46. Boileau P, Watkinson D, Hatzidakis AM, Hovorka I. Neer Award 2005: The Grammont reverse shoulder prosthesis: results in cuff tear arthritis, fracture sequelae, and revision arthroplasty. *J Shoulder Elbow Surg.* 2006;15(5):527-540. doi:10.1016/j.jse.2006.01.003.
47. Frankle M, Siegal S, Pupello D, Saleem A, Mighell M, Vasey M. The reverse shoulder prosthesis for glenohumeral arthritis associated with severe rotator cuff deficiency. A minimum two-year follow-up study of sixty patients. *J Bone Joint Surg Am.* 2005;87(8):1697-1705. doi:10.2106/JBJS.D.02813.
48. Seebauer L. Total reverse shoulder arthroplasty: European lessons and future trends. *Am J Orthop (Belle Mead NJ).* 2007;36(12 Suppl 1):22-28.
49. Sirveaux F, Favard L, Oudet D, Huquet D, Walch G, Molé D. Grammont inverted total shoulder arthroplasty in the treatment of glenohumeral osteoarthritis with massive rupture of the cuff. Results of a multicentre study of 80 shoulders. *J Bone Joint Surg Br.* 2004;86(3):388-395. doi:10.1302/0301-620x.86b3.14024.
50. Namdari S, Skelley N, Keener JD, Galatz LM, Yamaguchi K. What is the role of arthroscopic debridement for glenohumeral arthritis? A critical examination of the literature. *Arthroscopy.* 2013;29(8):1392-1398. doi:10.1016/j.arthro.2013.02.022.
51. Skelley NW, Namdari S, Chamberlain AM, Keener JD, Galatz LM, Yamaguchi K. Arthroscopic debridement and capsular release for the treatment of shoulder osteoarthritis. *Arthroscopy.* 2015;31(3):494-500. doi:10.1016/j.arthro.2014.08.025.
52. Mitchell JJ, Horan MP, Greenspoon JA, Menge TJ, Tahal DS, Millett PJ. Survivorship and patient-reported outcomes after comprehensive arthroscopic management of glenohumeral osteoarthritis: minimum 5-year follow-up. *Am J Sports Med.* 2016;44(12):3206-3213. doi:10.1177/0363546516656372.
53. Levine WN, Fischer CR, Nguyen D, Flatow EL, Ahmad CS, Bigliani LU. Long-term follow-up of shoulder hemiarthroplasty for glenohumeral osteoarthritis. *J Bone Joint Surg Am.* 2012;94(22):e164
54. Weldon EJ III, Boorman RS, Smith KL, Matsen FA III. Optimizing the glenoid contribution to the stability of a humeral hemiarthroplasty without a prosthetic glenoid. *J Bone Joint Surg Am.* 2004;86(9):2022-2029. doi:10.2106/00004623-200409000-00022.
55. Saltzman MD, Chamberlain AM, Mercer DM, Warme WJ, Bertelsen AL, Matsen FA III. Shoulder hemiarthroplasty with concentric glenoid reaming in patients 55 years old or less. *J Shoulder Elbow Surg.* 2011;20(4):609-615. doi:10.1016/j.jse.2010.08.027.
56. Getz CL, Kearns KA, Padegimas EM, Johnston PS, Lazarus MD, Williams GR Jr. Survivorship of hemiarthroplasty with concentric glenoid reaming for glenohumeral arthritis in young, active patients with a biconcave glenoid. *J Am Acad Orthop Surg.* 2017;25(10):715-723. doi:10.5435/JAAOS-D-16-00019.

57. Ball CM, Galatz LM, Yamaguchi K. Meniscal allograft interposition arthroplasty for the arthritic shoulder: description of a new surgical technique. *Tech Shoulder Elb Surg.* 2001;2(4):247-254. doi:10.1097/00132589-200112000-00004.
58. Nicholson GP, Goldstein JL, Romeo AA, et al. Lateral meniscus allograft biologic glenoid arthroplasty in total shoulder arthroplasty for young shoulders with degenerative joint disease. *J Shoulder Elbow Surg.* 2007;16(5 suppl):S261-S266. doi:10.1016/j.jse.2007.03.003.
59. Namdari S, Alosh H, Baldwin K, Glaser D, Kelly JD. Biological glenoid resurfacing for glenohumeral osteoarthritis: a systematic review. *J Shoulder Elbow Surg.* 2011;20(7):1184-1190. doi:10.1016/j.jse.2011.04.031.
60. Puskas GJ, Meyer DC, Lebschi JA, Gerber C. Unacceptable failure of hemiarthroplasty combined with biological glenoid resurfacing in the treatment of glenohumeral arthritis in the young. *J Shoulder Elbow Surg.* 2015;24(12):1900-1907. doi:10.1016/j.jse.2015.05.037.
61. Iannotti JP, Gabriel JP, Schneck SL, Evans BG, Misra S. The normal glenohumeral relationships. An anatomical study of one hundred and forty shoulders. *J Bone Joint Surg Am.* 1992;74(4):491-500.
62. Williams GR Jr, Wong KL, Pepe MD, et al. The effect of articular malposition after total shoulder arthroplasty on glenohumeral translations, range of motion, and subacromial impingement. *J Shoulder Elbow Surg.* 2001;10(5):399-409. doi:10.1067/mse.2001.116871.
63. Karduna AR, Williams GR, Williams JL, Iannotti JP. Joint stability after total shoulder arthroplasty in a cadaver model. *J Shoulder Elbow Surg.* 1997;6(6):506-511. doi:10.1016/s1058-2746(97)90082-3.
64. Walch G, Edwards TB, Boulahia A, Boileau P, Mole D, Adeleine P. The influence of glenohumeral prosthetic mismatch on glenoid radiolucent lines: results of a multicenter study. *J Bone Joint Surg Am.* 2002;84(12):2186-2191. doi:10.2106/00004623-200212000-00010.
65. Clavert P, Millett PJ, Warner JJ. Glenoid resurfacing: what are the limits to asymmetric reaming for posterior erosion? *J Shoulder Elbow Surg.* 2007;16(6):843-848. doi:10.1016/j.jse.2007.03.015.
66. Nowak DD, Bahu MJ, Gardner RT, et al. Simulation of surgical glenoid resurfacing using three-dimensional computed tomography of the arthritic glenohumeral joint: the amount of glenoid retroversion that can be corrected. *J Shoulder Elbow Surg.* 2009;18(5):680-688. doi: doi:10.1016/j.jse.2009.03.019.
67. Matsen FA III, Clinton J, Lynch J, Bertelsen A, Richardson ML. Glenoid component failure in total shoulder arthroplasty. *J Bone Joint Surg Am.* 2008;90(4):885-896. doi:10.2106/JBJS.G.01263.
68. Boyd AD Jr, Thomas WH, Scott RD, Sledge CB, Thornhill TS. Total shoulder arthroplasty versus hemiarthroplasty. Indications for glenoid resurfacing. *J Arthroplasty.* 1990;5(4):329-336. doi:10.1016/s0883-5403(08)80092-7.
69. Wright TW, Grey SG, Roche CP, Wright L, Flurin PH, Zuckerman JD. Preliminary results of a posterior augmented glenoid compared to an all polyethylene standard glenoid in anatomic total shoulder arthroplasty. *Bull Hosp Jt Dis (2013).* 2015;73(suppl 1):S79-S85.
70. Stephens SP, Spencer EE, Wirth MA. Radiographic results of augmented all-polyethylene glenoids in the presence of posterior glenoid bone loss during total shoulder arthroplasty. *J Shoulder Elbow Surg.* 2017;26(5):798-803. doi:10.1016/j.jse.2016.09.053.
71. De Wilde LF, Audenaert EA, Berghs BM. Shoulder prostheses treating cuff tear arthropathy: a comparative biomechanical study. *J Orthop Res.* 2004;22(6):1222-1230. doi:10.1016/j.orthres.2004.03.010.
72. Florschütz AV, Lane PD, Crosby LA. Infection after primary anatomic versus primary reverse total shoulder arthroplasty. *J Shoulder Elbow Surg.* 2015;24(8):1296-1301. doi:10.1016/j.jse.2014.12.036.
73. Morris BJ, O'Connor DP, Torres D, Elkousy HA, Gartsman GM, Edwards TB. Risk factors for periprosthetic infection after reverse shoulder arthroplasty. *J Shoulder Elbow Surg.* 2015;24(2):161-166. doi:10.1016/j.jse.2014.05.020.
74. Werner CM, Steinmann PA, Gilbart M, Gerber C. Treatment of painful pseudoparesis due to irreparable rotator cuff dysfunction with the Delta III reverse-ball-and-socket total shoulder prosthesis. *J Bone Joint Surg Am.* 2005;87(7):1476-1486. doi:10.2106/JBJS.D.02342.
75. Kelly JD II, Humphrey CS, Norris TR. Optimizing glenosphere position and fixation in reverse shoulder arthroplasty, Part one: the twelve-mm rule. *J Shoulder Elbow Surg.* 2008;17(4):589-594. doi:10.1016/j.jse.2007.08.013.
76. Wong MT, Langohr GDG, Athwal GS, Johnson JA. Implant positioning in reverse shoulder arthroplasty has an impact on acromial stresses. *J Shoulder Elbow Surg.* 2016;25(11):1889-1895. doi:10.1016/j.jse.2016.04.011.
77. Teusink MJ, Otto RJ, Cottrell BJ, Frankle MA. What is the effect of postoperative scapular fracture on outcomes of reverse shoulder arthroplasty? *J Shoulder Elbow Surg.* 2014;23(6):782-790. doi:10.1016/j.jse.2013.09.010.
78. Lawrence C, Williams GR, Namdari S. Influence of Glenosphere Design on Outcomes and Complications of Reverse Arthroplasty: A Systematic Review. *Clin Orthop Surg.* 2016;8(3):288-297
79. Al-Hadithy N, Domos P, Sewell MD, Pandit R. Reverse shoulder arthroplasty in 41 patients with cuff tear arthropathy with a mean follow-up period of 5 years. *J Shoulder Elbow Surg.* 2014;23(11):1662-1668. doi:10.1016/j.jse.2014.03.001.
80. Bacle G, Nové-Josserand L, Garaud P, Walch G. Long-term outcomes of reverse total shoulder arthroplasty: a follow-up of a previous study. *J Bone Joint Surg Am.* 2017;99(6):454-461. doi:10.2106/JBJS.16.00223.

15

Scapular Disorders

Eric M. Padegimas, MD and Charles L. Getz, MD

Scapular Winging

- Normal scapular motion
  - The scapulothoracic joint is complex, with the medial border of the scapula articulating with the posterior aspect of the second through seventh ribs.
  - There are 3 scapular motions (retraction/protraction, lateral/medial rotation, and anterior/posterior tilt).
  - The ratio of glenohumeral to scapulothoracic motion during shoulder abduction is 2:1.[1]
  - As the arm elevates, the center of rotation of the scapula moves superiorly and medially with lateral displacement of the inferior angle (lateral rotation).
  - Cranial elevation (anterior tilt) of the scapula is accomplished by the trapezius and countered by gravity and the latissimus dorsi (the primary scapular depressor). The serratus anterior, pectoralis minor, and lower trapezius also act to depress (posterior tilt) the scapula. Additionally, at 45 degrees of scapular abduction, the serratus anterior acts to pull the inferior angle of the scapula laterally (lateral rotation).
  - Downward rotators (medial rotators) of the scapula include the rhomboid major/minor and levator scapulae. Lateral rotators of the scapula include the lower and middle trapezius.
  - Protractors of the scapula include the serratus anterior and pectoralis major and minor.
  - Retractors of the scapula include the middle trapezius and rhomboid major and minor.
  - There are 2 major scapulothoracic bursae (infraserratus and supraserratus) and 4 minor/adventitial bursae (infraserratus at superomedial border, supraserratus at superomedial border, infraserratus at inferomedial border, and trapezoid).
- Overview: Winging of the scapula was first described more than 250 years ago.[2] Scapular winging can be primary, secondary (from glenohumeral or subacromial pathology), or volitional (in setting of psychological disorders). Sprengel deformity should also be considered in

Namdari S, Zmistowski B, Omid R, eds.
The Foundations of Shoulder and Elbow Surgery (pp 285-298).

the differential diagnosis. Sprengel deformity presents with a small and undescended scapula leading to superior positioning, medial rotation and limited scapulothoracic motion leading to deficiencies both in forward elevation and abduction.[3] Primary scapular winging can be divided into 3 categories:

1. Neurologic
    - Long thoracic nerve (serratus anterior)
    - Spinal accessory nerve (trapezius)
    - Dorsal scapular nerve (rhomboids)
2. Osseous
    - Osteochondromas
    - Fracture malunion
3. Soft tissue
    - Contracture
    - Muscle avulsion or agenesis
    - Scapulothoracic bursitis
    - Glenohumeral instability (posterior instability)

- Serratus anterior winging (medial winging)
    - In the setting of long thoracic nerve palsy[4]
    - Presentation
        - Patients complain of pain and easy fatigability secondary to the other periscapular muscles attempting to compensate.
        - More severe pain can be indicative of brachial plexus neuritis with long thoracic nerve involvement (Parsonage-Turner syndrome).[5]
        - On physical examination, the scapula is elevated superiorly (anterior tilt) and medially translated with the inferior pole rotated medially. The inferior angle of the scapula will displace and wing medially (Figure 15-1).[4,6] Patients tend to have difficulty with arm elevation above 120 degrees. Patients may develop signs of subacromial impingement due to poor acromial elevation.
        - This winging is most pronounced by forward elevation in the sagittal plane. Can also be exacerbated with resisted forward elevation (seen while attempting wall push-ups). A "rope-like" lower trapezius muscle can be seen due to compensation.
        - Resolution/improvement seen with "scapular compression test" (manual compression of the scapula against the chest wall)
    - Incidence and etiology
        - Damage to the long thoracic nerve (C5 to C7 nerve roots) is the most common neurologic cause of scapular winging.[7-9]
        - Injury to the long thoracic nerve with associated serratus anterior palsy is often associated with blunt trauma or stretching in athletes and those who use their shoulder for repetitive motion.[4,7,10,11] This nerve is susceptible to trauma because of its superficial course. Additionally, a fascial band from the inferior aspect of the brachial plexus to the first rib was found to be a source of compression with bowstringing of the nerve across this band with shoulder abduction and external rotation.[12]
        - Injury can also occur from a number of a non-traumatic etiologies such as viral illness,[11] drug reaction,[13] Parsonage-Turner syndrome,[5] iatrogenically from positioning in the operating room,[4] and post–radical mastectomy[14] among a number of other potential causes. One significant etiology is C7 nerve root compression (C7 radiculopathy) because the long thoracic nerve has a substantial C7 component.[15]

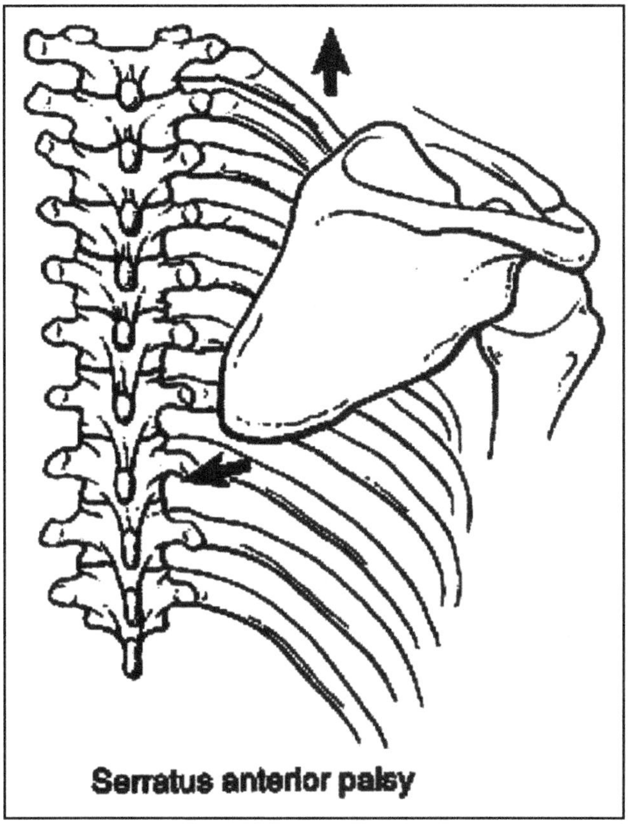

Figure 15-1. Medial scapular winging. (Reprinted with permission from Williams GR, Ramsey ML, Wiesel BB. Pectoralis Major Transfer for Long Thoracic Nerve Palsy. In: *Operative Techniques in Shoulder and Elbow Surgery.* 2nd ed. Philadelphia, PA: Wolters Kluwer; 2016:466.)

- Diagnosis
  - Confirmation of long thoracic nerve/serratus anterior palsy is done by electromyography (EMG).[16] It is important to ask the electromyographer performing the study to specifically test the serratus anterior so that this is evaluated.
- Treatment
  - Initial treatment is nonoperative for most patients, with physical therapy for strengthening of the periscapular muscles and passive stretching of the glenohumeral joint to prevent adhesive capsulitis. Most patients recover spontaneously within 1 year, but may take up to 2 years for full recovery. Up to 25% of patients will require surgery.
  - Patients with suspected transection of the nerve from lacerations or trauma may warrant earlier intervention.
  - Surgical treatment typically involves scapulothoracic fusion or dynamic stabilization by muscle transfers. However, nerve exploration with neurolysis or long thoracic nerve transfer have shown early promising results and therefore may be favorable as an option before muscle transfer.[17-19]
    - Marmor-Bechtol procedure: The sternocostal head of the pectoralis major with a fascia lata graft extension is inserted into the inferior-lateral aspect of the scapula. This can be complicated by pneumothorax or fracture of the inferior border of the scapula.[20,21]
    - A more recent variation of this procedure includes the use of semitendinosus autograft to reinforce the pectoralis major insertion on the scapula.

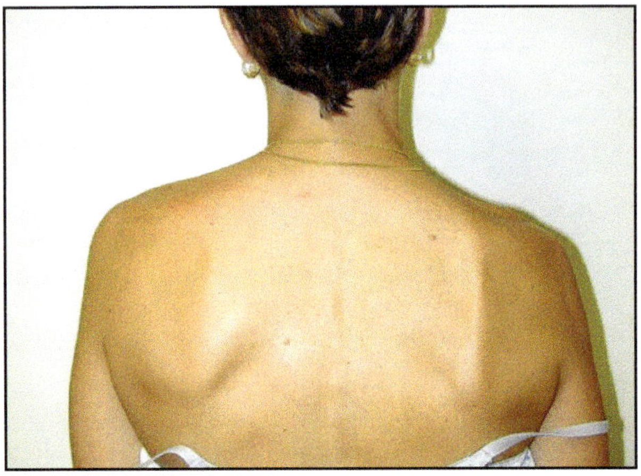

Figure 15-2. Lateral scapular winging.

- Direct and indirect transfers have been described. Originally, an indirect transfer was described and involved removal of the pectoralis major tendon (split or whole) with augmentation using fascia lata autograft. Direct transfers were popularized in 2000, where emphasis was placed on direct contact of the pectoralis major tendon on the scapula (as opposed to indirect attachment with autograft extension).[22]
- Up to 25% failure rates are noted in the literature.
- Static fascial slings have been used in the past with poor results due to graft stretching.
- Scapulothoracic fusion is less commonly used because patients can lose up to one-third total elevation as well as up to 50% pseudoarthrosis.

- Trapezius winging (lateral winging)
    - Defined in setting of spinal accessory nerve palsy[23]
    - Presentation
        - Compensation by straining other muscles of the shoulder girdle (levator scapulae and rhomboid major/minor) leading to pain and spasm. This is worse with prolonged activity and overhead activity.[23,24]
        - On physical examination, patient may have an asymmetric neckline with the affected shoulder depressed (angel-wing deformity). The inferior angle of the scapula will displace and wing laterally (Figure 15-2).[6,25,26] Additionally, winging is worsened with abduction in the coronal plane and may improve with forward elevation.[27]
        - Trapezius winging is also worsened with resisted external rotation.
        - Active-elevation lag sign and triangle sign have been described.[28]
    - Incidence and etiology
        - Damage to the spinal accessory nerve (branch of cranial nerve XI) may occur as a result of the subcutaneous location of the spinal accessory nerve in the posterior triangle of the neck.[29]
        - Though this nerve can be injured as a result of trauma, iatrogenic injury during cervical lymph node or cervical mass excisions is far more common.[26,27,30,31]
        - Neurologic amyotropy (Parsonage-Turner syndrome) is the most common medical cause of trapezius palsy.[32]
        - Difficulty with shoulder abduction is a consistent finding in these patients.[26]

- Diagnosis
  - Confirmation of trapezius palsy is made by EMG.[33] It is important to ask the electromyographer performing the study to specifically test the trapezius and shoulder girdle muscles so that this is excluded.
- Treatment
  - Initial treatment is nonoperative with physical therapy for strengthening of the periscapular muscles and passive stretching of the glenohumeral joint to prevent adhesive capsulitis. Patients who have more than 1 year of symptoms are unlikely to benefit from nonoperative management.
  - Surgical treatment involves neurolysis and repair if possible. The largest series of patients treated with nerve salvage surgery exhibited good or excellent results in approximately two-thirds of cases.[31,34] If nerve salvage is not possible, scapulothoracic fusion or dynamic stabilization by muscle transfers are potential surgical options.
    - Dewar-Harris procedure: Stabilization of the medial border of the scapula to the spinous processes of T1 and T2 with fascia lata strips (static) to compensate for the middle and lower thirds of the trapezius and transfer of the levator scapulae laterally to the spine of the scapula to compensate for the upper third of the trapezius.[35] *Recommended reading for historical context and surgical description of a novel procedure* This is no longer as common since the development of the Eden-Lange procedure.
    - Eden-Lange procedure: Transfer of the levator scapulae and rhomboid insertions laterally to effectively position the scapula medially and thus improve the mechanical advantage of these periscapular muscles and eliminate winging. The levator scapulae substitutes for the upper third of the trapezius, the rhomboid major for the middle third, and the rhomboid minor for the lower third. The surgery is performed through 2 incisions (1 along medial border of the scapula and 1 over the spine of the scapula). Drill holes are placed 5 cm lateral to the medial border of the scapula and the levator scapulae is sutured to the scapular spine (Figure 15-3). The failure rate is approximately 15%.[36,37] *Recommended reading for understanding treatment options for scapular winging* Results are variable at best (excellent outcomes reported in 57% to 75% of patients).
    - Recently a "T3 transfer" altering the line of pull on the scapula to approximate the pull of the lower trapezius better for lateral rotation was described by transferring the rhomboid major and minor to the scapular spine and levator scapulae to the posterior acromion.[38]
    - Spira's partial fusion: A mostly historical procedure in which a hole is made in the inferior angle of the scapula and the sixth rib is cut and passed through the hole

- Rhomboid major/minor winging (lateral winging)
  - This is a less common cause of scapular winging[39,40] than serratus anterior or trapezius dysfunction.
  - Presentation
    - Patients mostly complain of pain along the medial border of the scapula, and it appears similar to trapezius winging. The scapula is slightly depressed and translated with the inferior angle rotated laterally. There may be atrophy along the medial border.
    - Rhomboid winging is typically not as severe as other forms and may be less symptomatic.
  - Incidence and etiology
    - Damage to the dorsal scapular nerve, which arises from the C5 nerve root. Therefore C5 radiculopathy must be assessed as a potential etiology.[39-41]

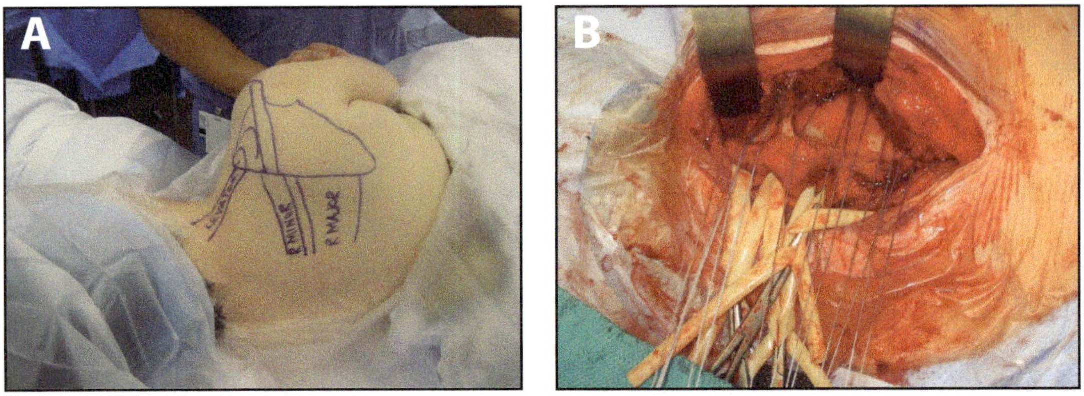

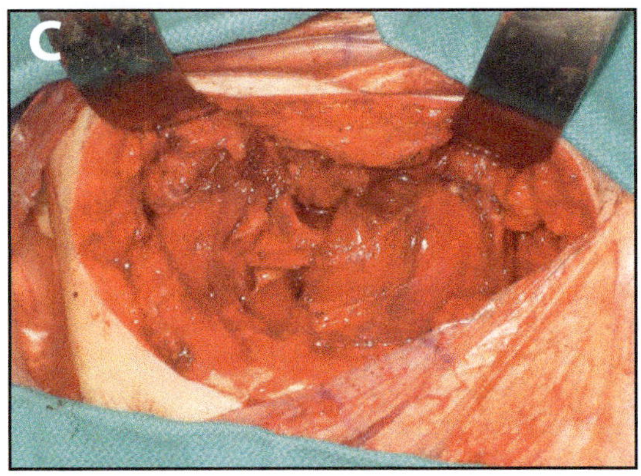

Figure 15-3. Eden-Lange procedure. (A) Surface anatomy. (B) Drill holes through medial scapula with suture passed through and tendons marked with Penrose drains. (C) Final transfer.

- Diagnosis
  - Confirmation of rhomboid palsy is made by EMG.[42] It is important to ask the physician performing the EMG study to specifically test the rhomboids muscles so that this is excluded.
- Treatment
  - Initial treatment is nonoperative with physical therapy for trapezius strengthening. Unlike other forms of neuropraxic scapular winging, rhomboid winging is not likely to improve spontaneously. However, it does tend to be less symptomatic.
  - Surgical treatment involves a fascial sling procedure in which 2 fascia lata grafts are tubularized and used to connect the lower vertebral border of the scapula to the spinal muscles and inferior angle of the scapula to the fibers of the latissimus dorsi. The teres major is transferred from its insertion on the humerus to a spinous process.[43] Neurolysis and nerve exploration of the dorsal scapular nerve has been previously described,[44] but this has not been as well studied as these same techniques for long thoracic and spinal accessory nerve palsy.

- Primary scapular winging secondary to muscle disorders
  - Traumatic ruptures of periscapular muscles can lead to winging, the presentation of which depends on the specific injury.[45,46]
    - Kibler et al have described reattachment of the lower trapezius and rhomdoid through drill holes in the setting of traumatic avulsion with significant improvement in American Shoulder and Elbow Surgeons scores.[47]
  - Congenital absence of the serratus anterior[48] and trapezius[49] have been reported and are tolerated well without significant scapular dysfunction.

- Sprengel deformity
  - Sprengel deformity is a congenital anomaly of scapular development in which the scapula remains small and undescended secondary to an interruption of the embryonic subclavian blood supply. This leads to scapular hypoplasia and winging with limited scapulothoracic motion. Patients typically have deficiencies both in forward elevation and abduction.[3]
  - It may require surgical correction for severe functional deformities with surgery ideally being performed between 3 and 8 years old (patients older than 8 years old have an increased risk of nerve injury). Advanced imaging should be performed to asses for presence of an omovertebral bar connecting the superomedial border of the scapulae to one of the lower cervical vertebrae.[50,51]
    - Woodward procedure: This procedure includes resection of any omovertebral bar division of the vertebral attachments of the trapezius, rhomboids and levator scapulae with correction of scapular rotation, and reattachment of these muscular origins to more caudal vertebrae. This may be combined with clavicular osteotomy to prevent compression of the brachial plexus.[50-52]
    - Green procedure: Resection of the prominent superior border of the scapula, subperiosteal division of the medial scapular muscle attachments, displacement of the scapula inferiorly, and reattachment after appropriate translation.[50,53,54]
- Fascioscapulohumeral dystrophy
  - Fascioscapulohumeral dystrophy is a genetic neuromuscular dystrophy presenting in the second decade of life with shoulder girdle weakness, scapulothoracic instability, and limitations in flexion and abduction. The deltoid is typically spared and disease progression is slow.[55]
  - Given the involvement of multiple periscapular muscles, dynamic muscle transfers are not as effective as scapulothoracic fusion. If stability of the scapulothoracic articulation is achieved, the deltoid is typically is sufficiently functional for elevation and improved function.[56] Scapulothoracic fusion results in one-third loss of total elevation and up to 50% pseudoarthrosis rates.
- Primary scapular winging secondary to osseous abnormalities
  - Scapular winging can occur secondary to osteochondromas of the scapula[57] (the most common scapular bony tumor) or malunion of a prior scapula fracture.[4]
- Secondary scapular winging
  - Physical examination of any patient with shoulder dysfunction should include evaluation for secondary scapular winging at rest, with dynamic forward elevation, and resisted forward elevation. Normal EMG findings are suggestive of secondary winging.
  - A common cause of secondary medial winging is posterior glenohumeral instability. As the shoulder subluxates out posteriorly, the scapula attempts to capture the humeral head by winging medially.
  - Contractural winging is an example of when soft-tissue contracture can produce secondary scapular winging. Contractural winging is found when patients exhibit the "scapular sign of Putti"—the superior corner of the scapula projects away from the chest wall as the shoulder is forcibly adducted to the chest wall.[58] Contractural winging can also occur in the setting of fibrosis of the deltoid in which cases winging decreases with arm elevation and increases with lowering of the arm.
  - Glenohumeral motion is reflexively limited in the setting of a painful shoulder, thus leading to increased work of the periscapular muscles. As the periscapular muscles fatigue with this increased workload, secondary winging occurs.
  - The treatment for secondary scapular winging is to address the primary pathology; the scapular winging is not likely to improve until the primary source is corrected.

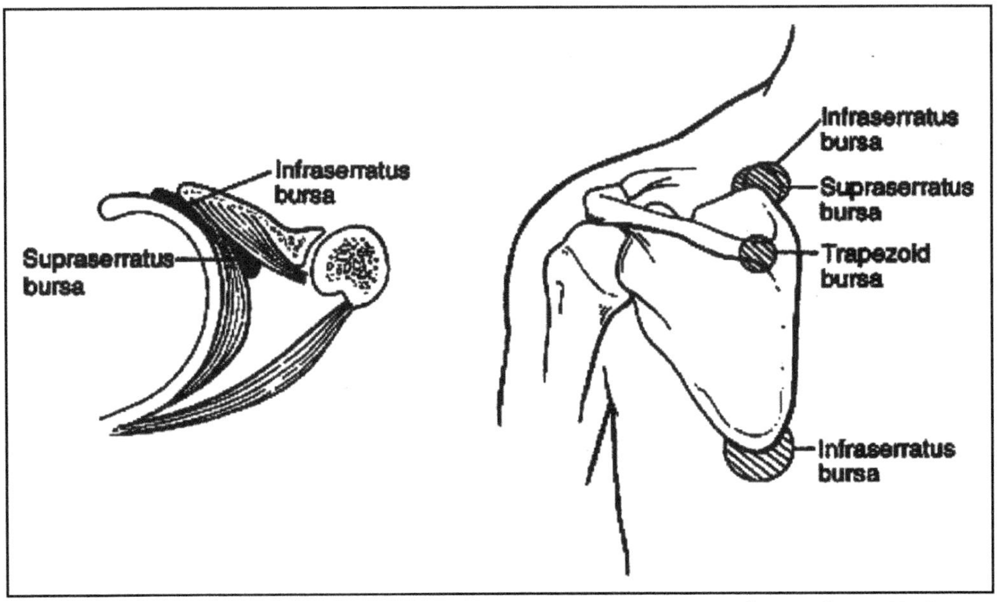

Figure 15-4. Bursae of the scapulothoracic joint. (Reprinted with permission from Williams GR, Ramsey ML, Wiesel BB. Snapping Scapula Syndrome. In: *Operative Techniques in Shoulder and Elbow Surgery*. 2nd ed. Philadelphia, PA: Wolters Kluwer; 2016:466.)

Snapping Scapula

- Presentation
  - Snapping scapula is also known as scapulothoracic crepitus or bursitis. This phenomenon is characterized by a tactile-acoustic sensation occurring with anomalous tissue between the chest wall and the scapula. This is typically a painless presentation though some patients report pain that correlates with this phenomenon.[59] This may occur following trauma (either a single episode or repetitive motion of the scapulothoracic joint) and is believed to be caused by abnormal motion between the anterior surface of the scapula and the chest wall.[59-61]
  - Patients should be evaluated for any scoliosis because this may alter scapular motion by changing the contour of the chest wall. Additionally, lesions such as osteochondroma (of the rib or scapula) and elastofibroma dorsi may lead to snapping scapula.
- Incidence and etiology
  - The articulation between the scapula and the chest wall is incongruent and made up of 3 layers (superficial, intermediate, and deep) with associated muscles and bursae (Figure 15-4).[62]
    - Superficial layer: Contains the trapezius and latissimus dorsi as well as the inferior angle bursa. The inferior angle bursa is between the inferomedial angle of the scapula and the superficial fibers of the latissimus dorsi, measuring on average 1.9 by 2.4 cm.[62]
    - Intermediate layer: Contains the rhomboid major, rhomboid minor, and levator scapulae muscles as well as the trapezial bursa. The trapezial bursa lies between the trapezius and the base of the scapular spine measuring on average 4.3 by 2.7 cm. This bursa importantly provides a smooth surface over which the scapula rotates. Importantly, this layer contains the spinal accessory nerve (crosses the superior border of the scapula approximately 2.7 cm lateral to the superomedial angle), the dorsal scapular nerve (deep to the levator scapulae, parallel to the medial border of the scapula), the transverse

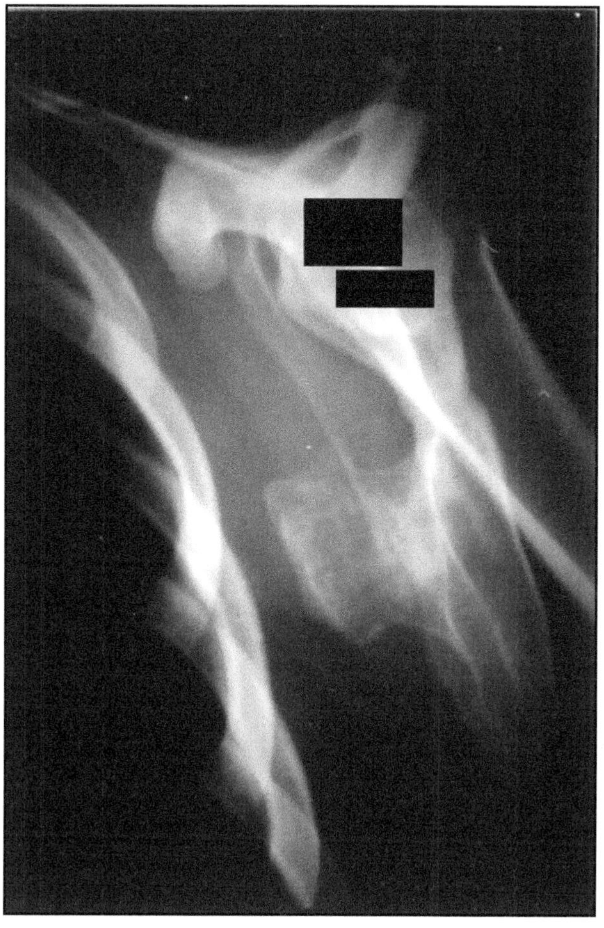

Figure 15-5. Osteochondroma of the scapula leading to snapping scapula syndrome.

cervical artery (divided by the levator scapulae into the dorsal scapular artery and a branch that runs with the spinal accessory nerve), and the suprascapular nerve (travels obliquely across the superomedial angle and superior border of the scapula). These structures are all at risk during surgical dissection within this level.[62]

- Deep layer: Contains the serratus anterior and subscapularis muscles along with 2 major bursae—the scapulothoracic (supraserratus) bursa and the subscapularis (infraserratus) bursa. The scapulothoracic bursa averages 9 by 7.4 cm in size and is located between the serratus anterior and the chest wall. The subscapularis bursa averages 5.3 by 5.3 cm in size and is located between the serratus anterior and the subscapularis. The subscapularis bursa is inconsistently present.[59]

- Approximately 6% of scapulae have a hooked shape prominence known as Luschka tubercle at the superomedial angle. This may enlarge and cause irritation by articulation with the chest wall.[61,63]
- Osteochondromas are a common cause of snapping scapula syndrome and can be excised if symptomatic (Figure 15-5).[64] However, chondrosarcoma must be considered in the differential diagnosis when evaluating lesions in the scapulothoracic articulation.[65]
- Elastofibromas are a result of friction between the chest wall and the scapula that can present with snapping scapula. These are circumscribed, but not encapsulated, benign lesions formed of collagen, adipose, and elastin. These can be excised surgically as symptoms dictate.[66]

  - Scapulothoracic bursitis may also be a result of abnormal scapular motion in the setting of muscle overuse, muscle imbalance, or glenohumeral pathology. Baseball pitchers may exhibit similar symptoms in the setting of overuse fatigue leading to Scapular malposition, Inferior medial border prominence, Coracoid pain and malposition, and dysKinesis of scapular movement (SICK) scapular syndrome.[67-69]
- Diagnosis
  - Standard radiographs should be performed to evaluate any potential osseous pathology. These include an anteroposterior view, a true anteroposterior (scapula flat against the cassette and the beam tilted to account for the scapular angle), a scapular-Y view (beam parallel to the spine of the scapula), and an axillary view (assessment of the glenohumeral joint). Routine computed tomography scan is not indicated and magnetic resonance imaging is useful if suspicious for a soft-tissue lesion.
- Treatment
  - The majority of patients with scapulothoracic crepitus or bursitis can be managed nonoperatively. Nonoperative management includes physical therapy, anti-inflammatories, and corticosteroid injections with local anesthetics. Injection of the scapulothoracic bursa is diagnostic as well as therapeutic. Injections are most easily placed with the shoulder extended and internally rotated to lift the medial border of the scapula away from the chest wall.[70]
  - Operative intervention is usually reserved for those with a clearly identifiable osseous or soft-tissue lesion.[65]
    - Skin incision is vertical, in line with the medial border of the scapula.
    - The incision should be centered (superior or inferior) on the area of pathology.
    - At the superomedial angle of the scapula, the trapezius may be split in line with its fibers over the scapular spine. Care must be taken to protect the spinal accessory nerve crossing the superior border of the scapula lateral to the superomedial angle (just lateral to levator scapulae).
    - The rhomboids and levator scapulae can be released subperiosteal to expose the anteromedial scapular border. The dorsal scapular nerve runs 2 cm medial to the medial scapular edge and care must be taken to avoid injury.
    - The soft-tissue or osseous lesion can be removed through this window.
    - The rhomboids may be reattached through drill holes.
  - Arthroscopic scapulothoracic bursectomy has also been described (Figure 15-6).[71,72]
    - Positioning can be either prone with the arm extended and internally rotated (opens the medial border of the scapula) or lateral decubitus (allowing for concomitant glenohumeral and subacromial arthroscopy).
    - Portals must be placed at least 3 cm medial to the medial border of the scapula to avoid injury to the dorsal scapular nerve and vessels.
    - The superior visualization portal should be placed just inferior to the scapular spine to access both the superomedial and inferomedial angle of the scapula.
    - The inferior working portal should be placed under direct visualization, with the starting point approximately between the scapular spine and inferomedial angle of the scapula.
    - Taking care to point the instruments away from the coracoid process will help prevent injury of the suprascapular nerve and vessels that travel just medial to the base of the coracoid.
    - The incision should be centered (superior or inferior) on the area of pathology.

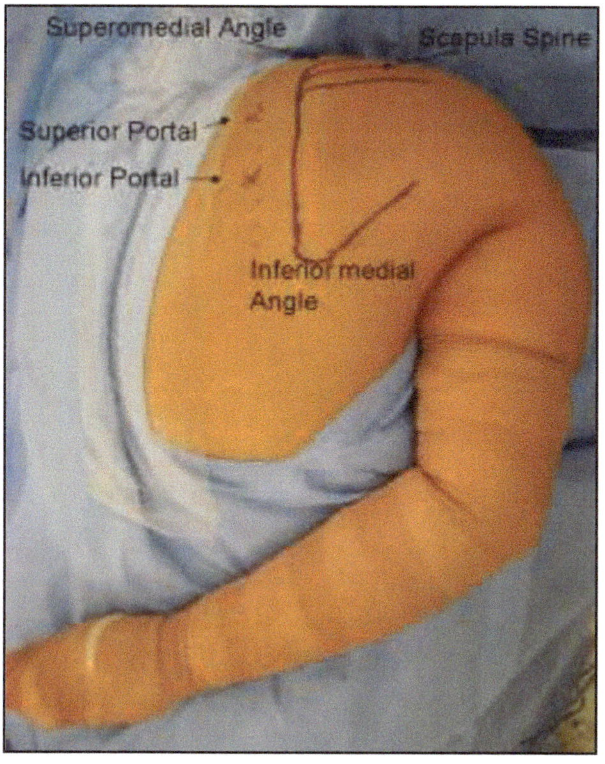

Figure 15-6. Landmarks and portal placement for scapulothoracic arthroscopy.

- Portals superior to the scapular spine should be avoided because of the risk of injury to the dorsal scapular nerve or spinal accessory nerve. If access to the superomedial angle is limited, a second superolateral working portal can be placed inside out. This can be placed safely at one-third the distance from the superomedial angle and the acromion.
- Arthroscopically, the scapulothoracic bursa can be excised and the shoulder may be ranged by the surgeon with visualization of the superomedial angle. Any prominence can then be resected arthroscopically. The amount of bony resection that can be tolerated has been debated, but most recommend 2 to 3 cm of resection.[71,72]
- Arthroscopic technique preserves the rhomboid insertion and mitigates the need for postoperative immobilization of open surgery.
- Following debridement, the surgeon should examine the patient under anesthesia to ensure adequate elimination of impingement.

References

1. Inman VT, Saunders JB, Abbott LC. Observations of the function of the shoulder joint. 1944. *Clin Orthop Relat Res.* 1996;(330):3-12.
2. Winslow J. Observations anatomiques sur, quelques mouvements extraordinaires des omoplates et des bras, et sur une nouveau espece de muscles. *Mem Acad Royale Sci.* 1719;IV(486):98-112.
3. Leibovic SJ, Ehrlich MG, Zaleske DJ. Sprengel deformity. *J Bone Joint Surg Am.* 1990;72(2):192-197.
4. Wiater JM, Flatow EL. Long thoracic nerve injury. *Clin Orthop Relat Res.* 1999;(368):17-27.
5. Feinberg JH, Radecki J. Parsonage-Turner syndrome. *HSS J.* 2010;6(2):199-205. doi:10.1007/s11420-010-9176-x.
6. Martin RM, Fish DE. Scapular winging: anatomical review, diagnosis, and treatments. *Curr Rev Musculoskelet Med.* 2008;1(1):1-11. doi:10.1007/s12178-007-9000-5.
7. Gregg JR, Labosky D, Harty M, et al. Serratus anterior paralysis in the young athlete. *J Bone Joint Surg Am.* 1979;61(6A):825-832.

8. Fardin P, Negrin P, Dainese R. The isolated paralysis of the serratus anterior muscle: clinical and electromyographical follow-up of 10 cases. *Electromyogr Clin Neurophysiol.* 1978;18(5):379-386.
9. Overpeck DO, Ghormley RK. Paralysis of the serratus magnus muscle: caused by lesions of the long thoracic nerve. *JAMA.* 1940;114(20):1994-1996. doi:10.1001/jama.1940.02810200022006.
10. Gozna ER, Harris WR. Traumatic winging of the scapula. *J Bone Joint Surg Am.* 1979;61(8):1230-1233.
11. Foo CL, Swann M. Isolated paralysis of the serratus anterior. A report of 20 cases. *J Bone Joint Surg Br.* 1983;65(5):552-556.
12. Erdogmus S, Govsa F. Mapping the course of long thoracic nerve. *Neuroanatomy.* 2004;(3):2-7.
13. Goodman CE, Kenrick MM, Blum MV. Long thoracic nerve palsy: a follow-up study. *Arch Phys Med Rehabil.* 1975;56(8):352-358.
14. Kauppila LI, Vastamäki M. Iatrogenic serratus anterior paralysis. Long-term outcome in 26 patients. *Chest.* 1996;109(1):31-34. doi:10.1378/chest.109.1.31.
15. Makin GJ, Brown WF, Ebers GC. C7 radiculopathy: importance of scapular winging in clinical diagnosis. *J Neurol Neurosurg Psychiatry.* 1986;49(6):640-644. doi:10.1136/jnnp.49.6.640.
16. Kaplan PE. Electrodiagnostic confirmation of long thoracic nerve palsy. *J Neurol Neurosurg Psychiatry.* 1980;43(1):50-52. doi:10.1136/jnnp.43.1.50.
17. Tomaino MM. Neurophysiologic and clinical outcome following medial pectoral to long thoracic nerve transfer for scapular winging: a case report. *Microsurgery.* 2002;22(6):254-257. doi:10.1002/micr.10046.
18. Disa JJ, Wang B, Dellon AL. Correction of Scapular winging by supraclavicular neurolysis of the long thoracic nerve. *J Reconstr Microsurg.* 2001;17(02):79-84. doi:10.1055/s-2001-12694.
19. Novak CB, Mackinnon SE. Surgical treatment of a long thoracic nerve palsy. *Ann Thorac Surg.* 2002;73(5):1643-1645. doi:10.1016/S0003-4975(01)03372-0.
20. Connor PM, Yamaguchi K, Manifold SG, Pollock RG, Flatow EL, Bigliani LU. Split pectoralis major transfer for serratus anterior palsy. *Clin Orthop Relat Res.* 1997;(341):134-142.
21. Post M. Pectoralis major transfer for winging of the scapula. *J Shoulder Elbow Surg.* 1995;4:1-9. doi:10.1016/s1058-2746(10)80001-1.
22. Povacz P, Resch H. Dynamic stabilization of winging scapula by direct split pectoralis major transfer: a technical note. *J Shoulder Elbow Surg.* 2000;9(1):76-78. doi:10.1016/s1058-2746(00)90015-6.
23. Wiater JM, Bigliani LU. Spinal accessory nerve injury. *Clin Orthop Relat Res.* 1999;(368):5-16.
24. Bigliani LU, Compito CA, Duralde XA, Wolfe IN. Transfer of the levator scapulae, rhomboid major, and rhomboid minor for paralysis of the trapezius. *J Bone Joint Surg Am.* 1996;78(10):1534-1540. doi:10.2106/00004623-199610000-00011.
25. Bigliani LU, Perez-Sanz JR, Wolfe IN. Treatment of trapezius paralysis. *J Bone Joint Surg Am.* 1985;67(6):871-877.
26. Williams WW, Twyman RS, Donell ST, Birch R. The posterior triangle and the painful shoulder: spinal accessory nerve injury. *Ann R Coll Surg Engl.* 1996;78(6):521-525.
27. Saeed MA, Gatens PF Jr, Singh S. Winging of the scapula. *Am Fam Physician.* 1981;24(4):139-143.
28. Levy O, Relwani JG, Mullett H, Haddo O, Even T. The active elevation lag sign and the triangle sign: new clinical signs of trapezius palsy. *J Shoulder Elbow Surg.* 2009;18(4):573-576. doi:10.1016/j.jse.2009.02.015.
29. Kierner AC, Zelenka I, Heller S, Burian M. Surgical anatomy of the spinal accessory nerve and the trapezius branches of the cervical plexus. *Arch Surg.* 2000;135(12):1428-1431. doi:10.1001/archsurg.135.12.1428.
30. Donner TR, Kline DG. Extracranial spinal accessory nerve injury. *Neurosurgery.* 1993;32(6):907-910; discussion 911. doi:10.1227/00006123-199306000-00004.
31. Teboul F, Bizot P, Kakkar R, Sedel L. Surgical management of trapezius palsy. *J Bone Joint Surg Am.* 2004;86(9):1884-1890. doi:10.2106/00004623-200409000-00005.
32. Seror P, Stojkovic T, Lefevre-Colau MM, Lenglet T. Diagnosis of unilateral trapezius muscle palsy: 54 cases. *Muscle Nerve.* 2017;56(2):215-223. doi:10.1002/mus.25481.
33. Petrera JE, Trojaborg W. Conduction studies along the accessory nerve and follow-up of patients with trapezius palsy. *J Neurol Neurosurg Psychiatry.* 1984;47(6):630-636. doi:10.1136/jnnp.47.6.630.
34. Kim DH, Cho YJ, Tiel RL, Kline DG. Surgical outcomes of 111 spinal accessory nerve injuries. *Neurosurgery.* 2003;53(5):1106-1112; discussion 1102-1103. doi:10.1227/01.neu.0000089058.82201.3d.
35. Dewar FP, Harris RI. Restoration of function of the shoulder following paralysis of the trapezius by fascial sling fixation and transplantation of the levator scapulae. *Ann Surg.* 1950;132(6):1111-1115. doi:10.1097/00000658-195012000-00010.
36. Langenskiöld A, Ryöppy S. Treatment of paralysis of the trapezius muscle by the Eden-Lange operation. *Acta Orthop Scand.* 1973;44(4):383-388. doi:10.3109/17453677308989074.
37. Galano GJ, Bigliani LU, Ahmad CS, Levine WN. Surgical treatment of winged scapula. *Clin Orthop Relat Res.* 2008;466(3):652-660. doi:10.1007/s11999-007-0086-2.
38. Elhassan BT, Wagner ER. Outcome of triple-tendon transfer, an Eden-Lange variant, to reconstruct trapezius paralysis. *J Shoulder Elbow Surg.* 2015;24(8):1307-1313. doi:10.1016/j.jse.2015.01.008.
39. Meininger AK, Figuerres BF, Goldberg BA. Scapular winging: an update. *J Am Acad Orthop Surg.* 2011;19(8):453-462. doi:10.5435/00124635-201108000-00001.

40. Sultan HE, Younis El-Tantawi GA. Role of dorsal scapular nerve entrapment in unilateral interscapular pain. *Arch Phys Med Rehabil.* 2013;94(6):1118-1125. doi:10.1016/j.apmr.2012.11.040.
41. Benedetti M, Zati A, Stagni S, Fusaro I, Monesi R, Rotini R. Winged scapula caused by rhomboid paralysis: a case report. *Joints.* 2016;04(04):247-249. doi:10.11138/jts/2016.4.4.247.
42. Sultan HE, Younis El-Tantawi GA. Role of dorsal scapular nerve entrapment in unilateral interscapular pain. *Arch Phys Med Rehabil.* 2013;94(6):1118-1125. doi:10.1016/j.apmr.2012.11.040.
43. Dickson FD. Fascial transplants in paralytic and other conditions. *J Bone Joint Surg Am.* 1937;19(2):405-412.
44. Chen D, Gu Y, Lao J, Chen L. Dorsal scapular nerve compression. Atypical thoracic outlet syndrome. *Chin Med J (Engl).* 1995;108(8):582-585.
45. Hayes JM, Zehr DJ. Traumatic muscle avulsion causing winging of the scapula. A case report. *J Bone Joint Surg Am.* 1981;63(3):495-497.
46. Lee SG, Kim JH, Lee SY, Choi IS, Moon ES. Winged scapula caused by rhomboideus and trapezius muscles rupture associated with repetitive minor trauma: a case report. *J Korean Med Sci.* 2006;21(3):581. doi:10.3346/jkms.2006.21.3.581.
47. Kibler WB, Sciascia A, Uhl T. Medial scapular muscle detachment: clinical presentation and surgical treatment. *J Shoulder Elbow Surg.* 2014;23(1):58-67. doi:10.1016/j.jse.2013.05.008.
48. Chernev I, Pessina MA. Unilateral complete congenital serratus anterior muscle aplasia: a case report. *PM R.* 2009;1(6):587-589. doi:10.1016/j.pmrj.2009.01.025.
49. Vajramani A, Witham FM, Richards RH. Congenital unilateral absence of sternocleidomastoid and trapezius muscles: a case report and literature review. *J Pediatr Orthop B.* 2010;19(5):462-464. doi:10.1097/BPB.0b013e32833ce404.
50. Kadavkolan A, Bhatia D, Dasgupta B, Bhosale P. Sprengel's deformity of the shoulder: current perspectives in management. *Int J Shoulder Surg.* 2011;5(1):1-8. doi:10.4103/0973-6042.80459.
51. Carson WG, Lovell WW, Whitesides TE Jr. Congenital elevation of the scapula. Surgical correction by the Woodward procedure. *J Bone Joint Surg Am.* 1981;63(8):1199-1207.
52. Borges JL, Shah A, Torres BC, Bowen JR. Modified Woodward procedure for Sprengel deformity of the shoulder: long-term results. *J Pediatr Orthop.* 1996;16(4):508-513. doi:10.1097/00004694-199607000-00018.
53. Andrault G, Salmeron F, Laville JM. Green's surgical procedure in Sprengel's deformity: cosmetic and functional results. *Orthop Traumatol Surg Res.* 2009;95(5):330-335. doi:10.1016/j.otsr.2009.04.015.
54. Gonen E, Simsek U, Solak S, Bektaser B, Ates Y, Aydin E. Long-term results of modified Green method in Sprengel's deformity. *J Child Orthop.* 2010;4(4):309-314. doi:10.1007/s11832-010-0265-7.
55. Tawil R. Facioscapulohumeral muscular dystrophy. *Neurotherapeutics.* 2008;5(4):601-606. doi:10.1016/j.nurt.2008.07.005.
56. Rhee YG, Ha JH. Long-term results of scapulothoracic arthrodesis of facioscapulohumeral muscular dystrophy. *J Shoulder Elbow Surg.* 2006;15(4):445-450. doi:10.1016/j.jse.2005.10.015.
57. Tomo H, Ito Y, Aono M, Takaoka K. Chest wall deformity associated with osteochondroma of the scapula: a case report and review of the literature. *J Shoulder Elbow Surg.* 2005;14(1):103-106. doi:10.1016/j.jse.2004.03.007.
58. Eismann EA, Little KJ, Laor T, Cornwall R. Glenohumeral abduction contracture in children with unresolved neonatal brachial plexus palsy. *J Bone Joint Surg Am.* 2015;97(2):112-118. doi:10.2106/JBJS.N.00203.
59. Gaskill T, Millett PJ. Snapping scapula syndrome: diagnosis and management. *J Am Acad Orthop Surg.* 2013;21(4):214-224. doi:10.5435/JAAOS-21-04-214.
60. Aggarwal A, Wahee P, Harjeet, Aggarwal AK, Sahni D. Variable osseous anatomy of costal surface of scapula and its implications in relation to snapping scapula syndrome. *Surg Radiol Anat.* 2011;33(2):135-140. doi:10.1007/s00276-010-0723-4.
61. Edelson JG. Variations in the anatomy of the scapula with reference to the snapping scapula. *Clin Orthop Relat Res.* 1996;(322):111-115.
62. Kuhn JE. The scapulothoracic articulation: anatomy, biomechanics, pathophysiology, and management. In: Iannotti JP, Williams GR, eds. *Disorders of the Shoulder: Diagnosis and Management.* Philadelphia, PA: Lippincott Williams & Wilkins; 1999:817-845.
63. Dietrich TJ, Agten CA, Fürnstahl P, Vlachopoulos L, Pfirrmann CWA. The legend of the Luschka tubercle and its association with snapping scapulae: osseous morphology of snapping scapulae on CT images. *AJR Am J Roentgenol.* 2017;209(1):159-166. doi:10.2214/AJR.16.17232.
64. Clarke DO, Crichlow A, Christmas M, et al. The unusual osteochondroma: a case of snapping scapula syndrome and review of the literature. *Orthop Traumatol Surg Res.* 2017;103(8):1295-1298. doi:10.1016/j.otsr.2017.01.019.
65. Ford LT, Ramsey RH. Chondrosarcoma of the pelvis and shoulder girdle. *South Med J.* 1962;55:901-906. doi:10.1097/00007611-196209000-00008.
66. Majó J, Gracia I, Doncel A, Valera M, Núñez A, Guix M. Elastofibroma dorsi as a cause of shoulder pain or snapping scapula. *Clin Orthop Relat Res.* 2001;(388):200-204. doi:10.1097/00003086-200107000-00027.
67. Seroyer ST, Nho SJ, Bach BR Jr, Bush-Joseph CA, Nicholson GP, Romeo AA. Shoulder Pain in the overhead throwing athlete. *Sports Health.* 2009;1(2):108-120. doi:10.1177/1941738108331199.
68. Kibler WB. The role of the scapula in athletic shoulder function. *Am J Sports Med.* 1998;26(2):325-337. doi:10.1177/03635465980260022801.

69. Meister K. Injuries to the shoulder in the throwing athlete. Part one: Biomechanics/pathophysiology/classification of injury. *Am J Sports Med.* 2000;28(2):265-275. doi:10.1177/03635465000280022301.
70. Chang WH, Im SH, Ryu JA, Lee SC, Kim JS. The effects of scapulothoracic bursa injections in patients with scapular pain: a pilot study. *Arch Phys Med Rehabil.* 2009;90(2):279-284. doi:10.1016/j.apmr.2008.07.027.
71. Saper M, Kasik C, Dietzel D. Arthroscopic scapulothoracic decompression for snapping scapula syndrome. *Arthrosc Tech.* 2015;4(6):e631-e636. doi:10.1016/j.eats.2015.07.002.
72. Tashjian RZ, Granger EK, Barney JK, Partridge DR. Functional outcomes after arthroscopic scapulothoracic bursectomy and partial superomedial angle scapulectomy. *Orthop J Sports Med.* 2013;1(5):2325967113505739. doi:10.1177/2325967113505739.

16

Acromioclavicular Disorders

Jason E. Hsu, MD

Anatomy and Pathophysiology

- Anatomy of the acromioclavicular (AC) joint
  - The AC joint is formed by the junction of concave surface of the anteromedial acromion and the convex surface of the lateral clavicle with an intervening fibrocartilaginous disc.
  - Static stabilizers include the overlying capsule and ligaments.[1-4]
    - AC ligaments are restraints to smaller displacements at the joint, primarily in the anterior and posterior direction.
    - Coracoclavicular (CC) ligaments include the conoid ligament (4.5 cm from the AC joint) and trapezoid ligament (2.5 cm from the AC joint), which resist larger displacements; primary restraints in vertical and axial translation and secondary restraints to anterior and posterior displacement in the absence of AC ligaments (Figure 16-1).
  - Dynamic stabilizers include the anterior deltoid, trapezius, and serratus anterior.
- AC degenerative joint disease occurs as a result of degeneration of the fibrocartilaginous disc as a result of mechanical stress and aging.[5]
- Distal clavicle osteolysis may be a result of repetitive microtrauma and increased osteoclastic activity.[6]
- AC separations typically occur as a result of fall directly onto the shoulder and injury to the AC and CC ligaments.
  - The Rockwood classification[7] is the most commonly referenced classification for AC injuries (Figure 16-2). *Recommended reading for historical context and understanding classification*
    - Type I: sprain or partial tear of joint capsule
    - Type II: complete tear of AC ligaments; intact CC ligaments

Namdari S, Zmistowski B, Omid R, eds.
The Foundations of Shoulder and Elbow Surgery (pp 299-307).

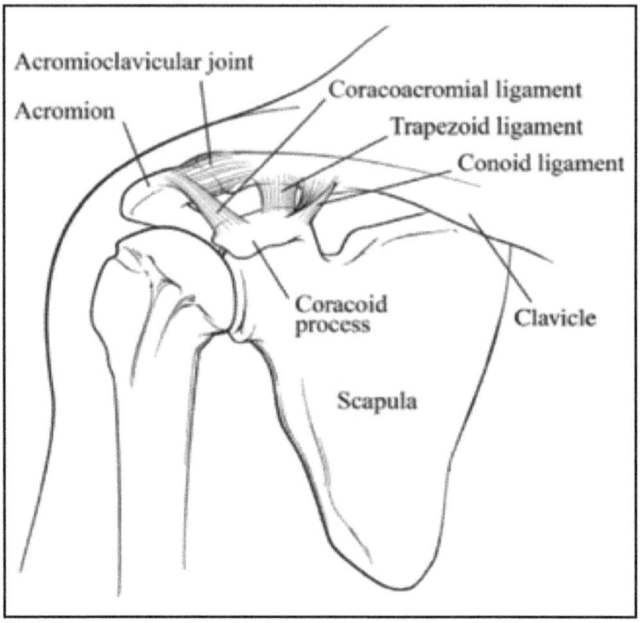

Figure 16-1. The CC ligaments include the conoid ligament and the trapezoid ligament and resist superior displacement of the clavicle relative to the acromion. (Reprinted with permission from Beitzel K, Obopilwe E, Chowaniec DM, et al. Biomechanical comparison of arthroscopic repairs for acromioclavicular joint instability: suture button systems without biological augmentation. *Am J Sports Med.* 2011;39[10]:2218-2225. doi: 10.1177/0363546511416784.)

- Type III: complete disruption of AC and CC ligaments; CC interval up to 100% greater than uninjured side
- Type IV: posterior displacement
- Type V: complete disruption of AC and CC ligaments; CC interval 100% to 300% greater than uninjured side
- Type VI: inferior displacement of distal clavicle into the subcoracoid position

- Distal clavicle fractures also can result from a fall onto the shoulder or blunt trauma to the distal clavicle.
  - Multiple classification of clavicle fractures exist, including the Allman,[8] Neer,[9,10] Craig,[11] and Robinson[12] classifications.
  - Stability of the fracture is based on the location of the fracture relative to the CC ligaments.

Diagnosis

- AC osteoarthritis and distal clavicle osteolysis are diagnosed by a combination of clinical and radiographic findings.
  - History
    - Patients will typically complain of pain over the anterosuperior shoulder with activity, particularly with motions requiring cross-body adduction.
    - History of inflammatory arthropathies or risk factors for septic arthritis may be elicited.
    - Distal clavicle osteolysis should be considered in heavy laborers, weight lifters, and other individuals who participate in activities involving large forces across the AC joint.
  - Clinical examination
    - The patient will exhibit prominence and tenderness over the lateral clavicle.
    - Provocative testing includes the following[13]:

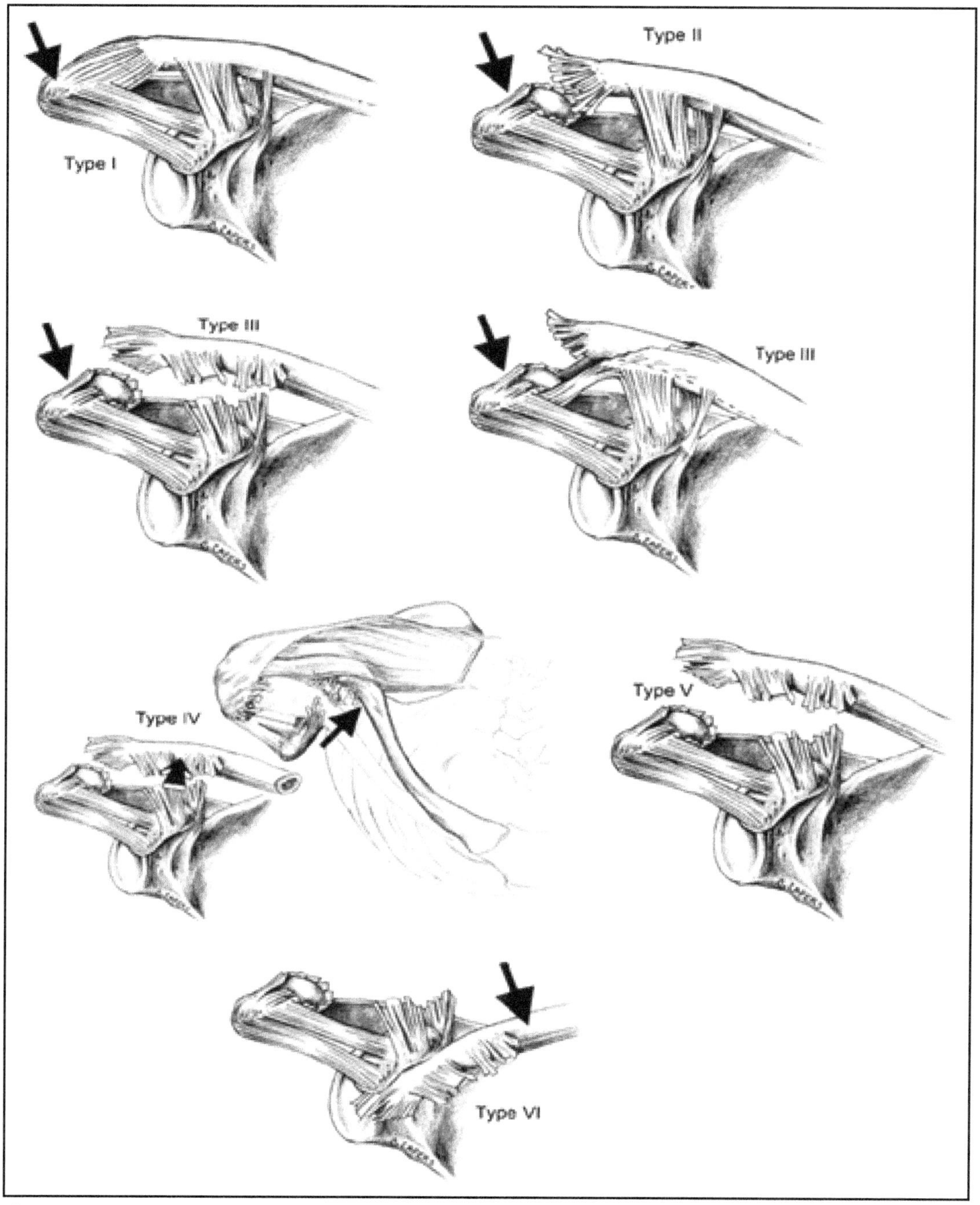

Figure 16-2. The Rockwood classification system of AC separation includes 6 different types. (Reprinted with permission from Beim GM. Acromioclavicular joint injuries. *J Athl Train.* 2000;35[3]:261-267.)

- Cross-body adduction test: pain with maximal adduction in 90 degrees of forward elevation
- AC resisted extension test: pain with resisted shoulder extension with arm in 90 degrees of forward elevation
- O'Brien active compression test: Pain with resisted shoulder flexion with shoulder in 90 degrees of forward flexion, 10 degrees of adduction, and with arm in maximal

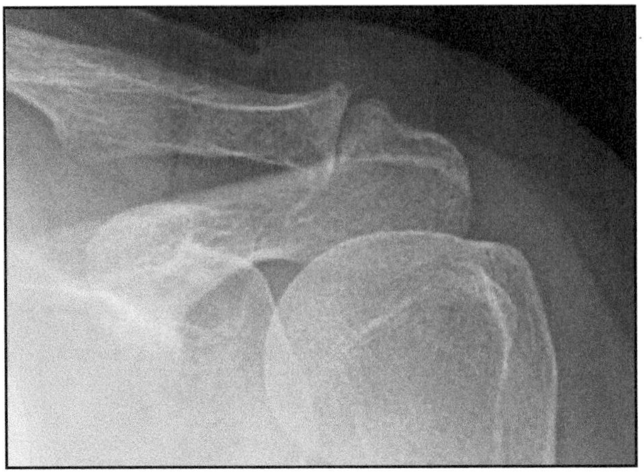

Figure 16-3. Radiographic appearance of AC degenerative disease includes joint space narrowing, subchondral cysts, osteophytes, and subchondral sclerosis.

supination. Pain with arm in maximal internal rotation is more consistent with a superior labrum anterior and posterior lesion.

- A comprehensive shoulder girdle examination to rule out glenohumeral and scapulothoracic pathologies must be conducted, because AC joint pain may be best treated by addressing the concomitant pathology rather than the AC joint itself.
  - Cyst formation (ie, "Geyser sign") may occur in older patients with concomitant full-thickness rotator cuff tears.
  - Glenohumeral capsular stiffness is commonly associated with AC joint pain.
- Given that the symptoms of AC joint arthritis overlap with symptoms of other common shoulder diagnoses, a diagnostic injection into the AC joint can be used if the clinician is uncertain of the source of pain.

- Imaging
  - Zanca view: anteroposterior view with 10 to 15 degrees of cephalad tilt[14]
  - Classic radiographic signs of osteoarthritis include joint space narrowing, subchondral cysts, osteophytes, and subchondral sclerosis (Figure 16-3).
  - Distal clavicle osteolysis will show lysis of the distal clavicle; magnetic resonance imaging may show increased T2 signal in the distal clavicle and medial acromion (Figure 16-4).
  - Many asymptomatic patients have radiographic findings of AC arthritis; diagnosis must be in the context of appropriate clinical findings.

- Diagnosis of AC separations are diagnosed with an appropriate injury mechanism, examination findings, and radiographic findings.
  - Tenderness at the AC joint with lower-grade AC separations
  - High-grade AC separations typically clinically obvious on inspection and palpation
  - Radiographs
    - Bilateral Zanca view should be used to compare CC intervals (Figure 16-5).
    - The typical CC interval is 11 to 13 mm.[15]
    - An axillary view should be performed to diagnose type IV injuries.
    - Some clinicians incorporate stress radiographs (holding 10-pound [4.5 kg] weights) to help differentiate between type II and III injuries.
- Diagnosis of distal clavicle fractures is typically made with radiographs.
  - Swelling, ecchymosis, and tenting of the skin over the proximal fragment may be seen.

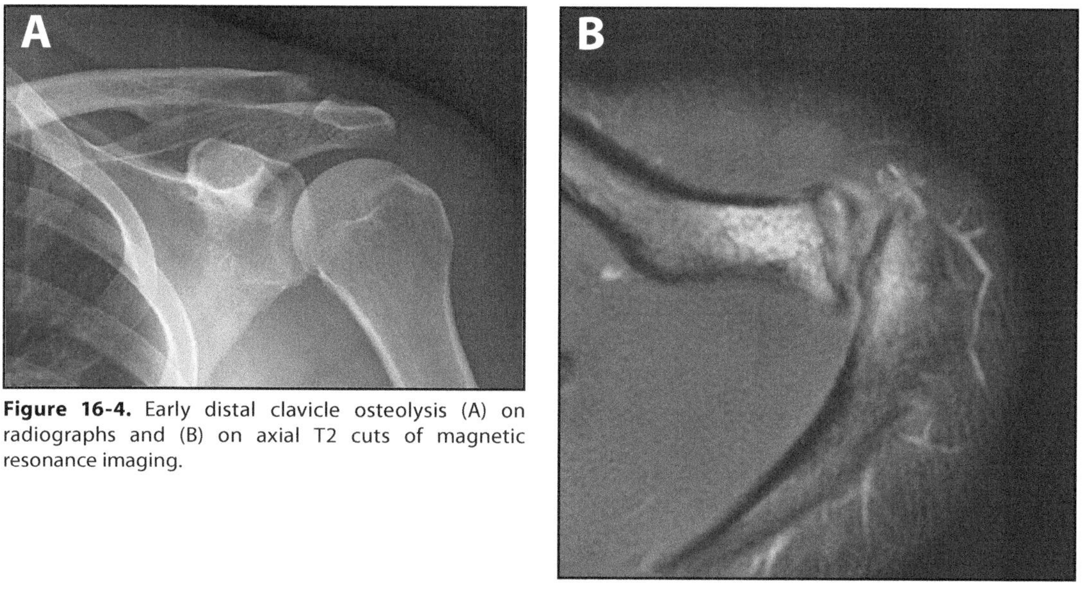

Figure 16-4. Early distal clavicle osteolysis (A) on radiographs and (B) on axial T2 cuts of magnetic resonance imaging.

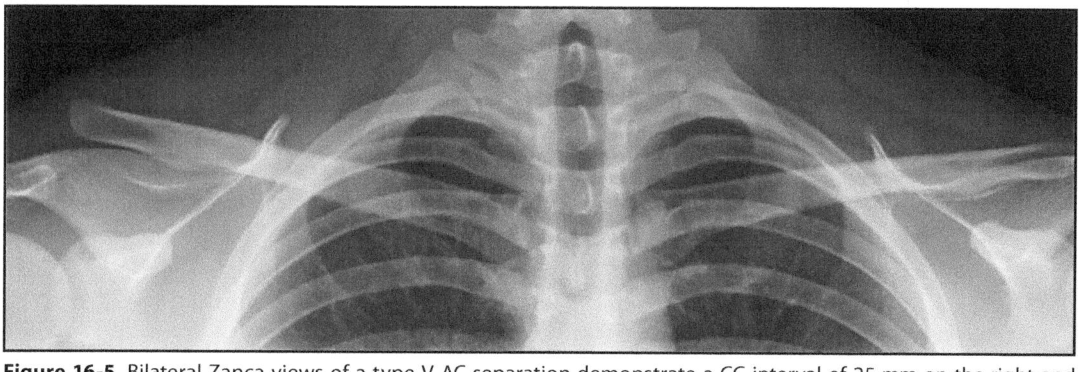

Figure 16-5. Bilateral Zanca views of a type V AC separation demonstrate a CC interval of 25 mm on the right and 11 mm on the left.

- Palpation of the scapula and ribs and a thorough neurovascular examination should be performed to rule out concomitant injuries.
- Radiographs can be used to determine amount of displacement and relationship or involvement of fracture fragments to CC ligaments (Figure 16-6A).

Treatment

- Treatment of AC arthritis and distal clavicle osteolysis beings with conservative modalities such as activity modification, nonsteroidal anti-inflammatory medications, and intra-articular injections, progressing to surgical options if nonoperative treatments provide inadequate control of symptoms.
  - Physical therapy may not be helpful for isolated AC joint pain but should be considered in patients with concomitant glenohumeral and scapulothoracic problems (eg, frozen shoulder or scapular dyskinesis) given the increased stresses across the AC joint in these pathologies.

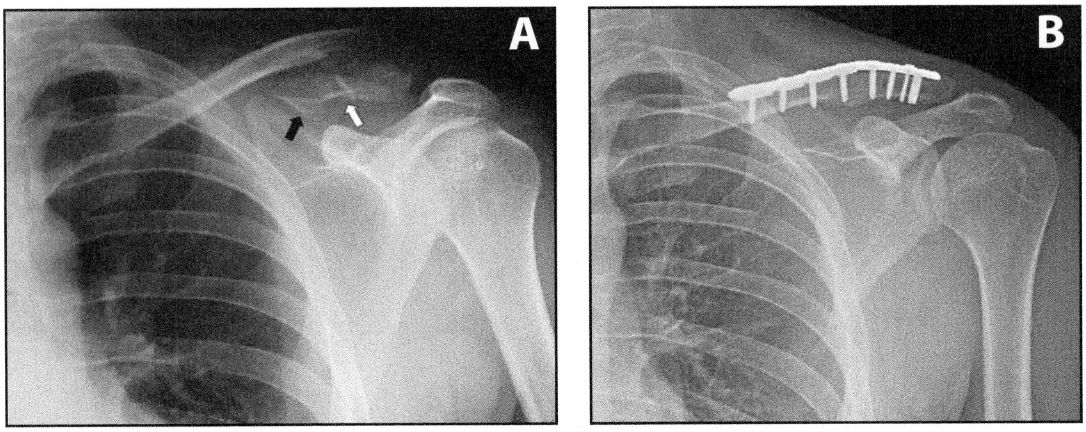

Figure 16-6. (A) Radiographs of a distal clavicle fracture demonstrate displaced fragments attached to the conoid (black arrow) and trapezoid (white arrow) ligaments. (B) Open reduction internal fixation with a distal clavicle locking plate; in this case, no CC ligament repair or reconstruction was necessary given the stable fixation of the fragments attached to the ligaments.

- Distal clavicle excision can be considered when nonoperative treatment fails.
  - Either an open or arthroscopic approach can be considered with comparable results.[16-18]
  - Open approach
    - A 3 to 4 cm saber incision just medial to the overlying joint down to the deltotrapezial fascia, which is split longitudinally
    - Resection using an oscillating sagittal saw is carried parallel to the medial border of the acromion.
    - Flexion-adduction maneuver is performed while palpating for residual bony contact to ensure adequate resection.
    - The capsule and deltotrapezial fascia must be closed to prevent subtle instability.
  - Arthroscopic approach
    - After appropriate subacromial bursectomy, the AC joint is visualized from a lateral portal and can be confirmed with palpation over the distal clavicle.
    - Resection of medial acromion and inferior joint capsule exposes the articular portion; ensure that posterior AC ligaments are not compromised
    - Through an anterior portal in line with the AC joint, the distal clavicle is excised from anterior to posterior and inferior to superior using a bur.
    - Downward force on the lateral clavicle can assist in ensuring that the superior distal clavicle is adequately resected; this can be confirmed by visualizing through the anterior portal.
  - The appropriate width of resection is controversial; it must be adequate to avoid residual bony contact, but excessive resection can lead to iatrogenic instability.[19]
    - It is generally accepted that resection should not exceed 10 mm to prevent iatrogenic instability.[20]
    - Resection of 2 to 3 mm of the medial acromion and 3 to 4 mm of the distal clavicle can be performed without compromising the ligamentous insertions.[1,21,22]
- Treatment of AC joint dislocation is controversial with regards to operative vs nonoperative management, early vs delayed treatment, and anatomic vs nonanatomic techniques.
  - Treatment of types I and II is nonoperative: a brief period of sling immobilization followed by early shoulder motion.

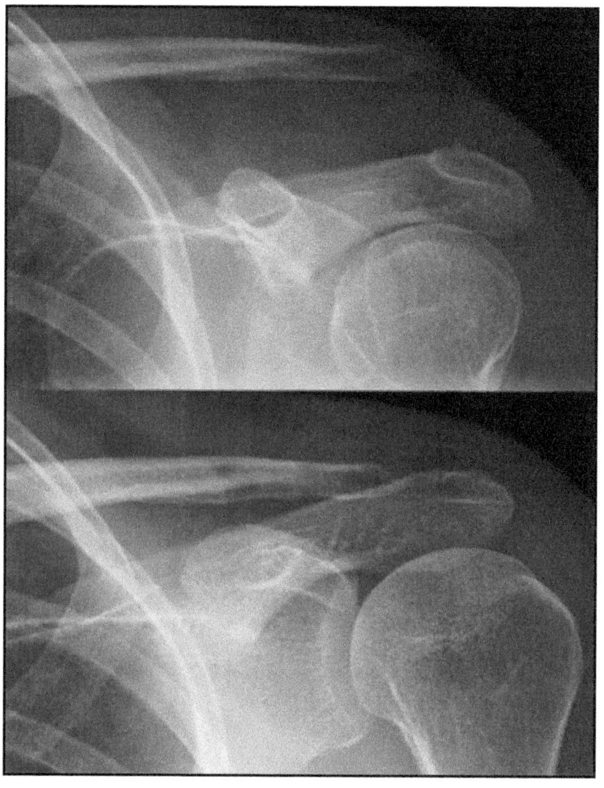

Figure 16-7. CC ligament reconstruction can be performed by numerous techniques, including a dual-tunnel configuration.

- Treatment of type III is controversial, and operative management is considered primarily in young patients with high functional demands or those that have failed nonoperative treatment.
- Treatment of types IV, V, and VI is generally accepted to be surgical, but nonoperative treatment can be considered in some cases given the high complication rate and failure associated with fixation.
- A large number of open and arthroscopic techniques have been described without evidence of superiority of any particular technique.
  - The Weaver-Dunn is a classic but outdated technique involving excision of the distal clavicle and transfer of the CC ligament from the acromion to the distal clavicle[23]; screw fixation between the clavicle and coracoid and pin fixation of the AC joint are techniques that are also largely outdated.
  - Autograft or allograft CC ligament reconstruction can be considered; the graft can be docked through or around the coracoid and looped around the clavicle, passed through a nonanatomic single tunnel,[24-26] or through an anatomic dual tunnel configuration[27-30] (Figure 16-7).
  - AC ligaments can be repaired or reconstructed with excess graft from the CC ligament reconstruction to provide enhanced stability.
  - A number of devices using heavy suture, button, and screws are available for open and arthroscopic techniques.
  - Hook plate fixation can be considered but requires subsequent removal.

- Treatment of distal clavicle fractures is typically nonoperative for stable and minimally displaced fractures and operative for unstable or displaced fractures.

- Stability of the fracture is determined by the location of the fracture fragments and the potential involvement of the coracoacromial ligaments.
- Operative treatment should be considered in unstable distal clavicle fractures because of the risk of nonunion.[31]
- Options for operative repair include CC reconstruction/repair (options discussed previously), internal fixation,[32] and hook plate constructs[33,34]; a combination of procedures may be required dependent on the fracture configuration and stability (Figure 16-6B).
- Guiding principles are stable fixation of the fracture fragments, fixation of fragments attached to the CC ligaments, and/or CC ligament repair or reconstruction if the CC ligaments are torn.

References

1. Stine IA, Vangsness CT Jr. Analysis of the capsule and ligament insertions about the acromioclavicular joint: a cadaveric study. *Arthroscopy* 2009;25(9):968-974. doi:10.1016/j.arthro.2009.04.072.
2. Fukuda K, Craig EV, An KN, Cofield RH, Chao EY. Biomechanical study of the ligamentous system of the acromioclavicular joint. *J Bone Joint Surg Am.* 1986;68(3):434-440.
3. Lee KW, Debski RE, Chen CH, Woo SL, Fu FH. Functional evaluation of the ligaments at the acromioclavicular joint during anteroposterior and superoinferior translation. *Am J Sports Med.* 1997;25(6):858-862. doi:10.1177/036354659702500622.
4. Rios CG, Arciero RA, Mazzocca AD. Anatomy of the clavicle and coracoid process for reconstruction of the coracoclavicular ligaments. *Am J Sports Med.* 2007;35(5):811-817. doi:10.1177/0363546506297536.
5. Petersson CJ. Degeneration of the acromioclavicular joint. A morphological study. *Acta Orthop Scand.* 1983;54(3):434-438. doi:10.3109/17453678308996597.
6. Cahill BR. Osteolysis of the distal part of the clavicle in male athletes. *J Bone Joint Surg Am.* 1982;64(7):1053-1058.
7. Rockwood, CA. Injuries to the acromioclavicular joint: subluxations and dislocations about the shoulder. In: Rockwood, CA, Green, DP, eds. *Fractures in Adults.* 2nd ed. Philadelphia: JB Lippincott; 1984:860-910.
8. Allman FL Jr. Fractures and ligamentous injuries of the clavicle and its articulation. *J Bone Joint Surg Am* 1967;49(4):774-784.
9. Neer CS II. Fractures of the distal third of the clavicle. *Clin Orthop Relat Res.* 1968;58:43-50.
10. Bishop JY, Jones GL, Lewis B, Pedroza A, Group MS. Intra- and interobserver agreement in the classification and treatment of distal third clavicle fractures. *Am J Sports Med.* 2015;43(4):979-984. doi:10.1177/0363546514563281.
11. Craig EV. Fractures of the clavicle. In: Rockwood Jr DP, Green CA, Bucholz RW, eds. *Fractures in Adults.* 3rd ed. Philadelphia, PA: JB Lippincott; 1991:928-990.
12. Robinson CM. Fractures of the clavicle in the adult. Epidemiology and classification. *J Bone Joint Surg Br.* 1998;80(3):476-484. doi:10.1302/0301-620x.80b3.8079.
13. Chronopoulos E, Kim TK, Park HB, Ashenbrenner D, McFarland EG. Diagnostic value of physical tests for isolated chronic acromioclavicular lesions. *Am J Sports Med.* 2004;32(3):655-661. doi:10.1177/0363546503261723.
14. Zanca P. Shoulder pain: involvement of the acromioclavicular joint. (Analysis of 1,000 cases). *Am J Roentgenol Radium Ther Nucl Med.* 1971;112(3):493-506. doi:10.2214/ajr.112.3.493.
15. Bearden JM, Hughston JC, Whatley GS. Acromioclavicular dislocation: method of treatment. *J Sports Med.* 1973;1(4):5-17. doi:10.1177/036354657300100401.
16. Elhassan B, Ozbaydar M, Diller D, Massimini D, Higgins LD, Warner JJ. Open versus arthroscopic acromioclavicular joint resection: a retrospective comparison study. *Arthroscopy.* 2009;25(11):1224-1232. doi:10.1016/j.arthro.2009.06.010.
17. Freedman BA, Javernick MA, O'Brien FP, Ross AE, Doukas WC. Arthroscopic versus open distal clavicle excision: comparative results at six months and one year from a randomized, prospective clinical trial. *J Shoulder Elbow Surg.* 2007;16(4):413-418. doi:10.1016/j.jse.2006.10.006.
18. Robertson WJ, Griffith MH, Carroll K, O'Donnell T, Gill TJ. Arthroscopic versus open distal clavicle excision: a comparative assessment at intermediate-term follow-up. *Am J Sports Med.* 2011;39(11):2415-2420. doi:10.1177/0363546511419633.
19. Strauss EJ, Barker JU, McGill K, Verma NN. The evaluation and management of failed distal clavicle excision. *Sports Med Arthrosc Rev.* 2010;18(3):213-219. doi:10.1097/JSA.0b013e3181e892da.
20. Corteen DP, Teitge RA. Stabilization of the clavicle after distal resection: a biomechanical study. *Am J Sports Med.* 2005;33(1):61-67. doi:10.1177/0363546504268038.

21. Edwards SL, Wilson NA, Flores SE, Koh JL, Zhang LQ. Arthroscopic distal clavicle resection: a biomechanical analysis of resection length and joint compliance in a cadaveric model. *Arthroscopy.* 2007;23(12):1278-1284. doi:10.1016/j.arthro.2007.07.004.
22. Renfree KJ, Riley MK, Wheeler D, Hentz JG, Wright TW. Ligamentous anatomy of the distal clavicle. *J Shoulder Elbow Surg.* 2003;12(4):355-359. doi:10.1016/s1058-2746(03)00029-6.
23. Weaver JK, Dunn HK. Treatment of acromioclavicular injuries, especially complete acromioclavicular separation. *J Bone Joint Surg Am.* 1972;54(6):1187-1194.
24. Banffy MB, van Eck CF, ElAttrache NS. Clinical outcomes of a single-tunnel technique for coracoclavicular and acromioclavicular ligament reconstruction. *J Shoulder Elbow Surg.* 2018;27(6S):S70-S75. doi:10.1016/j.jse.2017.11.032.
25. Choi NH, Lim SM, Lee SY, Lim TK. Loss of reduction and complications of coracoclavicular ligament reconstruction with autogenous tendon graft in acute acromioclavicular dislocations. *J Shoulder Elbow Surg.* 2017;26(4):692-698. doi:10.1016/j.jse.2016.09.014.
26. Cook JB, Shaha JS, Rowles DJ, Bottoni CR, Shaha SH, Tokish JM. Early failures with single clavicular transosseous coracoclavicular ligament reconstruction. *J Shoulder Elbow Surg.* 2012;21(12):1746-1752. doi:10.1016/j.jse.2012.01.018.
27. Carofino BC, Mazzocca AD. The anatomic coracoclavicular ligament reconstruction: surgical technique and indications. *J Shoulder Elbow Surg.* 2010;19(2 suppl):37-46. doi:10.1016/j.jse.2010.01.004.
28. Martetschläger F, Horan MP, Warth RJ, Millett PJ. Complications after anatomic fixation and reconstruction of the coracoclavicular ligaments. *Am J Sports Med.* 2013;41(12):2896-2903. doi:10.1177/0363546513502459.
29. Millett PJ, Horan MP, Warth RJ. Two-year outcomes after primary anatomic coracoclavicular ligament reconstruction. *Arthroscopy.* 2015;31(10):1962-1973. doi:10.1016/j.arthro.2015.03.034.
30. Mori D, Yamashita F, Kizaki K, Funakoshi N, Mizuno Y, Kobayashi M. Anatomic coracoclavicular ligament reconstruction for the treatment of acute acromioclavicular joint dislocation: minimum 10-year follow-up. *JB JS Open Access.* 2017;2(3):e0007. doi:10.2106/JBJS.OA.16.00007.
31. Neer CS II. Fracture of the distal clavicle with detachment of the coracoclavicular ligaments in adults. *J Trauma.* 1963;3:99-110. doi:10.1097/00005373-196303000-00001.
32. Andersen JR, Willis MP, Nelson R, Mighell MA. Precontoured superior locked plating of distal clavicle fractures: a new strategy. *Clin Orthop Relat Res.* 2011;469(12):3344-3350. doi:10.1007/s11999-011-2009-5.
33. Haidar SG, Krishnan KM, Deshmukh SC. Hook plate fixation for type II fractures of the lateral end of the clavicle. *J Shoulder Elbow Surg.* 2006;15(4):419-423. doi:10.1016/j.jse.2005.11.012.
34. Kashii M, Inui H, Yamamoto K. Surgical treatment of distal clavicle fractures using the clavicular hook plate. *Clin Orthop Relat Res.* 2006;447:158-164. doi:10.1097/01.blo.0000203469.66055.6a.

17

The Athlete's Shoulder and Elbow

Michael C. Ciccotti, MD and Michael G. Ciccotti, MD

- Athletes in many sports subject their upper extremities to tremendous forces and are at risk both for traumatic and overuse injuries. Many of those pathologies, both traumatic and overuse, are addressed elsewhere in this text.
- This chapter reviews the physiology and biomechanics of the throwing athlete and addresses additional shoulder and elbow pathologies that should be considered by clinicians in a differential diagnosis for this athletic population. Such a differential is broad and, although this chapter introduces many important concepts, it is not exhaustive.
    - Clinician treating athletes should avail themselves of the many additional resources available for the unique injuries sustained by throwing athletes.
- Proper management of all of these pathologies requires thoughtful history-taking, physical examination, and appropriate diagnostic imaging.
    - Obtaining a thorough history of any overhead athlete, including any past injuries and treatments to the involved area as well as the remainder of the kinetic chain (core, hips, and legs), is an essential starting point.
    - Physical examination of these athletes should involve evaluation of the neck/cervical spine, both shoulder girdles (clavicles with associated joints, scapulae, and glenohumeral joints), both elbows, and the remainder of the kinetic chain.
    - Diagnostic imaging includes plain radiographs and advanced modalities such as ultrasound, computed tomography, and magnetic resonance imaging.
- This thorough clinical evaluation will allow the clinician to confirm the suspected diagnosis as well as thoroughly exclude alternative or potential concomitant diagnoses.

Namdari S, Zmistowski B, Omid R, eds.
The Foundations of Shoulder and Elbow Surgery (pp 309-337).

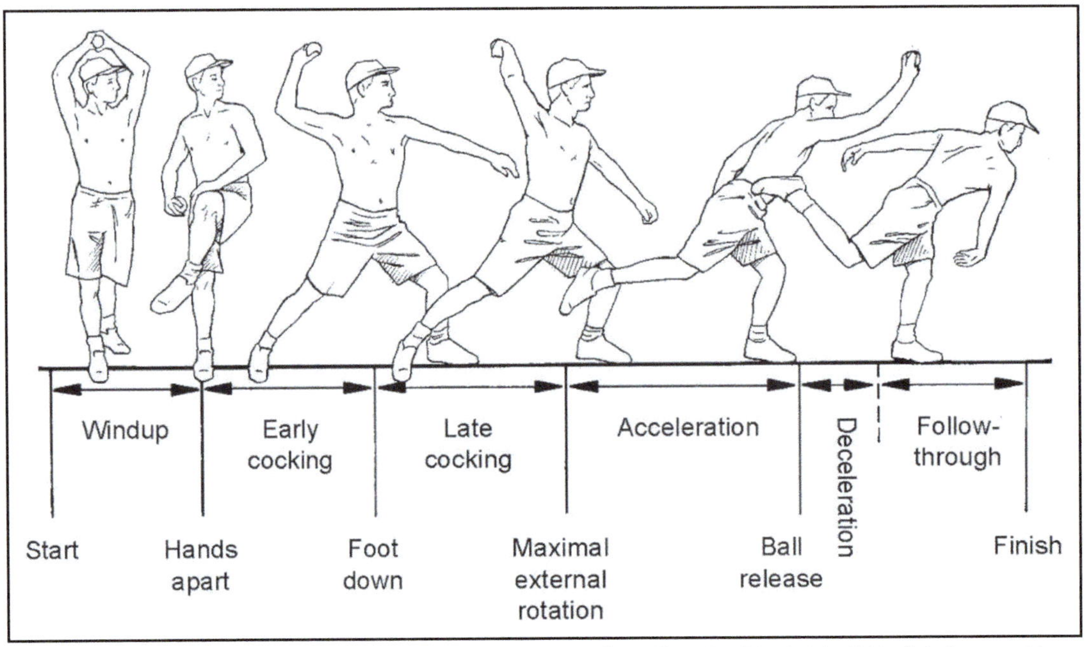

Figure 17-1. The 6 phases of throwing. (Reprinted with permission from Chen F, Rokito A, Jobe F. Medial elbow problems in the overhead-throwing athlete. *J Am Acad Orthop Surg*. 2001;9[2]:99-113. doi:10.5435/00124635-200103000-00004.)

Physiology of the Throwing Athlete

- Shoulder injuries can be career altering for the overhead athlete, such as baseball pitchers, football quarterbacks, tennis players, javelin throwers, and swimmers.
- The glenohumeral joint possesses tremendous range of motion in multiple planes as a result of the limited bony constraint imposed by its articular geometry, relying instead on the cartilaginous labrum and the associated glenohumeral ligaments as well as dynamic stabilizers such as the rotator cuff to prevent injury.
- The tremendous angular velocity and tensile forces experienced during the overhead-throwing motion subject each of these structures to substantial risk of injury with each throw.
- Although many complaints will be localized to the shoulder or elbow, an efficient throwing motion requires tremendous coordination from the toes to the fingertips.
- Energy is generated in the legs and then transferred through the core/trunk to the upper extremity.
- Kibler has termed this concept the "kinetic chain," and any deficiency in this chain can result in injury.[1,2]
- Although athletes may present with a shoulder or elbow complaints, it is critical to assess each link in the kinetic chain and to optimize the lower extremities, core, and cardiovascular conditioning along with the appropriate treatment of any upper extremity pathology.
- This complex throwing motion has been divided into 6 phases, all of which combined may occur in less than 2 seconds (Figure 17-1). The first 3 phases (wind-up, early-cocking, and late-cocking) account for approximately 1.5 seconds, acceleration (phase 4) occupies only approximately 0.05 seconds, whereas the final 2 phases (deceleration and follow-through) occur over approximately 0.35 seconds.[3-5] *Recommended reading for historical context and understanding shoulder physiology of the throwing athlete*

- Wind-up: This serves as a readying phase with the body's center of gravity raised with limited stress placed on the upper extremity.[6] The hips move forward to form a "V," in which the hips are the apex and the torso and stance leg are the 2 sides.
  - The upper extremity is essentially uninvolved in this phase with the shoulder remaining slightly abducted and minimally internally rotated.[6]
- Early-cocking: The "V" becomes more pronounced as the hips continue to move forward toward home plate and the stance foot is wedged into the pitching rubber. The shoulder moves into approximately 90 to 100 degrees of abduction (via activation of the deltoid and supraspinatus) and external rotation of approximately 45 degrees.[6]
  - The deltoid is activated early with late and lesser activation of the supraspinatus, infraspinatus, and teres minor.
- Late-cocking: The thrower's center of gravity is lowered to release stored energy and forward truncal rotation is delayed as long as possible. The upper extremity reaches maximum external rotation of 170 to 180 degrees through activation of the teres minor and infraspinatus.[6]
  - The scapular stabilizing muscles (trapezius, rhomboids, levator scapulae, and serratus anterior) are also active and retract the scapula to allow the glenoid to become a stable platform for humeral head motion, whereas the deltoid and supraspinatus activity diminishes.[7]
  - The terminal portion of the late-cocking phase is characterized by increased activation of the pectoralis major, latissimus dorsi, and serratus anterior muscles to generate adduction and internal rotation of the horizontally abducted and externally rotated upper extremity.
- Acceleration: Initiated when the humerus begins to internally rotate up angular velocities greater than 7000 degrees per second.[6]
  - The latissimus dorsi and the pectoralis major are the primary muscles contributing to the acceleration of the ball, with the latissimus dorsi showing the highest activity and oriented anatomically to provide the greatest torque.
  - Acceleration of the arm coincides with the deceleration of the rest of the body, producing efficient transfer of energy to the upper extremity and ball. Acceleration is terminated when the ball is released at approximately 90 degrees of rotation.
- Deceleration: The most violent phase of the throwing motion, in which the tremendous residual kinetic energy generated by acceleration must be arrested and dissipated.
  - Eccentric contraction of all muscle groups slows the arm and results in the greatest loads across the joint.
  - The teres minor contracts eccentrically and demonstrates the highest level of activity of all the muscles, whereas the subscapularis remains active to stabilize the humeral head.
- Follow-through: Rebalancing phase in which the body moves forward until upper extremity motion ceases.
  - Muscle firing returns to resting levels as the shoulder continues to horizontally adduct in from of the body while maintaining abduction

- The baseball pitch has traditionally been used as the prototype for the overhead-throwing motion. However, a smaller body of work has also examined that mechanics of the throwing motion in American football; although there are substantial similarities in the phases of the throw, the difference in weight between a football and a baseball appears to result in a number of alterations.
- In comparison to pitchers, quarterbacks rotate their shoulders sooner, achieve maximum external rotation sooner, lead with their elbow, and do not finish with a complete follow-through as seen in pitchers. Overall, throwing a football appears to generate lower torques

and forces on the upper extremity that may account for the lower incidence of shoulder and elbow injuries.[8]

- A number of physiologic adaptations have been identified in overhead-throwing athletes to answer the tremendous stresses subjected to the upper extremity.[9-12]
  - The dominant extremity may exhibit hypertrophy of the shoulder girdle muscles as well as that of the anterior and posterior chest walls.[6]
  - A loss of internal rotation at the shoulder is not uncommon and is accompanied by an increase in external rotation so the total arc of motion is roughly equivalent with the contralateral shoulder.
  - A substantial loss of total arc of motion compared to the contralateral shoulder should alert the clinician to potential pathology.
    - The decrease in internal rotation is often attributed to posterior capsular and soft-tissue contraction, whereas laxity of the axillary part of the inferior glenohumeral ligament and coracohumeral ligament may be responsible both for the increased external rotation as well as an increased sulcus sign often seen in pitchers.[6]
    - Further contributing to increased external rotation in acquired retroversion of the humeral head of 10 to 20 degrees; this is believed to occur principally in pitchers with substantial throwing prior to skeletal maturity with alteration of the proximal humeral physis.[13-15]
      - Humeral retroversion at birth is approximately 78 degrees and with age the proximal humerus derotates to a less retroverted position (approximately 20 degrees) in adulthood. The process occurs most rapidly up to 8 years old and then slows down. Rotational forces seen at the proximal humerus during throwing can alter the derotation process and if begun early enough can have a profound effect on humeral version.
      - Increased retroversion of the humerus is thought to be somewhat protective of the anterior soft-tissue structures during throwing (the anterior tissues do not need to stretch excessively to obtain the same amount of external rotation necessary for pitching).
      - However, increased retroversion of the humeral head can also lead to posterior capsular contracture, which can lead to a shift in the humeral head posteriorly and superiorly, predisposing the patient to an increased risk of internal impingement and subsequent labral and rotator cuff pathology.

Shoulder Pathology

External (Subacromial) Impingement

- Throwing athletes may infrequently develop shoulder pathology as a result of classic external subacromial impingement similar to nonthrowers and nonathletes.
- This classic form of impingement described by Neer in 1983 is characterized by a narrowing in the available subacromial space between the coracoacromial arch and the humeral head.[16] *Recommended reading for historical context*
  - This leads to compression of the rotator cuff and may result from anatomic variants such as a hooked acromion, acromioclavicular joint arthritis with osteophyte formation, and a laterally sloping acromion (Figure 17-2).
- As described by Neer, classical external subacromial impingement occurs in 3 stages: Stage I involves edema and hemorrhage of the subacromial bursa and rotator cuff, stage II progresses

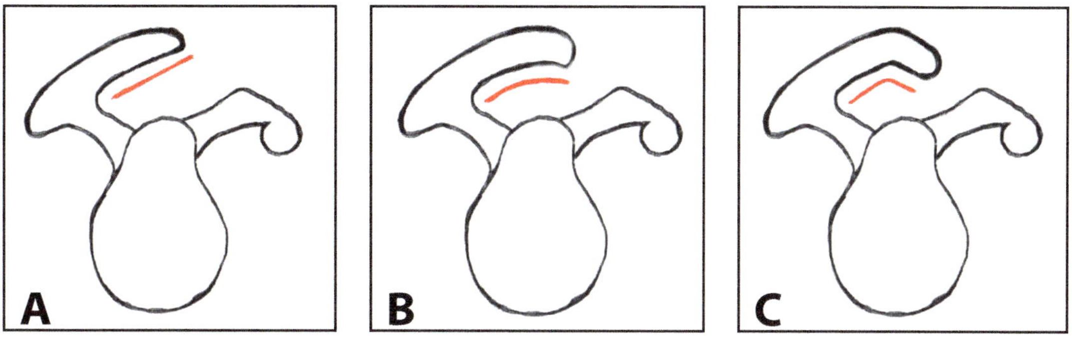

Figure 17-2. Schematic demonstrating the 3 classic acromial types described by Bigliani and Morrison and associated with impingement. (A) straight, (B) curved, and (C) hooked.

to fibrosis and tendinitis of the rotator cuff, and stage III is characterized by partial or complete rotator cuff tears.[16]

- These athletes have a history of insidious pain developing over a prolonged period of time that may be localized to the anterolateral acromion and may radiate laterally toward the deltoid tuberosity of the humerus.
- Physical exam findings noted with external impingement syndrome include the Neer sign (pain with forced flexion) and the Hawkins sign (symptoms or pain replicated by internal rotation with the arm abducted 90 degrees).
  - However, such maneuvers lack specificity and their diagnostic value has been called into question.[17]
- Plain radiographs may be negative or may show changes associated with rotator cuff disease: subacromial osteophytes, subacromial sclerosis, greater tuberosity cystic change, and narrowing of the acromiohumeral distance.[18,19]
- Magnetic resonance imaging may be more valuable, demonstrating bursal thickening, fluid medial to the acromioclavicular joint, fluid within the bursa, or evidence of rotator cuff tendinopathy and tearing.
- Initial treatment is nonoperative including physical therapy both for range of motion and strengthening, modalities such as ultrasound and phonopheresis, and nonsteroidal anti-inflammatory medications. Injections of corticosteroid have diagnostic and potentially therapeutic benefit.
- Recalcitrant or recurrent symptoms for 3 months or more are to be managed most commonly by arthroscopic subacromial decompression including bursectomy with or without acromioplasty.
- Return to play, however, has remained a concern among elite athletes following subacromial decompression, suggesting that classic primary subacromial impingement is infrequently the primary diagnosis in this specific population.[20]

Internal Impingement

- Walch et al first described internal impingement in 1992 as a cause of posterior shoulder pain among overhead athletes distinct from traditional external subacromial impingement.[21] *Recommended reading for historical context*
- Internal impingement differs from external impingement in that a true anatomic stenosis of the shoulder outlet is not present, rather internal impingement occurs as a result of glenohumeral instability, posterior capsular contracture, or scapular muscle dysfunction leading to impingement symptoms.

- In this disorder, the articular undersurface of the posterior supraspinatus and/or anterior infraspinatus tendons impinge on the posterior glenoid margin as the arm moves into a position of abduction and maximal external rotation. Repetitive abutment of these structures can result in fraying and tearing of both the posterosuperior labrum as well as the articular side of the rotator cuff.
- Anatomic factors such as excessive glenoid anteversion and reduced humeral retroversion may also contribute.[21,22]
- Andrews and colleagues and Bigliani et al have both documented that glenohumeral joint laxity is common among these throwing athletes, and Conway et al and Paley and colleagues have posited that this plays a role in the development of internal impingement by allowing abnormal anterior humeral head translation and subsequent impingement of posterior structures.[9,23-25] Such instability may not necessarily manifest as clinically appreciable glenohumeral laxity; the repetitive stresses of throwing may accumulate as progressive microtrauma to the glenohumeral ligaments resulting in attenuation.[26-28]
- Such microinstability can alter scapulohumeral kinematics or may cause secondary symptoms by increasing demand on the rotator cuff.
- The history of internal impingement is often one of decreased throwing velocity, control, and performance among overhead athletes with pain most pronounced in the abducted and maximally externally rotated position (eg, late-cocking and early-acceleration phases).
- Physical examination may be notable for posterior glenohumeral joint line tenderness with the increased external rotation and diminished internal rotation common among overhead-throwing athletes.
    - Meister et al[6] have described the "posterior impingement sign" as deep posterior pain when the late-cocking phase of the overhead-throwing motion is replicated (ie, abduction of 90 to 110 degrees, extension of 10 to 15 degrees, and maximal external rotation).
    - Jobe and colleagues have described the value of the apprehension-relocation test for internal impingement in which on abduction and maximum external rotation produces posterior shoulder pain (as opposed to apprehensive symptoms) and the relocation portion of the maneuver relieves this pain with posteriorly directed force.[26,29,30]
- Plain radiographs may be normal or may demonstrate rounding of the posterior glenoid rim, sclerosis of the greater tuberosity, and posterior humeral head cystic changes. A Bennett lesion, or calcification at the insertion of the posterior inferior glenohumeral ligament, may also be seen although this may be an incidental finding in many athletes.
- Magnetic resonance imaging findings consistent with internal impingement include articular-sided partial-thickness rotator cuff tears and posterior or posterosuperior labral lesions (Figure 17-3). As with any overhead athlete, magnetic resonance imaging abnormalities may be asymptomatic incidental findings and must be carefully correlated with history and physical examination findings.
- Principal management remains nonoperative for internal impingement and is aimed at correcting instability, scapular stabilization, and proprioception through targeted physical therapy and posterior capsular stretching. Nonsteroidal anti-inflammatory medications and corticosteroid injection may be provided.
- A thorough assessment of the athlete's kinetic chain should be carried out with all deficits corrected.
- Operative management is rarely performed and reserved for those athletes with persistent symptoms for 6 or more months recalcitrant to all nonoperative management. Indications for surgical management are failure to improve with prolonged conservative treatment and inability to return to prior level of competition.

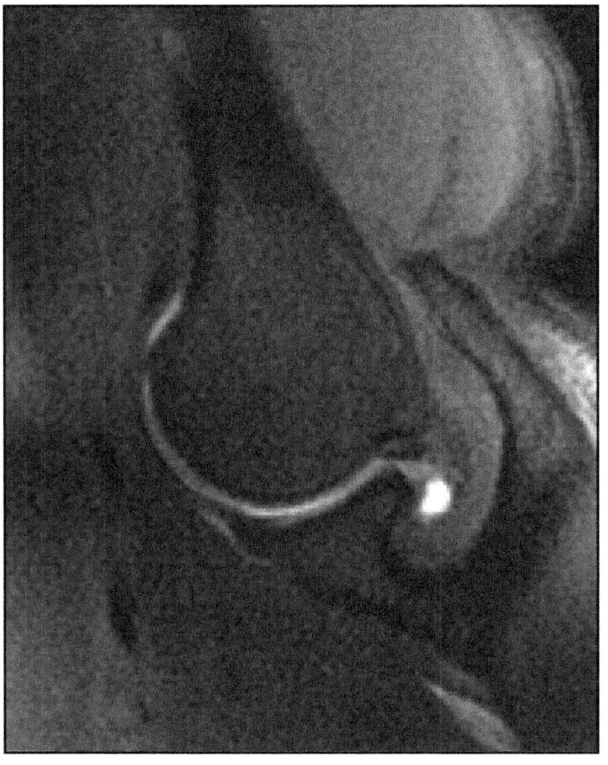

Figure 17-3. Magnetic resonance image capture in the abducted external rotation position demonstrating internal impingement of the posterior superior glenoid on the rotator cuff insertion. (Reprinted with permission from Adam Zoga, MD.)

- Any surgical approach should begin with a bilateral examination under anesthesia as well as a thorough diagnostic arthroscopy to identify all associated pathology.
- Traditionally, repair has been indicated in partial-thickness rotator cuff tears involving greater than 50% to 75% tendon thickness.[31]
- Labral pathology can be debrided or repaired as indicated with extreme care not to iatrogenically tighten the capsule. The entire labrum should be carefully evaluated because athletes may present with posterosuperior/superior labrum anterior and posterior (SLAP) lesions, posterior/Kim lesions, or anterior/Bankart lesions.

Regardless of the procedure performed, significant care must be exercised with operative treatment of impingement in overhead-throwing athletes, because return to play has been unpredictable.[20]

Subcoracoid Impingement

- A far less common cause of impingement type symptoms among athletes is coracoid or subcoracoid impingement.[32-36]
- The etiology of subcoracoid impingement may be idiopathic, iatrogenic (such as postoperative change from Bristow/Latarjet procedures or glenoid osteotomies) or traumatic (lesser tuberosity malunion or anterior instability).
- This form of impingement is characterized by anterior shoulder pain exacerbated by forward elevation, internal rotation, and cross-arm abduction and is believed to occur as a result of compression of the subscapularis tendon between the lesser tuberosity of the humerus and the coracoid tip.[33,36,37]

- Dines et al described the coracoid impingement test in which the shoulder is placed in cross-arm abduction, forward elevation, and abduction as a means of provoking the symptoms of coracoid impingement.[32]
- Furthermore, these authors advocated diagnostic lidocaine injection as a useful modality for distinguishing coracoid impingement from other forms of impingement.
- On axial magnetic resonance imaging, the coracohumeral distance can be measured as the minimal distance from the coracoid process and lesser tuberosity with the humerus in maximum internal rotation. Friedman and colleagues noted an average coracohumeral distance of 5.5 mm in symptomatic patients compared to an average of 11 mm in asymptomatic patients, but these values are not well defined.[38]
- First-line treatment remains nonoperative with activity modification, physical therapy, and anti-inflammatory medications. However, surgical decompression of the subcoracoid space via coracoplasty has been described.[32]

  However, any surgical intervention should take care to address the presumed etiology of coracoid impingement, such as instability or fracture malunion, if present.

Glenohumeral Internal Rotation Deficit

- As noted above, throwers may demonstrate asymptomatic adaptations, including changes in internal and external rotation while preserving overall total arc of motion. Glenohumeral internal rotation deficit (GIRD) describes an excessive, pathologic reduction in internal rotation in the throwing shoulder.[39-43]
- Although there is some disagreement over the precise definition, GIRD should be considered with concurrent deficits of internal rotation greater than or equal to 15 degrees and total arc of motion greater than or equal to 10 degrees.[44]
- A number of factors may contribute to the development of GIRD, including humeral retroversion, posteroinferior capsular contracture, and posterior rotator cuff tightness.[41]
- These adaptations can affect the deceleration phase of overhead throwing with increased eccentric loading of the posterior rotator cuff, resulting in tensile failure of these tissues, in contrast to the compressive failure seen in impingement syndromes.
- These tensile forces may also be transmitted via the long head of the biceps tendon to the labral complex, resulting in SLAP lesions via the so-called "peel-back" mechanism.
- Initial management is focused on stretching the tight posterior capsule to increase internal rotation; however, attention should also be paid to carefully normalizing the total arc of motion. Posterior capsular stretching is accomplished with both cross-body stretching and the sleeper stretch.
- Operative management in the form of careful arthroscopic posterior soft-tissue release is reserved only for the small percentage of athletes unresponsive to 3 to 6 months of nonoperative management.

Scapular Dyskinesia

- Smooth function of the shoulder joint relies on normal scapulohumeral rhythm. The integration of scapular and humeral motion such that the scapula provides a stable platform throughout humeral head motion was first described by Codman as a 2:1 ratio of glenohumeral motion to scapular motion.[45]
  - This may, however, oversimplify a complex coordinated motion between the scapula and humerus.[46]

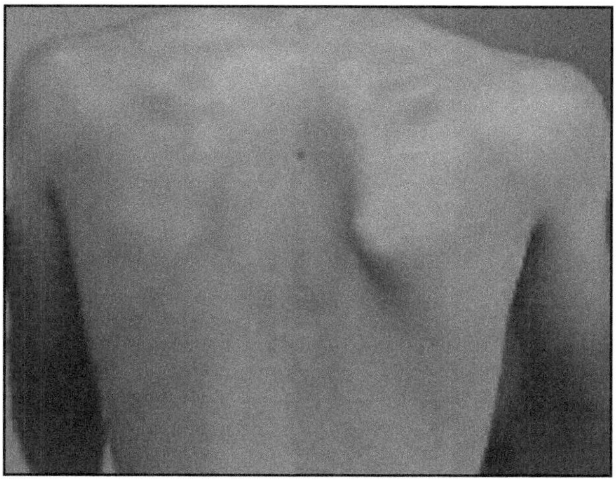

Figure 17-4. Scapular dyskinesia with medial border prominence. (Reprinted with permission from Uhl TL, Kibler WB, Gecewich B, Tripp BL. Evaluation of clinical assessment methods for scapular dyskinesis. *Arthroscopy.* 2009;25[11]:1240-1248. doi:10.1016/j.arthro.2009.06.007.)

- To reach the extremes of motion needed by overhead athletes, elevation of the acromion is necessary to prevent impingement.
  - Pull from the lower trapezius causes lateral rotation of the scapula (acromial elevation), whereas the serratus anterior stabilizes the medial border of the scapula against the chest wall to allow for full elevation of the arm without premature subacromial impingement.
- Scapular dyskinesia results from imbalances of the periscapular musculature secondary to fatigue, direct trauma, or nerve injury disrupting this normal scapulohumeral rhythm.
- Normal function of the serratus anterior, trapezius, and rhomboid muscles is required to achieve the necessary scapular positioning. Loss of function from nerve injury, weakness, and/or fatigue leads to scapular protraction and a relative increase in glenoid anteversion, placing the anterior capsular structures at risk.
- Some degree of scapular dyskinesis may be present in 67% to 100% of patients with shoulder injuries.[47,48]
- Physical examination to detect scapular dyskinesia requires dynamic evaluation of scapular motion with forward elevation and descent of the arm This motion should be observed multiple times and may be supplemented with hand weights. Failure to maintain scapulohumeral rhythm results in increased scapular protraction, medial rotation and medial border prominence[49] (Figure 17-4).
  - The scapular assistance test (SAT) and scapular retraction test (SRT) are maneuvers designed to further elucidate the role of scapular dyskinesis in patient-reported symptoms.
  - The SAT is performed by applying gentle pressure to the scapula from behind to assist scapular upward rotation and posterior tilt as the patient elevates the arm. It is positive if the painful impingement symptoms are relieved and the total arc of motion is improved.[50]
  - The SRT involves stabilizing the scapula in a retracted position and assessing supraspinatus strength or evaluating impingement/labral symptoms. If strength or impingement symptoms improve with stabilized scapular retraction, the SRT is positive.[51]
  - Although concomitant pathology may exist, these maneuvers help establish scapular dyskinesia as a contributing factor to the patient's symptoms and a focus for correction.
- The large majority of scapula-related issues can be resolved by a focused physical therapy program directed at the scapular stabilizers.
- In rare circumstances, operative intervention may be required after failure of nonoperative management for specific entities such as scapular bursitis or a snapping scapula, which can

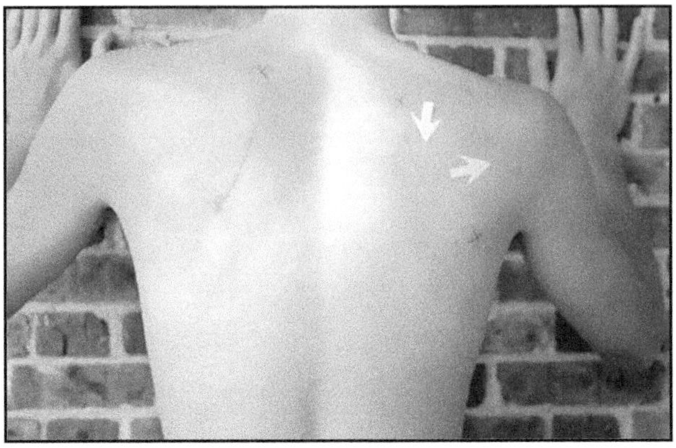

Figure 17-5. SICK scapula syndrome, with all 3 displacements: scapular infera, lateral protraction, and scapular abduction. (Reprinted with permission from Burkhart SS, Morgan CD, Kibler WB. The disabled throwing shoulder: spectrum of pathology part III: the SICK scapula, scapular dyskinesis, the kinetic chain, and rehabilitation. *Arthroscopy.* 2003;19[6]: 641-661. doi:10.1016/s0749-8063(03)00389-x.)

be treated by excision of the offending tissues at the inferior and/or superior margin of the scapula or excision of parts of the scapula itself.

Scapular Malposition, Inferior Medial Border Prominence, Coracoid Pain and Malposition, and Dyskinesia of Scapular Motion Scapula

- The Scapular malposition, Inferior medial border prominence, Coracoid pain and malposition, and dysKinesis of scapular movement (SICK) scapula syndrome represents an extreme form of scapular dyskinesis.[43] This represents an overuse syndrome in which the scapula appears inferiorly displaced or "dropped" as a result of exaggerated protraction and anteroinferior tilting of the upper scapula.[43]
- Symptomatic patients complain of any combination of anterior shoulder pain, posterosuperior scapular pain, superior shoulder pain, or proximal lateral arm pain. The insertion of the pectoralis minor tendon at the coracoid base may be particularly tender.
- Scapular position can be assessed objectively by 3 measurements with the patient standing with the arms relaxed in adduction at the side (Figure 17-5).
    - First, scapular "infera" is the difference in centimeters in the vertical height of the superomedial angle of the affected scapula in comparison to the contralateral asymptomatic scapula.
    - Second, scapular lateral displacement is the difference in centimeters in displacement of the superomedial angle of the affected scapula from the midline.
    - Finally, scapular abduction is the difference in angular degrees of the medial scapular margin and a plumb midline as measured by goniometer.[43]
    - Outlining the margins of both scapulae may aid in visualizing the degree of displacement.
- The SRT described previously may relieve coracoid pain with forward flexion and posterosuperior periscapular pain often observed in SICK scapula syndrome.
- Management of SICK scapula syndrome is nonoperative, including rest from the offending overhead activity and focused scapular muscle rehabilitation.
    - Burkhart et al recommend resumption of a tossing program in throwers when the scapula is 50% improved from its initial position, typically by 2 to 3 weeks with full normalization and return to play at 3 to 4 months.
    - In a series of 96 patients, they reported 100% return to preinjury play by 4 months.[43]

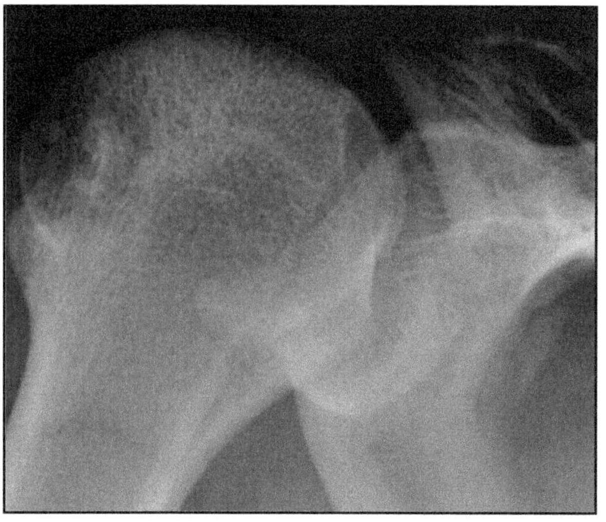

Figure 17-6. A plain radiograph demonstrating a Bennett lesion. (Reprinted with permission from Adam Zoga, MD.)

Bennett Lesion

- The Bennett lesion was first described in 1941 as a mineralization of the posterior inferior glenoid noted in overhead-throwing athletes, almost exclusively baseball players.[52]
- Initially believed to represent a traction of the long head of the triceps, it is now believed to be the result of capsular traction at the insertion of the posterior inferior glenohumeral ligament with subsequent enthesopathic changes.
- In many cases, such a finding is entirely asymptomatic and may be visualized incidentally on plain radiographs (Figure 17-6). It is best seen on the Stryker-Notch view.[53]
- Incidence among baseball players has been reported at approximately 20%.[53]
- Magnetic resonance imaging may show a bony excrescence along the posterior glenoid rim with concomitant posterior labral and/or capsular fraying or tearing.
- Treatment of Bennett lesions remains controversial because many clinicians believe the lesion itself is a rare cause of symptoms and is more likely an incidental finding in the presence of concomitant pathology.
- However, a symptomatic Bennett lesion is characterized by posterior shoulder pain, most notably in the follow-through phase of throwing.
- Targeted local injection may be both diagnostic and therapeutic.
- Although excision with labral and/or capsular repair have been described, care must be taken to avoid iatrogenic tightening of the posterior capsule and posterior band of the inferior glenohumeral ligament.
    - One series has suggested that only 55% of high-level throwers treated operatively returned to prior injury level of competition, suggesting that conservative management should be exhausted and alternative diagnoses excluded prior to proceeding with surgical treatment.[54]

Effort Thrombosis

- Upper extremity deep venous thrombosis is less common than its lower extremity counterpart. "Effort" or Paget-Schroetter syndrome describes the development of upper extremity deep venous thrombosis as a result of endothelial damage to the upper extremity venous system from recurrent vigorous exertion.[55,56]

- Many patients may additionally exhibit anatomic variants of the thoracic outlet such as cervical ribs, subclavius tendons, or hypertrophy of the scalenus anticus muscle, resulting in subclavian vein compression.
- History is significant for tiredness and heaviness of the involved extremity, whereas physical exam may demonstrate subtle discoloration, venous engorgement, side-to-side asymmetry with the uninvolved extremity, and swelling.
- The role of underlying thrombophilia such as activated protein C resistance, anticardiolipin antibodies, homocysteinemia, and the G21020A mutation in the prothrombin gene has been controversial but suggested by one retrospective study to be present in more than 60% of cases.[57]
- Venography or computed tomography (or magnetic resonance–based imaging) will demonstrate the presence of thrombosis of the subclavian vein.
- In the absence of anatomic abnormality, some patients may be adequately managed with anticoagulation alone.
- However in some cases, catheter-directed thrombolysis or balloon venoplasty may be required. Anatomic abnormalities of the thoracic outlet such as cervical ribs, subclavius tendons, or hypertrophy of the scalenus anticus muscle should be surgically corrected.

Thoracic Outlet Syndrome

- Thoracic outlet syndrome (TOS) was first described by Peet et al in 1956 as being caused by compression of the neurovascular structures passing through the thoracic outlet.[58]
- The thoracic outlet itself is defined as the interval between the first rib and the clavicle as the brachial plexus and subclavian vessels pass from the supraclavicular fossa into the axilla. Three anatomic regions for compression within the thoracic outlet have been described: the interscalene triangle (level of the brachial plexus trunks), the costoclavicular space (level of the divisions), and the retropectoralis minor space (level of the cords).[59]
- Most cases of TOS are thought to occur only after a superimposed trauma (either acute or chronic, repetitive stress) in an athlete with anatomic predisposition to compression.
    - Such anatomic predisposition may be due to soft-tissue abnormalities, such as an accessory scalenus minimus muscle, hypertrophy of the scalene muscles, congenital bands or ligaments, and post-traumatic scarring, or osseous abnormalities, such as cervical ribs, prominent C7 transverse processes, exostoses, tumors, or post-traumatic callus.
- TOS may manifest as neurogenic (greater than 90%) or vascular (approximately 4% to 6%).[60] Neurogenic symptoms include pain, paresthesias, and weakness in the affected upper extremity; vascular symptoms include activity-related claudication, pulse, or blood pressure asymmetries, temperature change, and discoloration in the affected upper extremity.
- Physical examination may employ a number of maneuvers designed to provoke symptoms.
    - The Wright test may detect a decrease in the radial pulse by placing the arm in hyperabduction and external rotation with the head turned to the opposite shoulder.[61]
    - The Adson test is performed by bringing the arm into extension, turning the head toward the affected extremity, and asking the patient to take a deep breath.
    - The Roos test involves provocation of dramatic symptoms by placing both arms in the 90-degree abducted position with the elbows flexed to 90 degrees and opening and closing the hands for 3 minutes.[62,63]
    - Chronic lower trunk neurogenic TOS may demonstrate the Gilliatt-Sumner hand, characterized by abductor pollicis brevis atrophy and lesser atrophy of the hypothenar and interossei muscles.[64,65]

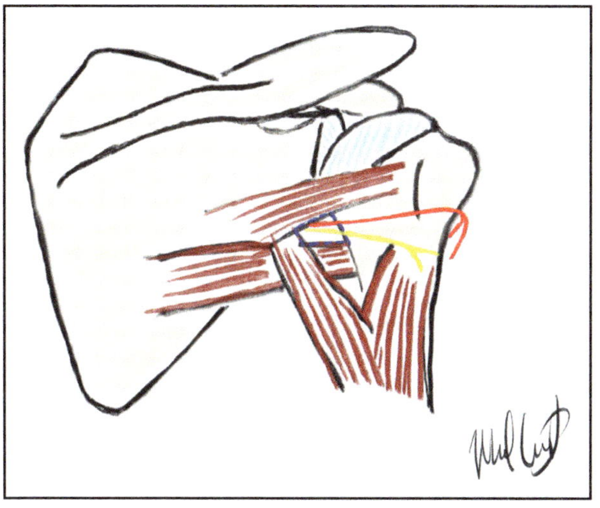

Figure 17-7. Anatomic borders of the quadrilateral space with a dashed blue line: the teres minor superiorly, the teres major inferiorly, the long head of the triceps medially, and the humeral shaft laterally. (Reprinted with permission from Michael C. Ciccotti, MD.)

- Further diagnostic testing begins with plain radiography of the chest and cervical spine to identify congenital abnormalities. Electrophysiologic testing may often be indicated in neurogenic TOS, whereas advanced imaging and angiography may be of use in vascular TOS.
- Neurogenic TOS may be managed initially with nonoperative treatments such as activity modification and physical therapy.
- Refractory neurogenic TOS and vascular TOS warrant surgical management directed at the anatomic source of compression, resulting in reliable improvement in symptoms but variable return to sport.[66,67]

Quadrilateral Space Syndrome

- Quadrilateral space syndrome results from compression of the axillary nerve and/or posterior humeral circumflex artery as they pass through the quadrilateral space.
  - This anatomic space is defined by the surgical neck of the humerus laterally, the long head of the triceps medially, the tendon of the teres major and latissimus dorsi muscles inferiorly, and the teres minor muscle superiorly (Figure 17-7).
- This syndrome has been reported among overhead athletes in numerous sports, including throwers.[68,69]
- Similar to TOS above, quadrilateral space syndrome may manifest with predominantly vascular or neurogenic manifestations.
  - Neurogenic symptoms include pain, numbness, and posterior shoulder/deltoid weakness and wasting.
  - Related vascular phenomena include pain, pallor, pulse asymmetry and may progress to thrombosis with distal embolism.
- Symptoms may be provoked or exacerbated by placing the arm in the flexion-abduction-external rotation position.
- Diagnostic imaging includes computed tomographic angiography, magnetic resonance angiography, and digital subtraction angiography and will demonstrate occlusion of the posterior humeral circumflex artery with the above arm positioning. Imaging may also reveal alternative sources of compression, including fracture callus or malunion, glenoid labral cysts, ganglion cysts, or osteochondromata.

- Electrophysiologic testing may demonstrate denervation in the deltoid and teres minor muscles with neurogenic quadrilateral space syndrome.
- Initial treatment is conservative in nature with activity modification, anti-inflammatories, and physical therapy.
- However, recalcitrant cases may require surgical decompression with neurolysis and excision/resection of any impinging lesions.[69-75]
- Thrombosis of the posterior humeral circumflex artery may require more urgent treatment with thrombolysis or ligation of the pathologic portion of the vessel to prevent embolization.[76-80]
- A recently described variation of quadrilateral space syndrome is called nerve to teres minor syndrome and presents with isolated involvement of the teres minor muscle belly with fatty degeneration noted on magnetic resonance imaging.[81,82]

Elbow Pathology

- Just as the throwing motion places tremendous stress on the shoulder, those forces are transmitted along the kinetic change to the athlete's elbow.
- During the acceleration phase of throwing, the elbow reaches an angular velocity of 3000 degrees per second as it extends from 110 degrees to 20 degrees of flexion. This speed corresponds to a 64 N/m valgus torque.
- This acceleration results in a predictable pattern of stresses on the 3 compartments of the elbow: tensile stress on the medial or ulnohumeral compartment, compressive stress on the lateral or radiocapitellar compartment, and shear on the posterior compartment as the olecranon articulates with the olecranon fossa of the humerus.

A variety of static and dynamic stabilizers exist to resist these stresses; however, the tremendous forces of the throwing motion may result in either acute, catastrophic failure or chronic injury to any of these structures.

Valgus Elbow Instability

- The valgus forces subjected to the elbow during the overhead-throwing motion result in significant tensile stresses.
- The primary restraint against these stresses is the ulnar collateral ligament (UCL), specifically the anterior band which is subdivided into reciprocally tightening anterior and posterior bundles.[83-85]
  - The primary restraint against valgus stress from 0 degrees to 20 degrees is the ulnohumeral joint, from 20 degrees to 120 degrees is the anterior band of the UCL, and from more than 120 degrees is the posterior band of the UCL.
- The maximum valgus torque (64 N/m) seen during throwing far exceeds the ultimate strength of the UCL (32 N/m), suggesting the importance of the secondary stabilizers of the medial elbow (flexor-pronator mass).[86]
- The valgus force exerted by throwing threatens to exceed the tensile strength of the UCL (32 N/m) on each throw and acute failure and chronic insufficiency both may result. Indeed, numerous studies have documented the high incidence of these injuries, particularly in the throwing athlete, as well as an increase both in primary and revision UCL reconstructions.[87-90]
- Although some athletes may complain of an acute injury with a "pop," most throwers will complain of insidious vague medial elbow pain or tightness accompanied by diminished velocity and control.

- Tenderness on examination should be localized to the course of the UCL between the medial epicondyle of the humerus and the sublime tubercle of the ulna.
- Special provocative tests to diagnose UCL injury include the milking maneuver and the moving valgus stress test, both of which elicit apprehension and pain localized to the ligament in the setting of injury.
    - The milking maneuver is performed by "milking" the thumb of the ipsilateral extremity while placing a valgus stress on the elbow as the ipsilateral shoulder is positioned in abduction and external rotation.[91]
    - The moving valgus stress test similarly involves applying valgus stress to the medial elbow but as the elbow is flexed from 30 to 120 degrees, simulating the late-cocking and acceleration phases of throwing.[92] Valgus stress will often elicit pain and apprehension in the setting of UCL injury; however, laxity may be more difficult to appreciate clinically.
- Although plain radiography should always be obtained, UCL injury or insufficiency is best appreciated on advanced imaging such as stress ultrasound and magnetic resonance arthrography (Figure 17-8).
    - Joyner et al have recently promulgated the first MR-based classification for UCL injury, which may prove to have prognostic value.[93]
    - Stress ultrasound provides a rapid, low-cost, nonradiating evaluation of the elbow with the dynamic application of valgus stress.
        - Although overhead throwers demonstrate changes over time including ligament thickening and increasing ulnohumeral joint gapping under stress, thresholds for gapping consistent with injury have been established and stress ultrasound combined with MR significantly increases the sensitivity and specificity of diagnosis.[85,94-98]
- Injury to the UCL was considered career ending until Dr. Frank Jobe performed the first reconstruction on Dodgers' pitcher Tommy John in 1974.
- Today, a number of procedures for reconstruction have been described that vary with respect to the placement of humeral and ulnar tunnels and fixation.[99] The modified Jobe and docking techniques are the most commonly performed, and they differ principally in the method of humeral attachment.[100,101] *Conway et al[100] is recommended reading for understanding the background of management of UCL injuries; Rohrbough et al[101] is recommended reading for change in management*
    - Detachment of the flexor-pronator mass has been abandoned in favor of a muscle-splitting approach (because of its importance as a secondary stabilizer), and obligatory transposition of the ulnar nerve, as originally described, is now typically performed only in the presence of persistent, preexisting symptoms (because of the higher rate of ulnar neuropathy).
- Primary repair with or without augmentation has been recently proposed in specific populations such as youth or adolescent throwers with limited throwing history, focal damage within the ligament or avulsion injury, without any chronic or degenerative changes in the remaining ligament.[102,103] *Recommended reading for change in management*
    - The results of repair, however, have traditionally been inferior to reconstruction, which provides well-documented, high rates of good-to-excellent results and return to play.[99,100,102,104,105]

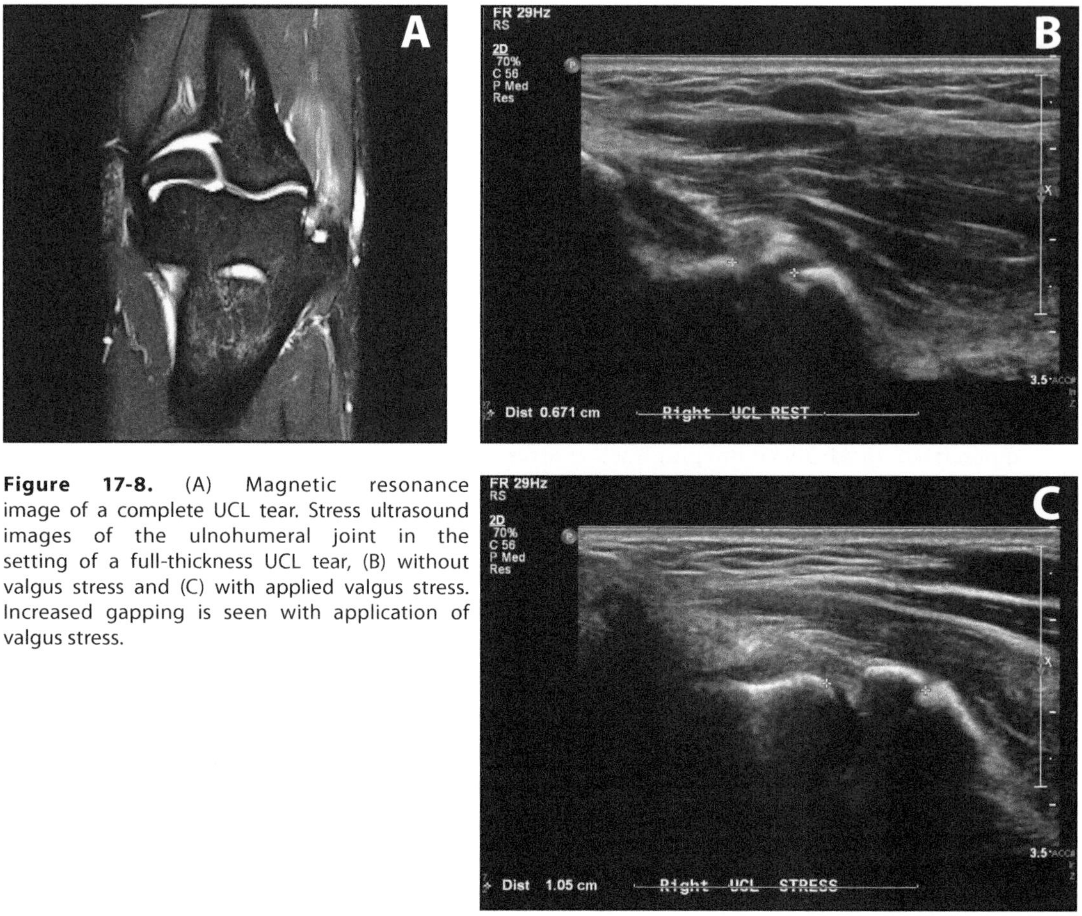

Figure 17-8. (A) Magnetic resonance image of a complete UCL tear. Stress ultrasound images of the ulnohumeral joint in the setting of a full-thickness UCL tear, (B) without valgus stress and (C) with applied valgus stress. Increased gapping is seen with application of valgus stress.

Valgus Extension Overload Syndrome and Posteromedial Impingement

- Valgus extension overload syndrome results from the tremendous forces the elbow is subjected to during the overhead-throwing motion: lateral compartment compression; medial compartment tension; and posterior compartment shear.
- The most common pathology observed is posteromedial olecranon osteophytes as a result of posteromedial impingement.[106]
- Ciccotti et al have demonstrated that medial ulnohumeral laxity increases over time in professional baseball pitchers, and any increase in laxity may subject the posterior compartment to increased shear with impingement of the olecranon on the medial wall of the olecranon fossa.[94,97,98]
- History is that of posterior elbow pain most pronounced at ball release near terminal extension. This should be carefully distinguished from distal triceps pathology; in valgus extension overload/posteromedial impingement, tenderness is located in the posteromedial elbow and worsened with the arm bar test.[107]
    - This test is performed by abducting the shoulder, extending the elbow, pronating the forearm and placing the patient's wrist on the examiner's shoulder, all while applying a hyperextension force on the posterior elbow to replicate the patient's symptoms.

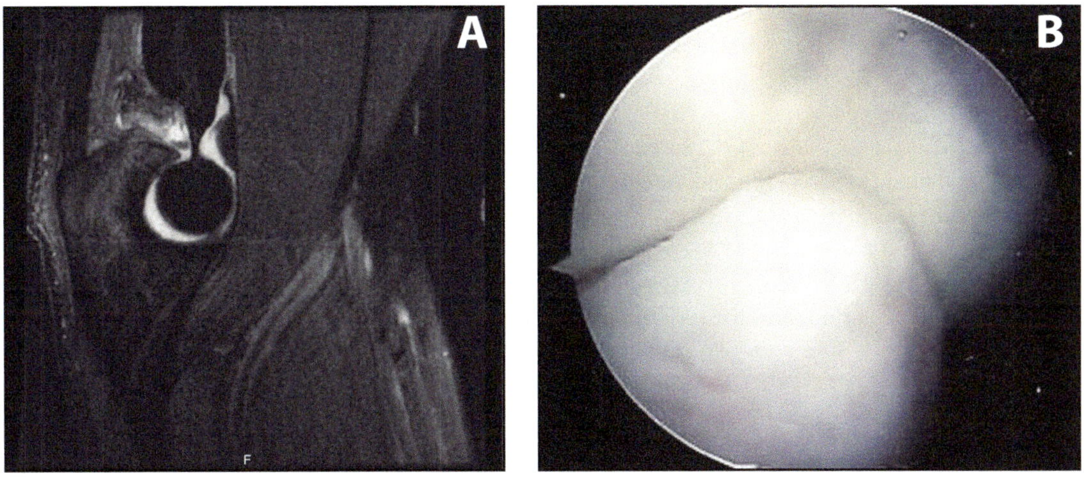

Figure 17-9. (A) Magnetic resonance image demonstrating the subchondral olecranon edema characteristic of posteromedial impingement in sagittal plane. (B) An arthroscopic view of spurring with posteromedial impingement.

- Concomitant injuries such UCL insufficiency, flexor-pronator tendinitis, and ulnar neuritis should be evaluated as well.
- Plain radiographs may reveal posteromedial olecranon osteophyte and/or loose bodies (Figure 17-9).
- Advanced imaging, such as magnetic resonance imaging, may not be necessary for diagnosis unless concomitant pathology such as UCL insufficiency is being considered.
- Initial conservative treatment involves rest, anti-inflammatories, and return via a graduated throwing program.
- Recalcitrant cases can be managed by arthroscopy with osteophyte resection and/or loose body removal; however, extreme care should be taken not to over-resect the olecranon.
    - Numerous studies have demonstrated an increased risk of subsequent UCL injury with over-resection of the olecranon; however, Levin et al have demonstrated that up to 8 mm may be safely resected.[106,108-110]
    - Andrews and Timmerman reported 92% good or excellent results at early follow-up after posteromedial olecranon resection for VEO; however, 41% developed recurrent medial elbow pain requiring surgery at 2 to 5 years, and 25% ultimately required UCL reconstruction.[104,106-111]

Ulnar Neuritis

- The ulnar nerve is at risk of compression as it courses down the arm because of numerous adjacent structures, including the following: the fascial hiatus in the medial intermuscular septum known as the *arcade of Struthers*; along the medial intermuscular septum; the medial head of the triceps; within the cubital tunnel between Osborne's ligament and the underlying UCL; in the presence of an accessory anconeus epitrochlearis muscle; between the 2 heads of the flexor carpi ulnaris muscle; and at the proximal edge of the flexor digitorum superficialis aponeurosis.[112-116]
- The ulnar nerve ultimately provides sensation to the small finger and ulnar aspect of the ring finger as well as motor innervation to the flexor carpi ulnaris, ulnar half of the flexor digitorum profundus, hypothenar eminence, and hand intrinsic musculature.

- The valgus stress placed on the medial elbow during many overhead athletic activities can result in traction injury to the ulnar nerve, generating both pain and neurologic symptoms such a numbness and tingling, cold intolerance, and motor weakness.
    - This may be further exacerbated by ulnar nerve instability with recurrent subluxation or dislocation of the nerve.[117]
- Physical examination should assess the ulnar nerve along its course, the presence and location of a Tinel sign, distal digital sensation, motor function of the hand intrinsics, and flexor digitorum profundus to the small finger.
    - The elbow flexion test is performed by placing the elbow in maximal flexion, the forearm in full pronation, and the wrist in extension with the shoulder in maximum external rotation and abduction for 30 seconds. It is considered positive if numbness and tingling occur in the ulnar nerve distribution with cubital tunnel pain.
- Electrodiagnostic testing should be obtained to document nerve conduction velocities bilaterally.
- Nonoperative treatment may involve rest, anti-inflammatories, and splinting.
- With failure of nonoperative treatment or physical examination or electrodiagnostic findings of severe disease, ulnar nerve neurolysis/decompression can be performed.
    - In the throwing athlete transposition (whether submuscular or subcutaneous) is most often performed.[118-120]

Olecranon Stress Fracture

- Olecranon stress fracture is an injury seen chiefly among overhead-throwing athletes. These stress fractures are often intractable, taking significant time to heal, and recur easily.
- Athletes will describe a history of repetitive overhead activity with progressive pain along the posterior elbow.
- Tenderness is present along the posterior olecranon.
- Plain radiography often demonstrates the fracture, but computed tomography and magnetic resonance imaging are both useful for supplementing the diagnosis (Figure 17-10).
    - Numerous patterns have been described, with Furushima et al proposing a classification system of 5 types of olecranon stress fracture:
        1. Physeal type: the most common adolescent type with delayed closure or nonunion of the physis
        2. Classic type: the most common adult type with an oblique fracture line
        3. Transitional type: with the appearance of a physeal type on anteroposterior radiograph but classic type on lateral radiograph
        4. Sclerotic type: in which only sclerosis is seen on plain radiography and magnetic resonance imaging reveals the diagnosis
        5. Distal type: with the fracture line originating from the cortical notch of the trochlear groove[121]
- Although no consensus exists for mechanism by which olecranon stress fractures occur, adult-type fractures are believed to represent the medial valgus and posterior shear forces of valgus extension overload, whereas pediatric-type fractures may occur via a triceps traction force on an immature olecranon physis.[12,122-128]
- An attempt at nonoperative management with rest should be attempted. However, these stress fractures are often intractable, taking significant time to heal, and recur easily.
- Fixation of the fracture may be necessary in athletes with recalcitrant symptoms, in which case the geometry of the fracture should be well understood prior to surgery.

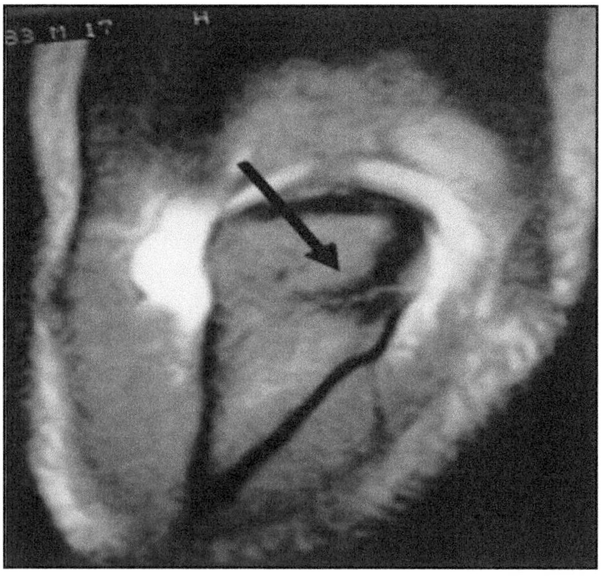

Figure 17-10. Magnetic resonance image demonstrating a stress fracture of the olecranon.

   - Fixation methods range from tension banding, to intramedullary screw placement to excision of small fragments.
- In some cases, olecranon stress fracture may be accompanied by medial elbow pathology such as UCL insufficiency or, in pediatric patients, medial epicondyle avulsion fracture, both of which should be addressed simultaneously.

Osteochondritis Dissecans of the Capitellum

- Osteochondritis dissecans of the capitellum is a focal, idiopathic disorder of subchondral bone of the capitellum, resulting in separation and fragmentation of the overlying articular surface.[129-133]
- Lesions are typically focal in nature with a limited capacity for healing and a propensity for fragmentation and formation of loose bodies.
- Although the etiology is idiopathic, repetitive microtrauma is believed to play a role because of the population in which this entity is seen, for whom the radiocapitellar joint is subjected to repeated compressive and shear forces.[126-134-138]
   - Furthermore the developing epiphysis of the capitellum has been demonstrated to have a vulnerable blood supply, further reducing its ability to respond to insult.[133]
- Typically, osteochondritis dissecans of the capitellum afflicts adolescent athletes 12 to 17 years old in sports subjecting the elbow to repetitive stress, including throwing and gymnastics.
- The most common presentation is pain with activity that is insidious in onset and relieved by rest.
- Physical examination may reveal tenderness of the radiocapitellar joint and crepitus with passive motion.
   - The active radiocapitellar compression test involves pronation and supination of the fully extended elbow in which dynamic muscle contraction reproduces symptoms.
   - Flexion contractures are not uncommon and may become significant.[137,139-143]
- Minami and colleagues have described a plain radiograph grading system in which grade 1 lesions demonstrate radiolucent cystic lesions in the middle or lateral capitellum, grade 2

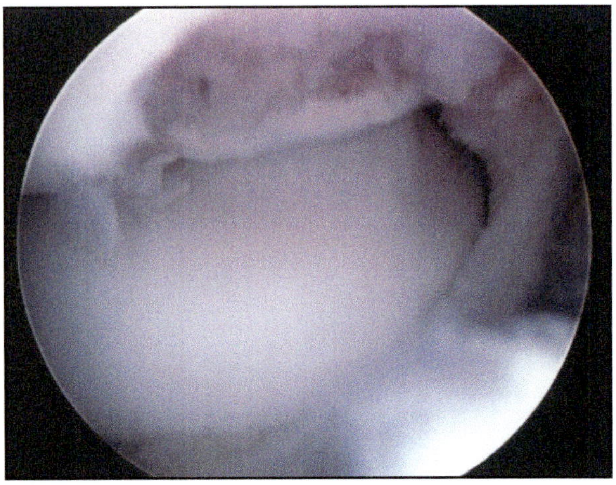

Figure 17-11. Arthroscopic view of an osteochondral lesion of the capitellum. (Reprinted with permission from John E. Conway, MD.)

lesions demonstrate a split or clear zone between the lesion and underlying subchondral bone, and grade 3 lesions are defined by the presence of loose bodies.[144]

- Magnetic resonance imaging with arthrography is valuable for further defining both the size and stability of lesions. Intravenous contrast during magnetic resonance imaging may provide additional benefit by demonstrating fragment viability by the presence or absence of blood supply.[129,145,146]
- Stable, viable lesions may be treated nonoperatively with extended rest. Nonoperative management has been most successful in patients with near-normal motion, an open physis, and absence of radiographic fragmentation.[141]
  - Some authors have advocated that pitchers be counseled to change positions or even consider changing sports.[133]
- Operative treatment is indicated for lesions failing to improve with appropriate nonoperative management. Numerous open and arthroscopic techniques have been described; however, residual symptoms have been noted in 42% to 65% of patients.[137,141,147-149]
- For athletes with early-stage lesions, nonoperative treatment including rest from throwing for 6 to 12 weeks, kinetic chain rehabilitation, and then a progressive throwing program, may be effective.
- Older athletes with more chronic symptoms and unstable or displaced fragments require operative treatment.
  - This may range from arthroscopic loose body removal and lesion debridement to microfracture and/or osteochondral grafting for lateral column deficiency (Figure 17-11).

Panner Disease

- Avascular necrosis of the humeral capitellum, or Panner disease, was first described in 1927 as resembling Calve-Perthe disease of the hip.
- The etiology of the avascular necrosis present in Panner disease is unknown and may result from acute trauma, repetitive microtrauma, or endocrine abnormalities leading to a failure of the local microcirculation and disordered endochondral ossification of the capitellum.[132,150,151]
- The typical symptoms of Panner disease are pain and tenderness localized to the lateral elbow and limited range of motion.
- It is critical to distinguish Panner disease from osteochondritis dissecans of the capitellum.

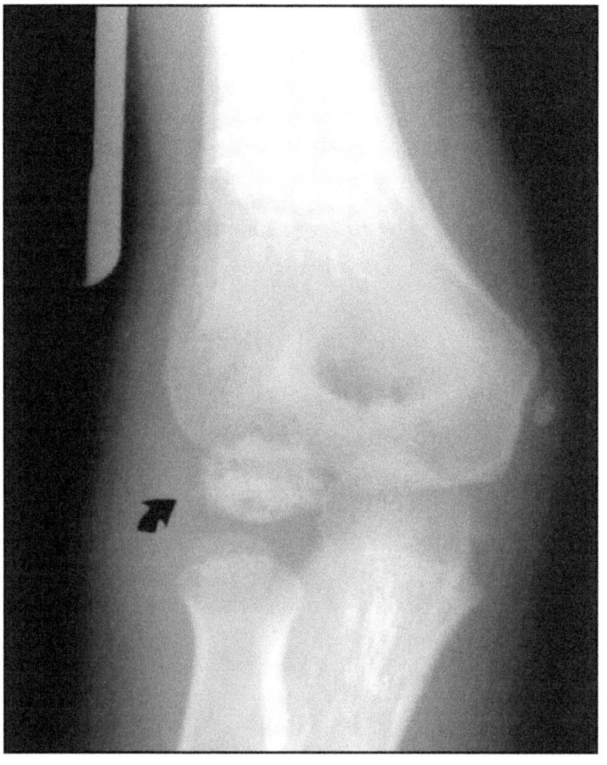

Figure 17-12. Plain radiograph demonstrating the global involvement of the capitellar epiphysis in Panner disease. (Reprinted with permission from Kobayashi K, Burton K, Rodner C, Smith B, Caputo AE. Lateral compression injuries in the pediatric elbow: Panner's disease and osteochondritis dissecans of the capitellum. *J Am Acad Orthop Surg.* 2004;12[4]: 246-254. doi:10.5435/00124635-200407000-00005.)

- Typically, Panner disease presents in athletes between 7 and 10 years old because ossification of the capitellum is generally complete by 10 years old.
- Plain radiography and magnetic resonance imaging both demonstrate more global involvement of the capitellum. In contrast, osteochondritis dissecans of the capitellum is characterized by a relatively older patient with more focal disease[132] (Figure 17-12).
- Furthermore, Panner disease is self-limited and well managed with rest and conservative measures, in distinction with the poorer prognosis associated with osteochondritis dissecans of the capitellum.
    - Long-term functional sequelae are generally not expected with Panner disease.[131,152]

Lateral Epicondylitis

- Commonly referred to as "tennis elbow," lateral epicondylitis has been recognized as a common source of elbow pain since the late 1800s.[153,154]
- It is characterized by insidious lateral elbow pain and diminished grip strength, exacerbated by resisted wrist extension.
- It is most common in the fourth through sixth decades and occurs 4 to 5 times more frequently in men than in women.[155]
- The most common source of pathology is microtearing of the origin of the extensor carpi radialis brevis, and microscopic evaluation of this tissue is classically characterized as "angiofibroblastic hyperplasia."[156]
- Physical examination is notable for reproducible, localized tenderness 1 to 2 cm distal and anterior to the extensor origin on the lateral epicondyle, worsened with resisted wrist and finger extension.
- Although the condition is typically self-limited, recovery make take as long as 2 years.

   - Treatment is predominantly aimed at conservative symptom management with activity modification, physical therapy for stretching, counterforce elbow bracing, and wrist bracing. One randomized, controlled trial demonstrated better pain relief with the wrist brace over the counterforce brace, but both were beneficial.[157]
   - Corticosteroid injections may provide short-term benefit but does not appear to alter the natural history.[158,159]
- Surgical treatment has been reported in 4% to 8% of cases, and the most common procedure involves excision of degenerative tissue within the extensor carpi radialis brevis tendon origin, creation of a bleeding bony bed, and reapproximation of the adjacent, normal common extensor tissue.[160]

Medial Epicondylitis

- Medial epicondylitis of the elbow, also known as "golfer's elbow," is more uncommon than its lateral counterpart.[161]
- This disorder is a similar overuse syndrome of the flexor-pronator mass due to activities involving repetitive forearm pronation and wrist flexion.
- Histologically, medial epicondylitis appears as an incomplete reparative process with similar "angiofibroblastic hyperplasia."[156]
- History is of insidious pain localized to the medial epicondyle and provoked on physical examination by resisted forearm pronation and wrist flexion.
- Careful physical examination should exclude alternative causes of medial elbow symptoms, including UCL insufficiency and ulnar neuritis.
- Nonsurgical management is similar to that of lateral epicondylitis and remains the mainstay of treatment, despite a lower efficacy than in lateral epicondylitis.[162,163]
- Surgical treatment is appropriate in athletes with acute traumatic disruption of the flexor-pronator tendon or chronic cases refractory to nonoperative treatment.
   - Surgical technique commonly involves debridement of the pathologic tissue and reattachment of the flexor-pronator mass to the medial epicondyle, with care not to damage the underlying anterior band of the UCL.

Radiocapitellar Plica

- Many joints exhibit synovial folds, or plica, which may represent remnants of embryologic development of the joint. Although less commonly seen in the elbow than in the knee, symptomatic plica may exist in the radiocapitellar articulation of the elbow joint.[164,165]
- Symptoms of radiocapitellar plica may be subtle and should be distinguished from lateral epicondylitis, loose bodies, elbow arthritis, or snapping triceps syndrome.[164,165]
- These athletes often have a history of repetitive overhead throwing and may describe a snapping or catching sensation in the posterolateral elbow.
- They exhibit focal tenderness in the posterolateral gutter worsened with hyperextension.
- Unfortunately, diagnostic imaging may have limited value in confirming the presence of plica.
- If the patient remains symptomatic despite conservative management including rest and gradual resumption of activities, diagnostic arthroscopy can be undertaken to confirm the presence of plica and resect the synovial thickening in the posterolateral gutter of the elbow.
   - The articular surfaces of the radial head and capitellum should be evaluated for the presence of "kissing lesions" of chondromalacia.[164]

Snapping Triceps Syndrome

- Snapping triceps syndrome is a rare condition of the elbow that can present with medial elbow pain.[166] The pain is related to irritation of the ulnar nerve from being subluxated over the medial epicondyle.
- The triceps has been reported to dislocate (or snap) over the lateral epicondyle as well but medial dislocation over the medial epicondyle is the most common variant.
- This is most often seen in men, laborers, and athletes and body builders. It can also be seen in patients with varus or valgus deformity due to altered triceps angle.
- Initially, conservative management is attempted to decrease the inflammation surrounding the ulnar nerve. If the patient fails conservative management, surgical treatment includes an ulnar nerve decompression and transposition with excision of a portion of the medial head of the triceps responsible for subluxation.

References

1. Kibler WB, McMullen J, Uhl T. Shoulder rehabilitation strategies, guidelines, and practice. *Orthop Clin North Am.* 2001;32(3):527-538. doi:10.1016/s0030-5898(05)70222-4.
2. Rubin BD, Kibler WB. Fundamental principles of shoulder rehabilitation: conservative to postoperative management. *Arthroscopy.* 2002;18(9 suppl 2):29-39. doi:10.1053/jars.2002.36507.
3. Dillman C, Fleisig G, Andrews J. Biomechanics of pitching with emphasis upon shoulder kinematics. *J Orthop Sports Phys Ther.* 1993;18(2):402-408. doi:10.2519/jospt.1993.18.2.402.
4. Fleisig GS, Andrews JR, Dillman CJ, Escamilla RF. Kinetics of Baseball pitching with implications about injury mechanisms. *Am J Sports Med.* 1995;23(2):233-239. doi:10.1177/036354659502300218.
5. Pappas AM, Zawacki RM, Sullivan TJ. Biomechanics of baseball pitching: a preliminary report. *Am J Sports Med.* 1985;13(4):216-222. doi:10.1177/036354658501300402.
6. Meister K. Injuries to the shoulder in the throwing athlete. Part one: biomechanics/pathophysiology/classification of injury. *Am J Sports Med.* 2000;28(2):265-275.
7. Harryman D, Sidles J, Clark J, McQuade K, Gibb T, Matsen F. Translation of the humeral head on the glenoid with passive glenohumeral motion. *J Bone Joint Surg Am.* 1990;72(9):1334-1343.
8. Fleisig GS, Barrentine SW, Zheng N, Escamilla RF, Andrews JR. Kinematic and kinetic comparison of baseball pitching among various levels of development. *J Biomech.* 1999;32(12):1371-1375. doi:10.1016/S0021-9290(99)00127-X.
9. Bigliani LU, Codd TP, Connor PM, Levine WN, Littlefield MA, Hershon SJ. Shoulder motion and laxity in the professional baseball player. *Am J Sports Med.* 1997;25(5):609-613. doi:10.1177/036354659702500504.
10. Brown LP, Niehues SL, Harrah A, Yavorsky P, Hirshman HP. Upper extremity range of motion and isokinetic strength of the internal and external shoulder rotators in major league baseball players. *Am J Sports Med.* 1988;16(6):577-585. doi:10.1177/036354658801600604.
11. Kibler WB, Chandler TJ, Livingston BP, Roetert EP. Shoulder range of motion in elite tennis players: effect of age and years of tournament play. *Am J Sports Med.* 1996;24(3):279-285. doi:10.1177/036354659602400306.
12. King J, Brelsford H, Tullos H. Analysis of the pitching arm of the professional baseball pitcher. *Clin Orthop Relat Res.* 1969;(67):116-123.
13. Reagan KM, Meister K, Horodyski MB, Werner DW, Carruthers C, Wilk K. Humeral Retroversion and its relationship to glenohumeral rotation in the shoulder of college baseball players. *Am J Sports Med.* 2002;30(3):354-360. doi:10.1177/03635465020300030901.
14. Fabricant PD, Lakomkin N, Sugimoto D, Tepolt FA, Stracciolini A, Kocher MS. Youth sports specialization and musculoskeletal injury: a systematic review of the literature. *Phys Sportsmed.* 2016;44(3):257-262. doi:10.1080/00913847.2016.1177476
15. Sabick MB, Kim Y-K, Torry MR, Keirns MA, Hawkins RJ. Biomechanics of the shoulder in youth baseball pitchers. *Am J Sports Med.* 2005;33(11):1716-1722. doi:10.1177/0363546505275347.
16. Neer CS II. Impingement lesions. *Clin Orthop Relat Res.* 1983;(173):70-77.

17. Hegedus EJ, Goode A, Campbell S, et al. Physical examination tests of the shoulder: a systematic review with meta-analysis of individual tests. *Br J Sports Med.* 2008;42(2):80. doi:10.1136/bjsm.2007.038406.
18. Weiner DS, Macnab I. Superior migration of the humeral head. *J Bone Joint Surg Br.* 1970;52-B(3):524-527. doi:10.1302/0301-620X.52B3.524.
19. House J, DO F, Mooradian A. Evaluation and management of shoulder pain in primary care clinics. *South Med J.* 2010;103(11):1129-1137. doi:10.1097/SMJ.0b013e3181f5e85f.
20. Burns TP, Turba JE. Arthroscopic treatment of shoulder impingement in athletes. *Am J Sports Med.* 1992;20(1):13-16. doi:10.1177/036354659202000104.
21. Walch G, Boileau P, Noel E, Donell ST. Impingement of the deep surface of the supraspinatus tendon on the posterosuperior glenoid rim: an arthroscopic study. *J Shoulder Elbow Surg.* 1992;1(5):238-245. doi:10.1016/S1058-2746(09)80065-7.
22. Riand N, Levigne C, Renaud E, Walch G. Results of derotational humeral osteotomy in posterosuperior glenoid impingement. *Am J Sports Med.* 1998;26(3):453-459. doi:10.1177/03635465980260032001.
23. Andrews JR, Broussard TS, Carson WG. Arthroscopy of the shoulder in the management of partial tears of the rotator cuff: a preliminary report. *Arthrosc J Arthrosc Relat Surg Off Publ Arthrosc Assoc N Am Int Arthrosc Assoc.* 1985;1(2):117-122.
24. Conway JE. Arthroscopic repair of partial-thickness rotator cuff tears and SLAP lesions in professional baseball players. *Orthop Clin North Am.* 2001;32(3):443-456.
25. Paley KJ, Jobe FW, Pink MM, Kvitne RS, ElAttrache NS. Arthroscopic findings in the overhand throwing athlete: evidence for posterior internal impingement of the rotator cuff. *Arthrosc J Arthrosc Relat Surg Off Publ Arthrosc Assoc N Am Int Arthrosc Assoc.* 2000;16(1):35-40.
26. Jobe FW, Kvitne RS, Giangarra CE. Shoulder pain in the overhand or throwing athlete. The relationship of anterior instability and rotator cuff impingement. *Orthop Rev.* 1989;18(9):963-975.
27. Fu F, Harner C, Klein A. Shoulder impingement syndrome: a critical review. *Clin Orthop Relat Res.* 1991;(269):162-173.
28. Arroyo JS, Hershon SJ, Bigliani LU. Special considerations in the athletic throwing shoulder. *Orthop Clin North Am.* 1997;28(1):69-78. doi:10.1016/S0030-5898(05)70265-0.
29. Davidson PA, Elattrache NS, Jobe CM, Jobe FW. Rotator cuff and posterior-superior glenoid labrum injury associated with increased glenohumeral motion: a new site of impingement. *J Shoulder Elbow Surg.* 1995;4(5):384-390.
30. Edelson G, Teitz C. Internal impingement in the shoulder. *J Shoulder Elbow Surg.* 2000;9(4):308-315. doi:10.1067/mse.2000.105449.
31. Heyworth BE, Williams RJ III. Internal impingement of the shoulder. *Am J Sports Med.* 2009;37(5):1024-1037. doi:10.1177/0363546508324966.
32. Dines D, Warren R, Inglis A, Pavlov H. The coracoid impingement syndrome. *J Bone Joint Surg Br.* 1990;72-B(2):314-316. doi:10.1302/0301-620X.72B2.2312576.
33. Gerber C, Terrier F, Ganz R. The role of the coracoid process in the chronic impingement syndrome. *J Bone Joint Surg Br.* 1985;67-B(5):703-708. doi:10.1302/0301-620X.67B5.4055864.
34. Gerber C, Terrier F, Zehnder R, Ganz R. The subcoracoid space: an anatomic study. *Clin Orthop Relat Res.* 1987;(215):132-138.
35. Patte D. The subcoracoid impingement. *Clin Orthop Relat Res.* 1990;(254):55-59.
36. Russo R, Togo F. The subcoracoid impingement syndrome: clinical, semeiologic and therapeutic considerations. *Ital J Orthop Traumatol.* 1991;17(3):351-358.
37. Ferrick MR. Coracoid impingement. A case report and review of the literature. *Am J Sports Med.* 2000;28(1):117-119. doi:10.1177/03635465000280010501.
38. Friedman RJ, Bonutti PM, Genez B. Cine magnetic resonance imaging of the subcoracoid region. *Orthopedics.* 1998;21(5):545-548.
39. Myers JB, Laudner KG, Pasquale MR, Bradley JP, Lephart SM. Glenohumeral range of motion deficits and posterior shoulder tightness in throwers with pathologic internal impingement. *Am J Sports Med.* 2006;34(3):385-391. doi:10.1177/0363546505281804.
40. Wilk KE, Macrina LC, Fleisig GS, et al. Correlation of glenohumeral internal rotation deficit and total rotational motion to shoulder injuries in professional baseball pitchers. *Am J Sports Med.* 2011;39(2):329-335. doi:10.1177/0363546510384223.
41. Burkhart SS, Morgan CD, Kibler WB. The disabled throwing shoulder: spectrum of pathology Part I: pathoanatomy and biomechanics. *Arthrosc J Arthrosc Relat Surg Off Publ Arthrosc Assoc N Am Int Arthrosc Assoc.* 2003;19(4):404-420. doi:10.1053/jars.2003.50128.
42. Burkhart SS, Morgan CD, Kibler WB. The disabled throwing shoulder: spectrum of pathology. Part II: evaluation and treatment of SLAP lesions in throwers. *Arthrosc J Arthrosc Relat Surg Off Publ Arthrosc Assoc N Am Int Arthrosc Assoc.* 2003;19(5):531-539. doi:10.1053/jars.2003.50139.

43. Burkhart SS, Morgan CD, Kibler WB. The disabled throwing shoulder: spectrum of pathology part III: the SICK scapula, scapular dyskinesis, the kinetic chain, and rehabilitation. *Arthroscopy.* 2003;19(6):641-661. doi:10.1016/s0749-8063(03)00389-x.
44. Noonan TJ, Shanley E, Bailey LB, et al. Professional pitchers with glenohumeral internal rotation deficit (GIRD) display greater humeral retrotorsion than pitchers without GIRD. *Am J Sports Med.* 2015;43(6):1448-1454. doi:10.1177/0363546515575020.
45. Codman E. *The Shoulder, Rupture of the Supraspinatus Tendon and Other Lesions on or about the Subacromial Bursa.* Boston, MA: Thomas Dodd Company; 1934.
46. Willmore EG, Smith MJ. Scapular dyskinesia: evolution towards a systems-based approach. *Shoulder Elb.* 2016;8(1):61-70. doi:10.1177/1758573215618857.
47. Warner JJ, Micheli LJ, Arslanian LE, Kennedy J, Kennedy R. Scapulothoracic motion in normal shoulders and shoulders with glenohumeral instability and impingement syndrome. A study using Moire topographic analysis. *Clin Orthop.* 1992;(285):191-199.
48. Paletta GAJ, Warner JJ, Warren RF, Deutsch A, Altchek DW. Shoulder kinematics with two-plane x-ray evaluation in patients with anterior instability or rotator cuff tearing. *J Shoulder Elbow Surg.* 1997;6(6):516-527.
49. Kibler WB, Uhl TL, Maddux JW, Brooks PV, Zeller B, McMullen J. Qualitative clinical evaluation of scapular dysfunction: a reliability study. *J Shoulder Elbow Surg.* 2002;11(6):550-556. doi:10.1067/mse.2002.126766.
50. Kibler WB, Sciascia A, Wilkes T. Scapular dyskinesis and its relation to shoulder injury. *J Am Acad Orthop Surg.* 2012;20(6):364-372. doi:10.5435/JAAOS-20-06-364.
51. Kibler WB, Sciascia A, Dome D. Evaluation of apparent and absolute supraspinatus strength in patients with shoulder injury using the scapular retraction test. *Am J Sports Med.* 2006;34(10):1643-1647. doi:10.1177/0363546506288728.
52. Bennett G. Shoulder and elbow lesions of the professional baseball pitcher. *J Am Med Assoc.* 1941;117:510-514.
53. Wright RW, Paletta GAJ. Prevalence of the Bennett lesion of the shoulder in major league pitchers. *Am J Sports Med.* 2004;32(1):121-124. doi:10.1177/0363546503260712.
54. Meister K, Andrews JR, Batts J, Wilk K, Baumgarten T. Symptomatic thrower's exostosis. Arthroscopic evaluation and treatment. *Am J Sports Med.* 1999;27(2):133-136. doi:10.1177/03635465990270020301.
55. Adams JT, DeWeese JA. "Effort" thrombosis of the axillary and subclavian veins. *J Trauma.* 1971;11(11):923-930.
56. Crowell DL. Effort thrombosis of the subclavian and axillary veins: review of the literature and case report with two-year follow-up with venography. *Ann Intern Med.* 1960;52:1337-1343.
57. Ellis MH, Manor Y, Witz M. Risk factors and management of patients with upper limb deep vein thrombosis. *Chest.* 2000;117(1):43-46.
58. Peet RM, Henriksen JD, Anderson TP, Martin GM. Thoracic-outlet syndrome: evaluation of a therapeutic exercise program. *Proc Staff Meet Mayo Clin.* 1956;31(9):281-287.
59. Hooper TL, Denton J, McGalliard MK, Brismee JM, Sizer PSJ. Thoracic outlet syndrome: a controversial clinical condition. Part 1: anatomy, and clinical examination/diagnosis. *J Man Manip Ther.* 2010;18(2):74-83. doi:10.1179/106698110X12640740712734.
60. Sanders RJ, Hammond SL, Rao NM. Diagnosis of thoracic outlet syndrome. *J Vasc Surg.* 2007;46(3):601-604. doi:10.1016/j.jvs.2007.04.050.
61. Brantigan CO, Roos DB. Diagnosing thoracic outlet syndrome. *Hand Clin.* 2004;20(1):27-36.
62. Atasoy E. A hand surgeon's further experience with thoracic outlet compression syndrome. *J Hand Surg.* 2010;35(9):1528-1538. doi:10.1016/j.jhsa.2010.06.025.
63. Klaassen Z, Sorenson E, Tubbs RS, et al. Thoracic outlet syndrome: a neurological and vascular disorder. *Clin Anat N Y N.* 2014;27(5):724-732. doi:10.1002/ca.22271.
64. Huang JH, Zager EL. Thoracic outlet syndrome. *Neurosurgery.* 2004;55(4):897-902; discussion 902-903.
65. Gilliatt RW, Le Quesne PM, Logue V, Sumner AJ. Wasting of the hand associated with a cervical rib or band. *J Neurol Neurosurg Psychiatry.* 1970;33(5):615-624.
66. Chang DC, Rotellini-Coltvet LA, Mukherjee D, De Leon R, Freischlag JA. Surgical intervention for thoracic outlet syndrome improves patient's quality of life. *J Vasc Surg.* 2009;49(3):630-635; discussion 635-637. doi:10.1016/j.jvs.2008.10.023.
67. Caputo FJ, Wittenberg AM, Vemuri C, et al. Supraclavicular decompression for neurogenic thoracic outlet syndrome in adolescent and adult populations. *J Vasc Surg.* 2013;57(1):149-157. doi:10.1016/j.jvs.2012.07.025.
68. Nuber GW, McCarthy WJ, Yao JS, Schafer MF, Suker JR. Arterial abnormalities of the shoulder in athletes. *Am J Sports Med.* 1990;18(5):514-519. doi:10.1177/036354659001800512.
69. Cormier PJ, Matalon TA, Wolin PM. Quadrilateral space syndrome: a rare cause of shoulder pain. *Radiology.* 1988;167(3):797-798. doi:10.1148/radiology.167.3.3363143.
70. Cahill BR, Palmer RE. Quadrilateral space syndrome. *J Hand Surg.* 1983;8(1):65-69.
71. Chautems RC, Glauser T, Waeber-Fey MC, Rostan O, Barraud GE. Quadrilateral space syndrome: case report and review of the literature. *Ann Vasc Surg.* 2000;14(6):673-676. doi:10.1007/s100169910120.

72. McKowen HC, Voorhies RM. Axillary nerve entrapment in the quadrilateral space. Case report. *J Neurosurg.* 1987;66(6):932-934. doi:10.3171/jns.1987.66.6.0932.
73. McAdams TR, Dillingham MF. Surgical decompression of the quadrilateral space in overhead athletes. *Am J Sports Med.* 2008;36(3):528-532. doi:10.1177/0363546507309675.
74. Francel TJ, Dellon AL, Campbell JN. Quadrilateral space syndrome: diagnosis and operative decompression technique. *Plast Reconstr Surg.* 1991;87(5):911-916.
75. Lester B, Jeong GK, Weiland AJ, Wickiewicz TL. Quadrilateral space syndrome: diagnosis, pathology, and treatment. *Am J Orthop Belle Mead NJ.* 1999;28(12):718-722, 725.
76. van de Pol D, Kuijer PPFM, Langenhorst T, Maas M. High prevalence of self-reported symptoms of digital ischemia in elite male volleyball players in the Netherlands: a cross-sectional national survey. *Am J Sports Med.* 2012;40(10):2296-2302. doi:10.1177/0363546512456973.
77. Atema JJ, Unlu C, Reekers JA, Idu MM. Posterior circumflex humeral artery injury with distal embolisation in professional volleyball players: a discussion of three cases. *Eur J Vasc Endovasc Surg Off J Eur Soc Vasc Surg.* 2012;44(2):195-198. doi:10.1016/j.ejvs.2012.05.018.
78. Reutter D, Hunziker R, Husmann M. Computed angiogram of the upper extremities for diagnosing a rare cause of brachial arterial embolism: the "Pitcher syndrome". *Eur Heart J.* 2010;31(22):2782. doi:10.1093/eurheartj/ehq269.
79. Duwayri YM, Emery VB, Driskill MR, et al. Positional compression of the axillary artery causing upper extremity thrombosis and embolism in the elite overhead throwing athlete. *J Vasc Surg.* 2011;53(5):1329-1340. doi:10.1016/j.jvs.2010.11.031.
80. McIntosh A, Hassan I, Cherry K, Dahm D. Posterior circumflex humeral artery aneurysm in 2 professional volleyball players. *Am J Orthop Belle Mead NJ.* 2006;35(1):33-36.
81. Chafik D, Galatz LM, Keener JD, Kim HM, Yamaguchi K. Teres minor muscle and related anatomy. *J Shoulder Elbow Surg.* 2013;22(1):108-114. doi:10.1016/j.jse.2011.12.005.
82. Kruse LM, Yamaguchi K, Keener JD, Chamberlain AM. Clinical outcomes after decompression of the nerve to the teres minor in patients with idiopathic isolated teres minor fatty atrophy. *J Shoulder Elbow Surg.* 2015;24(4):628-633. doi:10.1016/j.jse.2014.08.018.
83. Morrey B, Tanaka S, An KN. Valgus stability of the elbow: a definition of primary and secondary constraints. *Clin Orthop Relat Res.* 1991;(265):187-195.
84. Erickson BJ, Romeo AA. The ulnar collateral ligament injury: evaluation and treatment. *J Bone Joint Surg Am.* 2017;99(1):76-86. doi:10.2106/JBJS.16.01277.
85. Ciccotti MC, Hammoud S, Dodson CC, Cohen SB, Nazarian LN, Ciccotti MG. Stress ultrasound evaluation of medial elbow instability in a cadaveric model. *Am J Sports Med.* 2014;42(10):2463-2469. doi:10.1177/0363546514542805.
86. Park MC, Ahmad CS. Dynamic contributions of the flexor-pronator mass to elbow valgus stability. *J Bone Joint Surg Am.* 2004;86(10):2268-2274.
87. Cain EL, Andrews JR, Dugas JR, et al. Outcome of ulnar collateral ligament reconstruction of the elbow in 1281 athletes. *Am J Sports Med.* 2010;38(12):2426-2434. doi:10.1177/0363546510378100.
88. Ciccotti MG, Pollack KM, Ciccotti MC, et al. Elbow injuries in professional baseball: epidemiological findings from the Major League Baseball injury surveillance system. *Am J Sports Med.* 2017;45(10):2319-2328. doi:10.1177/0363546517706964.
89. Erickson BJ, Gupta AK, Harris JD, et al. Rate of return to pitching and performance after Tommy John surgery in Major League Baseball pitchers. *Am J Sports Med.* 2014;42(3):536-543. doi:10.1177/0363546513510890.
90. Marshall NE, Keller RA, Lynch JR, Bey MJ, Moutzouros V. Pitching performance and longevity after revision ulnar collateral ligament reconstruction in Major League Baseball pitchers. *Am J Sports Med.* 2015;43(5):1051-1056. doi:10.1177/0363546515579636.
91. Veltri DM, O'Brien SJ, Field LD, Deutsch A, Altchek DW, Potter HG. The milking manuever—a new test to evaluate the MCL of the elbow in the throwing athlete. *J Shoulder Elbow Surg.* 1995;4:S10. doi:10.1016/S1058-2746(95)80048-4.
92. O'Driscoll SWM, Lawton RL, Smith AM. The "Moving Valgus Stress Test" for medial collateral ligament tears of the elbow. *Am J Sports Med.* 2005;33(2):231-239. doi:10.1177/0363546504267804.
93. Joyner PW, Bruce J, Hess R, Mates A, Mills FB IV, Andrews JR. Magnetic resonance imaging-based classification for ulnar collateral ligament injuries of the elbow. *J Shoulder Elbow Surg.* 2016;25(10):1710-1716.
94. Nazarian LN, McShane JM, Ciccotti MG, O'Kane PL, Harwood MI. Dynamic US of the anterior band of the ulnar collateral ligament of the elbow in asymptomatic Major League Baseball pitchers. *Radiology.* 2003;227(1):149-154. doi:10.1148/radiol.2271020288.
95. Atanda A, Averill LW, Wallace M, Niiler TA, Nazarian LN, Ciccotti MG. Factors related to increased ulnar collateral ligament thickness on stress sonography of the elbow in asymptomatic youth and adolescent baseball pitchers. *Am J Sports Med.* 2016;44(12):3179-3187. doi:10.1177/0363546516661010.

96. Atanda A, Buckley PS, Hammoud S, Cohen SB, Nazarian LN, Ciccotti MG. Early anatomic changes of the ulnar collateral ligament identified by stress ultrasound of the elbow in young professional baseball pitchers. *Am J Sports Med.* 2015;43(12):2943-2949. doi:10.1177/0363546515605042.
97. Ciccotti M, Nazarian L, Ciccotti M. Ultrasound imaging of UCL injury. In: Dines J, Altchek, DW, eds. *Ulnar Collateral Ligament Injury: A Guide to Diagnosis and Treatment.* New York, NY: Springer; 2015:79-91.
98. Ciccotti MG, Atanda A, Nazarian LN, Dodson CC, Holmes L, Cohen SB. Stress sonography of the ulnar collateral ligament of the elbow in professional baseball pitchers. *Am J Sports Med.* 2014;42(3):544-551. doi:10.1177/0363546513516592.
99. Chang E, Dodson C, Ciccotti M. Comparison of surgical techniques for ulnar collateral ligament reconstruction in overhead athletes. *J Am Acad Orthop Surg.* 2016;24(3):135-149. doi:10.5435/JAAOS-D-14-00323.
100. Conway J, Jobe F, Glousman R, Pink M. Medial instability of the elbow in throwing athletes. Treatment by repair or reconstruction of the ulnar collateral ligament. *J Bone Joint Surg Am.* 1992;74(1):67-83.
101. Rohrbough JT, Altchek DW, Hyman J, Williams RJ, Botts JD. Medial collateral ligament reconstruction of the elbow using the Docking technique. *Am J Sports Med.* 2002;30(4):541-548. doi:10.1177/03635465020300041401.
102. Savoie FH, Trenhaile SW, Roberts J, Field LD, Ramsey JR. Primary repair of ulnar collateral ligament injuries of the elbow in young athletes. *Am J Sports Med.* 2008;36(6):1066-1072. doi:10.1177/0363546508315201.
103. Dugas JR, Walters BL, Beason DP, Fleisig GS, Chronister JE. Biomechanical comparison of ulnar collateral ligament repair with internal bracing versus modified Jobe reconstruction. *Am J Sports Med.* 2015;44(3):735-741. doi:10.1177/0363546515620390.
104. Vitale MA. Clinical sports medicine update: the outcome of elbow ulnar collateral ligament reconstruction in overhead athletes. *Am J Sports Med.* 2008;36(6):1193-1205. doi:10.1177/0363546508319053.
105. Watson JN, McQueen P, Hutchinson MR. A systematic review of ulnar collateral ligament reconstruction techniques. *Am J Sports Med.* 2013;42(10):2510-2516. doi:10.1177/0363546513509051.
106. Andrews JR, Timmerman LA. Outcome of elbow surgery in professional baseball players. *Am J Sports Med.* 1995;23(4):407-413. doi:10.1177/036354659502300406.
107. O'Driscoll SW. Valgus extension overload and plica. In: Levine WN, ed. *The Athlete's Elbow.* Rosemont, IL: American Academy of Orthopaedic Surgeons; 2008:71-83.
108. Levin JS, Zheng N, Dugas J, Cain EL, Andrews JR. Posterior olecranon resection and ulnar collateral ligament strain. *J Shoulder Elbow Surg.* 2004;13(1):66-71. doi:10.1016/S1058274603002532.
109. Kamineni S, ElAttrache NS, O'Driscoll SW, et al. Medial collateral ligament strain with partial posteromedial olecranon resection. A biomechanical study. *J Bone Joint Surg Am.* 2004;86(11):2424-2430.
110. Kamineni S, Hirahara H, Pomianowski S, et al. Partial posteromedial olecranon resection: a kinematic study. *J Bone Joint Surg Am.* 2003;85(6):1005-1011.
111. Osbahr DC, Cain EL, Raines BT, Fortenbaugh D, Dugas JR, Andrews JR. Long-term outcomes after ulnar collateral ligament reconstruction in competitive baseball players: minimum 10-year follow-up. *Am J Sports Med.* 2014;42(6):1333-1342. doi:10.1177/0363546514528870.
112. Gonzalez MH, Lotfi P, Bendre A, Mandelbroyt Y, Lieska N. The ulnar nerve at the elbow and its local branching: an anatomic study. *J Hand Surg Br.* 2001;26(2):142-144. doi:10.1054/jhsb.2000.0532.
113. Dahners LE, Wood FM. Anconeus epitrochlearis, a rare cause of cubital tunnel syndrome: a case report. *J Hand Surg.* 1984;9(4):579-580.
114. Glousman RE. Ulnar nerve problems in the athlete's elbow. *Clin Sports Med.* 1990;9(2):365-377.
115. Kleinman WB. Revision ulnar neuroplasty. *Hand Clin.* 1994;10(3):461-477.
116. Wojtys EM, Smith PA, Hankin FM. A cause of ulnar neuropathy in a baseball pitcher. A case report. *Am J Sports Med.* 1986;14(5):422-424. doi:10.1177/036354658601400518.
117. Childress HM. Recurrent ulnar-nerve dislocation at the elbow. *Clin Orthop Relat Res.* 1975;(108):168-173.
118. Bartels RH, Menovsky T, Van Overbeeke JJ, Verhagen WI. Surgical management of ulnar nerve compression at the elbow: an analysis of the literature. *J Neurosurg.* 1998;89(5):722-727. doi:10.3171/jns.1998.89.5.0722.
119. Stuffer M, Jungwirth W, Hussl H, Schmutzhardt E. Subcutaneous or submuscular anterior transposition of the ulnar nerve? *J Hand Surg Br.* 1992;17(3):248-250.
120. Macnicol MF. The results of operation for ulnar neuritis. *J Bone Joint Surg Br.* 1979;61-B(2):159-164.
121. Furushima K, Itoh Y, Iwabu S, Yamamoto Y, Koga R, Shimizu M. Classification of olecranon stress fractures in baseball players. *Am J Sports Med.* 2014;42(6):1343-1351. doi:10.1177/0363546514528099.
122. Ahmad CS, ElAttrache NS. Valgus extension overload syndrome and stress injury of the olecranon. *Clin Sports Med.* 2004;23(4):665-676. doi:10.1016/j.csm.2004.04.013.
123. Cain ELJ, Dugas JR, Wolf RS, Andrews JR. Elbow injuries in throwing athletes: a current concepts review. *Am J Sports Med.* 2003;31(4):621-635. doi:10.1177/03635465030310042601.
124. Nuber GW, Diment MT. Olecranon stress fractures in throwers. A report of two cases and a review of the literature. *Clin Orthop Relat Res.* 1992;(278):58-61.
125. Schickendantz MS, Ho CP, Koh J. Stress injury of the proximal ulna in professional baseball players. *Am J Sports Med.* 2002;30(5):737-741. doi:10.1177/03635465020300051801.

126. Slocum DB. Classification of elbow injuries from baseball pitching. *Tex Med.* 1968;64(3):48-53.
127. Suzuki K, Minami A, Suenaga N, Kondoh M. Oblique stress fracture of the olecranon in baseball pitchers. *J Shoulder Elbow Surg.* 1997;6(5):491-494.
128. Torg JS, Moyer RA. Non-union of a stress fracture through the olecranon epiphyseal plate observed in an adolescent baseball pitcher. A case report. *J Bone Joint Surg Am.* 1977;59(2):264-265.
129. Bradley JP, Petrie RS. Osteochondritis dissecans of the humeral capitellum. Diagnosis and treatment. *Clin Sports Med.* 2001;20(3):565-590.
130. Iwasaki N, Kato H, Ishikawa J, Saitoh S, Minami A. Autologous osteochondral mosaicplasty for capitellar osteochondritis dissecans in teenaged patients. *Am J Sports Med.* 2006;34(8):1233-1239. doi:10.1177/0363546506286343.
131. Schenck RCJ, Goodnight JM. Osteochondritis dissecans. *J Bone Joint Surg Am.* 1996;78(3):439-456.
132. Yadao MA, Field LD, Savoie FH III. Osteochondritis dissecans of the elbow. *Instr Course Lect.* 2004;53:599-606.
133. Baker CL III, Romeo AA, Baker CLJ. Osteochondritis dissecans of the capitellum. *Am J Sports Med.* 2010;38(9):1917-1928. doi:10.1177/0363546509354969.
134. Adams JE. Injury to the throwing arm. A study of traumatic changes in the elbow joints of boy baseball players. *Calif Med.* 1965;102:127-132.
135. Barnes DA, Tullos HS. An analysis of 100 symptomatic baseball players. *Am J Sports Med.* 1978;6(2):62-67. doi:10.1177/036354657800600205.
136. Bowen RE, Otsuka NY, Yoon ST, Lang P. Osteochondral lesions of the capitellum in pediatric patients: role of magnetic resonance imaging. *J Pediatr Orthop.* 2001;21(3):298-301.
137. McManama GBJ, Micheli LJ, Berry MV, Sohn RS. The surgical treatment of osteochondritis of the capitellum. *Am J Sports Med.* 1985;13(1):11-21. doi:10.1177/036354658501300103.
138. Tullos HS, Erwin WD, Woods GW, Wukasch DC, Cooley DA, King JW. Unusual lesions of the pitching arm. *Clin Orthop Relat Res.* 1972;88:169-182.
139. Baumgarten TE, Andrews JR, Satterwhite YE. The arthroscopic classification and treatment of osteochondritis dissecans of the capitellum. *Am J Sports Med.* 1998;26(4):520-523. doi:10.1177/03635465980260040801.
140. Ruch DS, Cory JW, Poehling GG. The arthroscopic management of osteochondritis dissecans of the adolescent elbow. *Arthroscopy.* 1998;14(8):797-803. doi:10.1016/s0749-8063(98)70013-1.
141. Takahara M, Mura N, Sasaki J, Harada M, Ogino T. Classification, treatment, and outcome of osteochondritis dissecans of the humeral capitellum. *J Bone Joint Surg Am.* 2007;89(6):1205-1214. doi:10.2106/JBJS.F.00622.
142. Tivnon MC, Anzel SH, Waugh TR. Surgical management of osteochondritis dissecans of the capitellum. *Am J Sports Med.* 1976;4(3):121-128. doi:10.1177/036354657600400305.
143. Woodward AH, Bianco AJJ. Osteochondritis dissecans of the elbow. *Clin Orthop.* 1975;(110):35-41.
144. Minami M, Nakashita K, Ishii S. Twenty-five cases of osteochondritis dissecans of the elbow [in Japanese]. *Rinsho Seikei Geka.* 1979;14:805-810.
145. Kijowski R, Tuite M, Sanford M. Magnetic resonance imaging of the elbow. Part I: normal anatomy, imaging technique, and osseous abnormalities. *Skeletal Radiol.* 2004;33(12):685-697. doi:10.1007/s00256-004-0853-z.
146. Peiss J, Adam G, Casser R, Urhahn R, Gunther RW. Gadopentetate-dimeglumine-enhanced MR imaging of osteonecrosis and osteochondritis dissecans of the elbow: initial experience. *Skeletal Radiol.* 1995;24(1):17-20.
147. Bauer M, Jonsson K, Josefsson PO, Linden B. Osteochondritis dissecans of the elbow. A long-term follow-up study. *Clin Orthop Relat Res.* 1992;(284):156-160.
148. Mitsunaga MM, Adishian DA, Bianco AJJ. Osteochondritis dissecans of the capitellum. *J Trauma.* 1982;22(1):53-55.
149. Takahara M, Ogino T, Sasaki I, Kato H, Minami A, Kaneda K. Long term outcome of osteochondritis dissecans of the humeral capitellum. *Clin Orthop Relat Res.* 1999;(363):108-115.
150. Panner H. An affection of the humeral capitellum resembling Calve-Perthe's disease of the hip. *Acta Radiol.* 1927;8:617-618.
151. Kobayashi K, Burton K, Rodner C, Smith B, Caputo AE. Lateral compression injuries in the pediatric elbow: Panner's disease and osteochondritis dissecans of the capitellum. *J Am Acad Orthop Surg.* 2004;12(4):246-254. doi:10.5435/00124635-200407000-00005.
152. Takahara M, Ogino T, Takagi M, Tsuchida H, Orui H, Nambu T. Natural progression of osteochondritis dissecans of the humeral capitellum: initial observations. *Radiology.* 2000;216(1):207-212. doi:10.1148/radiology.216.1.r00jl29207.
153. Bernhardt M. Ueber eine wenig bekannte Form der Beschaftigungsneuralgie. *Neurol Cent.* 1896;15:13-16.
154. Runge F. Genese und Behandlung des Schreibekrampfes. *Berl Klin Wchenschr.* 1873;10:245-248.
155. Gruchow HW, Pelletier D. An epidemiologic study of tennis elbow. Incidence, recurrence, and effectiveness of prevention strategies. *Am J Sports Med.* 1979;7(4):234-238. doi:10.1177/036354657900700405.
156. Nirschl RP, Pettrone FA. Tennis elbow. The surgical treatment of lateral epicondylitis. *J Bone Joint Surg Am.* 1979;61(6A):832-839.

157. Garg R, Adamson GJ, Dawson PA, Shankwiler JA, Pink MM. A prospective randomized study comparing a forearm strap brace versus a wrist splint for the treatment of lateral epicondylitis. *J Shoulder Elbow Surg.* 2010;19(4):508-512. doi:10.1016/j.jse.2009.12.015.
158. Assendelft WJ, Hay EM, Adshead R, Bouter LM. Corticosteroid injections for lateral epicondylitis: a systematic overview. *Br J Gen Pract.* 1996;46(405):209-216.
159. Hay EM, Paterson SM, Lewis M, Hosie G, Croft P. Pragmatic randomised controlled trial of local corticosteroid injection and naproxen for treatment of lateral epicondylitis of elbow in primary care. *BMJ.* 1999;319(7215):964-968. doi:10.1136/bmj.319.7215.964.
160. Cohen MS, Romeo AA. Open and arthroscopic management of lateral epicondylitis in the athlete. *Hand Clin.* 2009;25(3):331-338. doi:10.1016/j.hcl.2009.05.003.
161. Ciccotti MG, Ramani MN. Medial epicondylitis. *Tech Hand Up Extrem Surg.* 2003;7(4):190-196. doi:10.1097/00130911-200312000-00010.
162. Jobe FW, Ciccotti MG. Lateral and medial epicondylitis of the elbow. *J Am Acad Orthop Surg.* 1994;2(1):1-8. doi:10.5435/00124635-199401000-00001.
163. Binder AI, Hazleman BL. Lateral humeral epicondylitis—a study of natural history and the effect of conservative therapy. *Br J Rheumatol.* 1983;22(2):73-76. doi:10.1093/rheumatology/22.2.73.
164. Clarke RP. Symptomatic, lateral synovial fringe (plica) of the elbow joint. *Arthroscopy.* 1988;4(2):112-116. doi:10.1016/s0749-8063(88)80077-x.
165. Commandre FA, Taillan B, Benezis C, Follacci FM, Hammou JC. Plica synovialis (synovial fold) of the elbow. Report on one case. *J Sports Med Phys Fitness.* 1988;28(2):209-210.
166. Rioux-Forker D, Bridgeman J, Brogan DM. Snapping triceps syndrome. *J Hand Surg.* 2018;43(1):90.e1-90.e5. doi:10.1016/j.jhsa.2017.10.014.

SECTION III

Literature Review

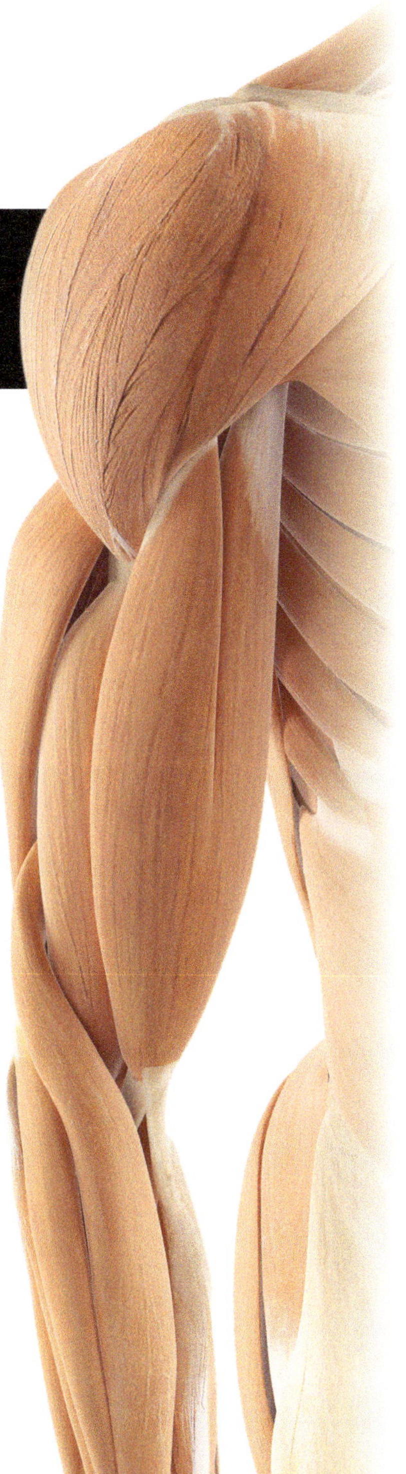

Recommended Reading by Chapter

Benjamin Zmistowski, MD; Surena Namdari, MD, MSc; and Reza Omid, MD

Elbow

Chapter 1 Elbow Anatomy and Physical Examination

- **Citation:** O'Driscoll SW, Bell DF, Morrey BF. Posterolateral rotatory instability of the elbow. *J Bone Joint Surg Am.* 1991;73(3):440-446.
    - **Recommended for:** historical context and description of common pathology
    - **Summary:** This article describes posterolateral rotator instability of the elbow for the first time. The pathophysiology is summarized as rotatory subluxation of the ulnohumeral joint with a transient subluxation of the radiohumeral joint secondary to lateral ulnar collateral ligament (UCL) laxity. In addition, the authors describe clinical exam maneuver and surgical treatment to identify and manage these injuries.
- **Citation:** O'Driscoll SW, Goncalves LB, Dietz P. The hook test for distal biceps tendon avulsion. *Am J Sports Med.* 2007;35(11):1865-1869. doi:10.1177/0363546507305016.
    - **Recommended for:** development and validation of a ubiquitous diagnostic test
    - **Summary:** This recent article describes for the first time the now commonly performed and referenced clinical test for distal biceps ruptures. A positive test is considered an inability to hook a cord-like structure while sweeping with a finger from lateral to medial in the antecubital fossa with the elbow supinated and flexed 90 degrees. The authors found the test to be 100% accurate for diagnosis of complete distal bicep tendon ruptures.

Namdari S, Zmistowski B, Omid R, eds.
The Foundations of Shoulder and Elbow Surgery (pp 341-353).

Chapter 2 Tendon Injuries

- **Citation:** Watson JN, Moretti VM, Schwindel L, Hutchinson MR. Repair techniques for acute distal biceps tendon ruptures: a systematic review. *J Bone Joint Surg Am.* 2014;96(24):2086-2090. doi:10.2106/JBJS.M.00481.
    - **Recommended for:** comparison of 1- vs 2-incision technique
    - **Summary:** Watson et al present a large systematic review of distal biceps tendon repair techniques. Their analysis includes 22 studies with 494 patients. They reported an overall complication rate of 24.5%; the complication rate following the 2-incision technique was 25.7% (44/171) compared with 23.9% (78/327) for the 1-incision technique. The majority of complications were lateral antebrachial cutaneous nerve neuropraxia, which was more common in 1-incision techniques.

Chapter 3 Elbow Instability

- **Citation:** Regan WD, Korinek SL, Morrey BF, An KN. Biomechanical study of ligaments around the elbow joint. *Clin Orthop Relat Res.* 1991;(271):170-179.
    - **Recommended for:** historical context
    - **Summary:** This cadaveric analysis of the ligaments around the elbow establishes the primary stabilizers of the elbow. The authors identified that the anterior medial collateral ligament (aMCL) and radial collateral ligament were taut throughout the entire flexion arc of the elbow. Furthermore, they found that the posterior medial collateral ligament became taut in higher degree of elbow flexion, whereas the lateral UCL was taut throughout the flexion arc when a varus stress was applied.
- **Citation:** Morrey BF, Tanaka S, An KN. Valgus stability of the elbow. A definition of primary and secondary constraints. *Clin Orthop Relat Res.* 1991;(265):187-195.
    - **Recommended for:** historical context
    - **Summary:** In this historically important cadaveric analysis, Morrey et al attempt to establish the stabilizers of the elbow against valgus stress. By sectioning cadaveric specimens, they find that removal of the radial head with an intact aMCL has little effect on the biomechanics of the elbow. However, removal of the aMCL demonstrated increased laxity even with an intact radial head. The combination of radial head excision and aMCL sectioning had the greatest impact on instability in this cadaveric model. They conclude that the aMCL is the primary stabilizer of the elbow against valgus stress while the radial head is a secondary stabilizer.
- **Citation:** Josefsson PO, Gentz CF, Johnell O, Wendeberg B. Surgical versus non-surgical treatment of ligamentous injuries following dislocation of the elbow joint. A prospective randomized study. *J Bone Joint Surg Am.* 1987;69(4):605-608.
    - **Recommended for:** historical context
    - **Summary:** This prospective, randomized analysis of treatment of the simple (nonfractured) elbow dislocation established that nonoperative management may be acceptable. After demonstrating that lateral elbow instability always and medial instability usually existed during examination under anesthesia following simple elbow dislocation, Joseffsson et al randomly assigned 30 patients to surgical vs nonsurgical management. In all surgically treated cases, disruption of the medial and lateral elbow ligaments was found. Despite this, no difference in the radiographic and clinical outcomes was noted.
- **Citation:** O'Driscoll SW, Bell DF, Morrey BF. Posterolateral rotatory instability of the elbow. *J Bone Joint Surg Am.* 1991;73(3):440-446.

- **Recommended for:** historical context
- **Summary:** See the previous summary for Chapter 1.

- **Citation:** O'Driscoll SW, Jupiter JB, Cohen MS, Ring D, McKee MD. Difficult elbow fractures: pearls and pitfalls. *Instr Course Lect.* 2003;52:113-134.
  - **Recommended for:** understanding of classification
  - **Summary:** This thorough review of fractures about the elbow provides an understanding of fracture patterns and their impact on elbow stability. This knowledge is directly applicable to treating the often complex fractures.
- **Citation:** Doornberg JN, Ring DC. Fracture of the anteromedial facet of the coronoid process. *J Bone Joint Surg Am.* 2006;88(10):2216-2224. doi:10.2106/JBJS.E.01127.
  - **Recommended for:** importance in change of practice
  - **Summary:** Through a review of 18 anteromedial facet coronoid fractures, the authors attempt to determine the impact of these fractures on long-term elbow function. All cases were treated surgically, although some in a delayed fashion. All but 3 patients had concomitant lateral elbow ligament injuries. Ultimately, the 6 patients who had displacement of the anteromedial facet of the coronoid either due to failed open reduction and internal fixation or benign neglect went on to develop arthrosis of the elbow. Alternatively, those patients who had successful healing of the anteromedial facet had superior outcomes without post-traumatic arthritis.

Chapter 4 Neuropathies of the Upper Extremity

- **Citation:** Johnson RK, Spinner M, Shrewsbury MM. Median nerve entrapment syndrome in the proximal forearm. *J Hand Surg Am.* 1979;4(1):48-51. doi:10.1016/s0363-5023(79)80104-5.
  - **Recommended for:** sites of compression and outcomes
  - **Summary:** In this early case series of median nerve compression in the proximal forearm, the authors provide a review of sites of compression and outcomes from surgical treatment. In the 51 cases treated surgically, compression occurred at the pronator teres, flexor superficialis arch, and the lacertus fibrosis. Frequency of compression at those sites occurred in decreasing order as listed. The authors also describe clinical tests to aid in localizing the site of compression.
- **Citation:** Stern MB. The anterior interosseous nerve syndrome (the Kiloh-Nevin syndrome). Report and follow-up study of three cases. *Clin Orthop Relat Res.* 1984;(187):223-227.
  - **Recommended for:** pathophysiology and surgical outcomes
  - **Summary:** The author describes 3 cases of a rare form of nerve compression that can be difficult to diagnose—anterior interosseous nerve syndrome. In all cases, patients had prolonged pain with weakness of the flexor policis longus, flexor digitorum longus to the index finger, and pronator quadratus. All patients underwent surgical exploration and were found to have compression of the anterior interosseous nerve as it branched from the median nerve between the 2 heads of the pronator teres. Following release, all patients had complete symptom resolution.
- **Citation:** McGowan AJ. The results of transposition of the ulnar nerve for traumatic ulnar neuritis. *J Bone Joint Surg Br.* 1950;32-B(3):293-301.
  - **Recommended for:** historical context and understanding of classification
  - **Summary:** For the time period of this paper, the author presents a large cohort of patients undergoing ulnar nerve transposition to treat multiple etiologies of cubital tunnel syndrome. The author reports good relief of pain and sensory deficits. Return of motor function appeared to be inveresly proportional to the degree of preoperative motor function.

Furthermore, 6 cases of revision ulnar transposition are described with good results following submuscular transposition.

- **Citation:** Roles NC, Maudsley RH. Radial tunnel syndrome: resistant tennis elbow as a nerve entrapment. *J Bone Joint Surg Br.* 1972;54(3):499-508.
    - **Recommended for:** historical context
    - **Summary:** This article provides a nearly 20-year review of treatment of a previously undescribed pathology: radial tunnel syndrome. The authors proposed that cases of recalcitrant tennis elbow were in fact compression neuropathies of the radial nerve. They describe treatment, with great success, of 38 elbows through an anterior approach to decompress the radial nerve. This paper established the diagnosis and treatment of radial tunnel syndrome.

Chapter 5 Fractures of the Elbow

- **Citation:** Pollock JW, Athwal GS, Steinmann SP. Surgical exposures for distal humerus fractures: a review. *Clin Anat.* 2008;21(8):757-768. doi:10.1002/ca.20720.
    - **Recommended for:** understanding of differences in surgical approaches to the distal humerus
    - **Summary:** This thorough review provides a relatively recent description of the advantages and disadvantages of each surgical approach to the distal humerus.
- **Citation:** O'Driscoll SW. Optimizing stability in distal humeral fracture fixation. *J Shoulder Elbow Surg.* 2005;14(1 suppl S):S186-S194. doi:10.1016/j.jse.2004.09.033.
    - **Recommended for:** further understanding of widely accepted surgical fixation principles
    - **Summary:** This review discusses the principles of construct stability in surgical management of distal humerus fractures. This includes a review of the existing literature and commentary on the varied constructs, such as perpindicular vs parrallel plating.

Chapter 6 Elbow Arthritis

- **Citation:** Miyake J, Shimada K, Oka K, et al. Arthroscopic debridement in the treatment of patients with osteoarthritis of the elbow, based on computer simulation. *Bone Joint J.* 2014;96-B(2):237-241. doi:10.1302/0301-620X.96B2.30714.
    - **Recommended for:** important change in best practices
    - **Summary:** This case series describes a novel way of assessing impinging osteophytes in the elbow and providing a visual guide to their subsequent arthroscopic removal. Using a 3-dimensional reconstruction of computed tomography scans of the elbow, the authors were able to identify osteophytes preventing flexion beyond 140 degrees or full extension of the elbow. Using these visual guides, the impinging osteophytes were arthroscopically excised. The authors report significant clinical success with this technique.
- **Citation:** Kelly EW, Morrey BF, O'Driscoll SW. Complications of elbow arthroscopy. *J Bone Joint Surg Am.* 2001;83(1):25-34. doi:10.2106/00004623-200101000-00004.
    - **Recommended for:** clinical relevance for surgeons new to elbow arthroscopy in this setting
    - **Summary:** This research reviews a large cohort of patients undergoing elbow arthroscopy for varied pathologies—osteoarthritis, loose bodies, or inflammatory arthritis. The authors focus on perioperative complications associated with an incidence of 0.8% for major complications (septic arthritis) and 11% for minor complications (eg, transient nerve palsy, portal site infection). The authors review measures necessary to minimize complications associated with elbow arthroscopy, which includes comfort with the neurovascular anatomy around the elbow.

Chapter 7 Humeral Shaft Fractures

- **Citation:** Sarmiento A, Zagorski JB, Zych GA, Latta LL, Capps CA. Functional bracing for the treatment of fractures of the humeral diaphysis. *J Bone Joint Surg Am*. 2000;82(4):478-486. doi:10.2106/00004623-200004000-00003.
    - **Recommended for:** historical importance
    - **Summary:** In this classic orthopedic article, Sarmiento and his coauthors demonstrate that nonoperative management with functional bracing is a viable, if not preferred, option in managing humeral shaft fractures. Despite poor long-term follow-up, the authors report that union was achieved in more than 97% of cases. The findings reported by these authors established standard of care for humeral shaft fractures.
- **Citation:** Gerwin M, Hotchkiss RN, Weiland AJ. Alternative operative exposures of the posterior aspect of the humeral diaphysis: with reference to the radial nerve. *J Bone Joint Surg Am*. 1996;78(11):1690-1695. doi:10.2106/00004623-199611000-00008.
    - **Recommended for:** understanding of humeral shaft approaches
    - **Summary:** This cadaveric study describes a new surgical approach for management of humeral shaft fractures. By studying the course of the radial nerve through the posterior arm, it was demonstrated that an approach elevating the triceps from lateral to medial after identification of the radial nerve by retrograde dissection of the lateral brachial cutaneous nerve provided the greatest exposure of the humeral shaft from a posterior approach.

SHOULDER

Chapter 8 Anatomy and Physical Examination

- **Citation:** Mochizuki T, Sugaya H, Uomizu M, et al. Humeral insertion of the supraspinatus and infraspinatus: new anatomical findings regarding the footprint of the rotator cuff. *J Bone Joint Surg Am*. 2008;90(5):962-969. doi:10.2106/JBJS.G.00427.
    - **Recommended for:** pertinent anatomic review
    - **Summary:** In this cadavaric study, the authors challenge the accepted insertion sites of the rotator cuff tendons. Using more than 100 cadavaric shoulders, they found that on removal of the overlying capsule and ligaments, the supraspinatus had a triangular footprint with an average length (medial to lateral) of 6.9 mm and medial width (anteroposterior) of 12.6 mm. They found the infraspinatus footprint to be larger than previously believed at 10.2 mm length and 32.7 mm maximum width. In addition, they found that more than one-fifth of the shoulders had supraspinatus insertion onto the lesser tuberosity.
- **Citation:** Hertel R, Ballmer FT, Lambert SM, Gerber CH. Lag signs in the diagnosis of rotator cuff rupture. *J Shoulder Elbow Surg*. 1996;5(4):307-313.
    - **Recommended for:** historical context
    - **Summary:** In this classic article, the authors describe and present the accuracy of 3 new clinical exams for rotator cuff pathology: the external rotation lag sign, drop sign, and internal rotation lag sign. In their analysis using a study group of 100 patients undergoing arthroscopy, they found that the internal and external rotation lag signs were accurate predictors of posterosuperior and subscap cuff pathology, respecitvely.

Chapter 9 Rotator Cuff Disease

- **Citation:** Yamaguchi K, Tetro AM, Blam O, Evanoff BA, Teefey SA, Middleton WD. Natural history of asymptomatic rotator cuff tears: a longitudinal analysis of asymptomatic tears detected sonographically. *J Shoulder Elbow Surg.* 2001;10(3):199-203. doi:10.1067/mse.2001.113086.
    - **Recommended for:** understanding of progression of asymptomatic tears
    - **Summary:** To determine the natural history of asymptomatic rotator cuff tears, these authors used a database of 58 patients who had asymptomatic rotator cuff tears identified by ultrasound at the time of diagnosis of contralateral symptomatic rotator cuff tear. In a survey follow-up of 45 patients, they found that more than half became symptomatic after an average of 2.8 years. Additionally, 23 patients returned for repeat imaging and 9 had tear progression. Onset of symptoms was associated with decreased functional scores and increased pain. This study established the high risk of future symptoms in currently asymptomatic rotator cuff tears.
- **Citation:** Yamaguchi K, Ditsios K, Middleton WD, Hildebolt CF, Galatz LM, Teefey SA. The demographic and morphological features of rotator cuff disease: a comparison of asymptomatic and symptomatic shoulders. *J Bone Joint Surg Am.* 2006;88(8):1699-1704. doi:10.2106/JBJS.E.00835.
    - **Recommended for:** understanding characteristics of asymptomatic tears
    - **Summary:** At the time of this study, it had been observed that an asymptomatic rotator cuff tear was not uncommon. However, the true prevelance, predictors, and progression of asymptomatic rotator cuff tears were unknown. By using ultrasound to image both shoulders of every patient presenting with unilateral shoulder pain, these authors were able to determine that 35.5% of the 183 patients with full-thickness rotator cuff tear in the painful shoulder had a contralateral full-thickness rotator cuff tear. The likelihood of bilateral tears increased with age. Furthermore, symptomatic rotator cuff tears were noted to be larger than asymptomatic rotator cuff tears.
- **Citation:** Kim DH, Elattrache NS, Tibone JE, et al. Biomechanical comparison of a single-row versus double-row suture anchor technique for rotator cuff repair. *Am J Sports Med.* 2006;34(3):407-414. doi:10.1177/0363546505281238.
    - **Recommended for:** understanding of single- vs double-row repair
    - **Summary:** In a cadaveric analysis, Kim et al evaluated the fixation strength of an established technique to recreate the supraspinatus footprint of the rotator cuff—double-row repair. In matched shoulders, they compared double-row (2 medial and 2 lateral anchors) repair to traditional repair with 2 lateral anchors. They found that a double-row repair provided a decreased initial strain, increased stiffness, and increased load to failure compared to single-row repair. However, the clinical impacts of this improved mechanical construct remain unknown.
- **Citation:** DeHaan AM, Axelrad TW, Kaye E, Silvestri L, Puskas B, Foster TE. Does double-row rotator cuff repair improve functional outcome of patients compared with single-row technique? A systematic review. *Am J Sports Med.* 2012;40(5):1176-1185. doi:10.1177/0363546511428866.
    - **Recommended for:** understanding of single-row vs transosseous-equivalent benefits
    - **Summary:** To fully evaluate the impact of surgical technique on functional outcome, these authors performed a systematic review. Included in their analysis were any level I or II studies prospectively comparing single- and double-row rotator cuff repair. In the 2011 review, they identified 7 studies for inclusion. The evaluation of more than 500 rotator cuff tears included in these 7 studies was unable to establish a difference in retear rate or functional outcome between single- or double-row repair.

- **Citation:** Iannotti JP, Deutsch A, Green A, et al. Time to failure after rotator cuff repair: a prospective imaging study. *J Bone Joint Surg Am.* 2013;95(11):965-971. doi:10.2106/JBJS.L.00708.
  - **Recommended for:** study design and understanding rotator cuff repair failure
  - **Summary:** This high-frequency radiographic analysis of rotator cuff integrity following arthroscopic repair of more than 100 shoulders provided a valuable understanding of the timing of rotator cuff repair failure. Patients younger than 75 years old with a rotator cuff tear sized between 1 and 4 cm with less than grade II fatty atrophy were imaged by magnetic resonanc imaging at 2, 6, 12, 16, 26, and 52 weeks after rotator cuff repair. In this highly selective group (low risk for retear), the authors identified a 17% rate of retear within 1 year. The mean time to retear was 19.2 weeks, and the vast majority (94.7%) of retears occurred within the first 6 months compared with the second 6 months. Between those with and those without retears, no patient reported functional outcomes were different.

Chapter 10 Shoulder Instability

- **Citation:** Bigliani LU, Kelkar R, Flatow EL, Pollock RG, Mow VC. Glenohumeral stability. Biomechanical properties of passive and active stabilizers. *Clin Orthop Relat Res.* 1996;(330):13-30.
  - **Recommended for:** understanding the role of static and dynamic stabilizers in shoulder stability
  - **Summary:** This classic article provides reviews and establishes the knowledge to date regarding glenohumeral stability and the mechanical properities of the dynamic and static glenohumeral stabilizers. The thorough review reinforces the importance of the static inferior glenohumeral ligament in glenohumeral stability. Furthermore, it demonstrates the impact of capsule tightness and glenohumeral congruity on humeral translation and glenohumeral contact pressures.
- **Citation:** Allain J, Goutallier D, Glorion C. Long-term results of the Latarjet procedure for the treatment of anterior instability of the shoulder. *J Bone Joint Surg Am.* 1998;80(6):841-852. doi:10.2106/00004623-199806000-00008.
  - **Recommended for:** long-term outcome of the Latarjet procedure
  - **Summary:** In this long-term follow-up of the Latarjet procedure for recurrent anterior shoulder stability, the authors establish low recurrence of glenohumeral dislocations. The authors were able to follow 58 of 95 (61%) Latarjet procedures performed between 1969 and 1983. With an average follow-up of 14.3 years (range, 10 to 23 years), they found no cases of recurrent dislocation. Though a large proportion of patients (43.1%) had grade 1 osteoarthritis on follow-up radiographis, this did not have clinical implications.

Chapter 11 Frozen Shoulder: Adhesive Capsulitis

- **Citation:** Neviaser JS. Adhesive capsulitis of the shoulder: a study of the pathological findings in periarthritis of the shoulder. *J Bone Joint Surg Am.* 1945;27(2):211-222.
  - **Recommended for:** historical context
  - **Summary:** In this classic article, Dr. Neviaser coins the term "adhesive capsulitis" for frozen shoulder. This term is based on the gross appearance of the capsule with findings of inflammation in the 10 patients surgically treated for frozen shoulder. This analysis established the "thickening and contraction of the capsule" as the pathology associated with idiopathic frozen shoulder.
- **Citation:** Zuckerman JD, Rokito A. Frozen shoulder: a consensus definition. *J Shoulder Elbow Surg.* 2011;20(2):322-325. doi:10.1016/j.jse.2010.07.008.

- **Recommended for:** understanding classifcation and process of consensus definitions
- **Summary:** In many orthopedic pathologies, a diagnosis relies on an assessment of many factors, including history, physical, and radiographic testing. To provide an accurate, consistent, and uniform diagnosis in such cases, the development of a definition for the diagnosis is beneficial. The authors of this analysis demonstrate such an effort. They provide a definition and classification of frozen shoulder to aid in diagnosis and research of this pathology. More important, the authors used a survey of specialists to confirm the consensus agreement of this definition.

Chapter 12 Injuries to the Biceps-Labral Complex

- **Citation:** Williams MM, Snyder SJ, Buford D. The Buford complex—the "cord-like" middle glenohumeral ligament and absent anterosuperior labrum complex: a normal anatomic capsulolabral variant. *Arthroscopy.* 1994;10(3):241-247. doi:10.1016/s0749-8063(05)80105-7.
  - **Recommended for:** historical context and understanding of variant anatomy
  - **Summary:** This study provides an important reminder of the "normal" anatomic variant. Williams et al established the normal anatomic variant of a "cord-like" middle glenohumeral ligament attached to the superior labrum and termed a "Burford complex." After review of 200 shoulder arthroscopies, the authors reported a 13.5% incidence of anterosuperior labral variants. Through use of a case report, they further cautioned against not fully identifying this normal anatomic variant and mistaking the cord-like middle glenohumeral ligament for labrum necessitating repair.
- **Citation:** Andrews JR, Carson WG Jr, McLeod WD. Glenoid labrum tears related to the long head of the biceps. *Am J Sports Med.* 1985;13(5):337-341. doi:10.1177/036354658501300508.
  - **Recommended for**: historical context
  - **Summary:** This now-classic article by Andrews et al formed the foundation for understanding superior labral tears of the throwing athlete. Through a review of 73 baseball pitchers undergoing surgical management of shoulder pathology, a high rate of superior labral tears were identified. Through testing in a subgroup of these patients, the long-head biceps was implicated as a potential source for the high incidence of superior labral tearing in the throwing athlete.
- **Citation:** Snyder SJ, Karzel RP, Del Pizzo W, Ferkel RD, Friedman MJ. SLAP lesions of the shoulder. *Arthroscopy.* 1990;6(4):274-279. doi:10.1016/0749-8063(90)90056-j.
  - **Recommended for:** historical context
  - **Summary:** With the understanding of superior labral pathology established by Andrews et al, Snyder et al further investigated superior labral pathology. Based on their retrospective review, they identified and coined the superior labrum anterior and posterior (SLAP) lesion in this paper. In addition, this paper provides the description of the 4 SLAP types based on the patterns observed in this review of 27 patients with SLAP tears. Further research would establish the treatment and clinical outcomes of SLAP tears.
- **Citation:** O'Brien SJ, Pagnani MJ, Fealy S, McGlynn SR, Wilson JB. The active compression test: a new and effective test for diagnosing labral tears and acromioclavicular joint abnormality. *Am J Sports Med.* 1998;26(5):610-613. doi:10.1177/03635465980260050201.
  - **Recommended for:** understanding development of diagnostic tests
  - **Summary:** As knowledge of superior labral pathology developed, physical exam tests for an accurate diagnosis were necessary. As such, O'Brien et al provided this description and validation of the active compression test to identify acromioclavicular or labral pathology. This prospective review of 318 patients found a sensitivity of 100% and specificity of 98.5%. This test has now become widely adopted.

Chapter 13 Shoulder Fractures

- **Citation:** Gstettner C, Tauber M, Hitzl W, Resch H. Rockwood type III acromioclavicular dislocation: surgical versus conservative treatment. *J Shoulder Elbow Surg.* 2008;17(2):220-225. doi:10.1016/j.jse.2007.07.017.
  - **Recommended for:** classic description of acromioclavicular injuries
  - **Summary:** This retrospective review compares operative vs nonoperative treatment of Rockwood type III acromioclavicular dislocations. Nonoperative treatment consisted of sling and functional therapy compared with operative treatment with a hook plate. Increased constant scores and radiologic results in the surgical treatment group make it a safe and viable treatment option especially when dealing with young, active patients.
- **Citation:** Canadian Orthopaedic Trauma Society. Nonoperative treatment compared with plate fixation of displaced midshaft clavicular fractures. A multicenter, randomized clinical trial. *J Bone Joint Surg Am.* 2007;89(1):1-10. doi:10.2106/JBJS.F.00020.
  - **Recommended for:** level-one evidence of clavicle fracture management
  - **Summary:** This study was a multicenter, prospective clinical trial. They randomly assigned 132 patients with displaced midshaft clavicle fractures into 2 treatment arms of operative with plate fixation and nonoperative with just a sling. Early primary plate fixation of displaced midshaft clavicle fractures had lower rate of malunion and nonunion. Patients in the operative treatment group also had higher patient satisfaction and patient-reported outcomes when compared with nonoperative.
- **Citation:** Williams GR Jr, Naranja J, Klimkiewicz J, Karduna A, Iannotti JP, Ramsey M. The floating shoulder: a biomechanical basis for classification and management. *J Bone Joint Surg Am.* 2001;83-A(8):1182-1187. doi:10.2106/00004623-200108000-00007.
  - **Recommended for:** providing an understanding in decision making of superior shoulder suspensory complex injuries
  - **Summary:** This cadaveric study evaluates the importance of stabilization of fractures in a floating shoulder. The authors determined that with an intact coracoacromial and acromioclavicular capsular ligament, it is not necessary to stabilize ipsilateral scapular neck and clavicular fractures. The scapula does not result in a floating shoulder unless all attachments of the distal fragment are disrupted from the proximal fragment.
- **Citation:** Neer CS II. Displaced proximal humeral fractures. I. Classification and evaluation. *J Bone Joint Surg Am.* 1970;52(6):1077-1089.
  - **Recommended for:** establishing classification and management of proximal humerus fractures
  - **Summary:** In this classic article, Neer evaluates 3-part and 4-part proximal humeral fractures, establishing classification and treatment recommendations. Of a total of 117 fractures, open reduction was recommended for 3-part fractures and prosthetic replacement for 4-part fractures.

Chapter 14 Shoulder Arthritis: Glenohumeral Arthritis

- **Citation:** Bercik MJ, Kruse K II, Yalizis M, Gauci MO, Chaoui J, Walch G. A modification to the Walch classification of the glenoid in primary glenohumeral osteoarthritis using three-dimensional imaging. *J Shoulder Elbow Surg.* 2016;25(10):1601-1606. doi:10.1016/j.jse.2016.03.010.
  - **Recommended for:** updated classification of glenoid morphology
  - **Summary:** This update on a classic article provides reproducibility of a modified classification for glenoid wear. Albeit a recent addition, this work provides an understanding for

an adapting classification despite already being widely used. In their update, the authors add B3 and D classifications with a more precise definition of the A2 classification. Furthermore, through review of 129 glenoid computed tomography images on 4 separate occasions, show a dramatic improvement both in intraobserver and interobserver reliability compared with the original classification.

- **Citation:** Neer CS II, Craig EV, Fukuda H. Cuff-tear arthropathy. *J Bone Joint Surg Am.* 1983;65(9):1232-1244.
    - **Recommended for:** historical context
    - **Summary:** This 1983 article provides one of the earliest thorough reviews of cuff-tear arthropathy. Now widely recognized, the presentation and etiology of this disease was not fully understood at the time of this publication. In this review, the authors provide a common history and physical for 26 patients treated surgically for cuff-tear arthropathy. In addition, they review their hypothesis for the pathophysiology of cuff-tear arthropathy. The authors discuss treatment of cuff-tear arthropathy while recognizing the struggles to adequately treat the disease with the available armamentarium.
- **Citation:** Hettrich CM, Boraiah S, Dyke JP, Neviaser A, Helfet DL, Lorich DG. Quantitative assessment of the vascularity of the proximal part of the humerus. *J Bone Joint Surg Am.* 2010;92(4):943-948. doi:10.2106/JBJS.H.01144.
    - **Recommended for:** study design and clinical importance
    - **Summary:** Prior to this publication, it had been well accepted that the anterior humeral circumflex artery was the predominant supplier of blood flow to the proximal humerus. Using 12 fresh-frozen cadavers, the authors ligated the anterior humeral circumflex or the posterior humeral circumflex prior to canulating and perfusing the axillary artery. Specimens with the anterior humeral circumflex ligated had 32% increased perfusion in the contralateral control shoulder. This is compared to 60% increased perfusion in the control vs shoulders with the posterior humeral circumflex artery ligated. Furthermore, they found that the posterior humeral circumflex artery accounted for 64% of the humeral head blood supply. The authors hypothesize that this explains the low rate of osteonecrosis observed in proximal humerus fractures.
- **Citation:** Boileau P, Watkinson D, Hatzidakis AM, Hovorka I. Neer Award 2005: The Grammont reverse shoulder prosthesis: results in cuff tear arthritis, fracture sequelae, and revision arthroplasty. *J Shoulder Elbow Surg.* 2006;15(5):527-540. doi:10.1016/j.jse.2006.01.003.
    - **Recommended for:** historical context and adoption of new technology
    - **Summary:** This article provides a midterm follow-up of Grammont reverse shoulder arthroplasties for various indications. In a review of 40 cases, the authors found favorable outcomes for previously difficult-to-treat pathologies, namely rotator cuff–deficient shoulders. Though promising, the authors did note a substantial complication rate, especially in patients undergoing conversion to a reverse shoulder for failed shoulder arthroplasty (47%).
- **Citation:** Frankle M, Siegal S, Pupello D, Saleem A, Mighell M, Vasey M. The reverse shoulder prosthesis for glenohumeral arthritis associated with severe rotator cuff deficiency: a minimum two-year follow-up study of sixty patients. *J Bone Joint Surg Am.* 2005;87(8):1697-1705. doi:10.2106/JBJS.D.02813.
    - **Recommended for:** historical context and adaptation of technology
    - **Summary:** As evidence of successfully managing complicated shoulder pathologies, such as cuff-tear arthropathy, with reverse arthroplasty became available, this report of a new lateralized glenosphere was published. The unique approach to reverse implant design violated principles championed by the Grammont design. However, this early report of

60 cases demonstrates successful outcomes of this design. This adaptation of existing technology demonstrated thoughtful design changes to minimize common complications (eg, scapular notching) of existing technology and provided documentation of new complications (eg, glenosphere dissociation) to be monitored and improved on.

- **Citation:** Weldon EJ III, Boorman RS, Smith KL, Matsen FA III. Optimizing the glenoid contribution to the stability of a humeral hemiarthroplasty without a prosthetic glenoid. *J Bone Joint Surg Am.* 2004;86(9):2022-2029. doi:10.2106/00004623-200409000-00022.
    - **Recommended for:** historical context and developing new techniques
    - **Summary:** Given the many restrictions placed on patients undergoing total shoulder arthroplasty, a method for managing severe arthritis in young, active patients was desirable. This work, a single-part of a large series, helped establish the rationale for performing shoulder hemiarthroplasty with glenoid reaming. Using cadaveric models, the authors were able to demonstrate that glenohumeral stability was decreased through removal of glenoid cartilage and labrum. However, stability, comparable to that achieved with a prosthetic implant, was restored with spherical reaming alone.

Chapter 15 Scapular Disorders

- **Citation:** Dewar FP, Harris RI. Restoration of function of the shoulder following paralysis of the trapezius by fascial sling fixation and transplantation of the levator scapulae. *Ann Surg.* 1950;132(6):1111-1115. doi:10.1097/00000658-195012000-00010.
    - **Recommended for:** historical context and surgical description of a novel procedure
    - **Summary:** This eloquently written case report provides an early description of the importance of the spinal accessory nerve and therefore the trapezius muscle in powering and stabilizing the scapula throughout shoulder range of motion. Dewar and Hariss describe a novel technique for providing scapular stabilization and motion in trapezius-deficient patients. Through transposition of the levator scapulae to the lateral scapula spine and tethering of the medial scapula to the dorsal spinal vertebra with a fascial sling, the patient's shoulder was no longer incapacitated and she was able to return to her prior activities of daily living.
- **Citation:** Galano GJ, Bigliani LU, Ahmad CS, Levine WN. Surgical treatment of winged scapula. *Clin Orthop Relat Res.* 2008;466(3):652-660. doi:10.1007/s11999-007-0086-2.
    - **Recommended for:** understanding treatment options for scapular winging
    - **Summary:** Treatment of a winging scapula, lateral or medial, can be challenging. Furthermore, cases for review are limited. In this case series, the authors present outcomes for 17 shoulders surgically treated for a winging scapula. Patients were treated with a split pectoralis transfer for long thoracic nerve palsy (medial scapula winging) or with an Eden-Lange (rhomboid and levator scapulae transfer) for spinal accessory nerve palsy (lateral scapula winging). In addition to describing their surgical technique, the authors report improved functional scores and decreased pain in the surgical cohort.

Chapter 16 Acromioclavicular Disorders

- **Citation:** Rockwood, CA. Injuries to the acromioclavicular joint: subluxations and dislocations about the shoulder. In: Rockwood, CA, Green, DP, eds. *Fractures in Adults.* 2nd ed. Philadelphia: JB Lippincott; 1984:860-910.
    - **Recommended for:** historical context and understanding classification
    - **Summary:** This chapter provides a review of fractures and dislocations about the shoulder, including acromioclavicular separation. The classification provided by Rockwood is the primary classification for clinical treatment and research of acromioclavicular

separation. Consisting of 6 types, the classification is defined by the ligaments damaged and the vector of separation.

Chapter 17 The Athlete's Shoulder and Elbow

- **Citation:** Pappas AM, Zawacki RM, Sullivan TJ. Biomechanics of baseball pitching: a preliminary report. *Am J Sports Med.* 1985;13(4):216-222. doi:10.1177/036354658501300402.
    - **Recommended for:** historical context and understanding shoulder physiology of the throwing athlete
    - **Summary:** To elucidate the etiology of shoulder pathology in the throwing athlete, it was first imperative to define the normal mechanics of throwing. This paper was one of the earliest to discuss the phases of throwing, credited to Tullos and King in 1973. In this work, the authors were able to establish the normal duration and arm position throughout the 3 primary phases of throwing: cocking, acceleration, and follow-through.
- **Citation:** Neer CS II. Impingement lesions. *Clin Orthop Relat Res.* 1983;(173):70-77.
    - **Recommended for:** historical context
    - **Summary:** In this review, Neer provides insight into his understanding of subacromial impingement, its role in rotator cuff pathology, and its diagnosis and treatment. Though routine subacromial decompression during rotator cuff repair has been challenged more recently, this article provides a thorough understanding of impingement and an early description of the Neer Impingement test with a thorough description of open subacromial decompression technique. In combination with more recent evidence, this review serves as an important guide to managing subacromial impingement.
- **Citation:** Walch G, Boileau P, Noel E, Donell ST. Impingement of the deep surface of the supraspinatus tendon on the posterosuperior glenoid rim: an arthroscopic study. *J Shoulder Elbow Surg.* 1992;1(5):238-245. doi:10.1016/S1058-2746(09)80065-7.
    - **Recommended for:** historical context
    - **Summary:** In this case series of 17 athletes (16 throwing athletes), Walch et al detailed the findings of internal impingement. This was the earliest description of internal impingement, characterized by impingement of the undersurface of the posterosuperior articular side of the rotator cuff and the posterior glenoid. In this series, the impingement was noted arthroscopically when the arm was abducted and externally rotated in the throwing position.
- **Citation:** Conway JE, Jobe FW, Glousman RE, Pink M. Medial instability of the elbow in throwing athletes. Treatment by repair or reconstruction of the ulnar collateral ligament. *J Bone Joint Surg Am.* 1992;74(1):67-83.
    - **Recommended for:** understanding of the background for management of UCL injuries
    - **Summary:** Jobe performed the first UCL reconstruction in 1974 on a professional pitcher. This paper details the results of a UCL repair or reconstruction in 68 athletes between 1974 and 1987. This manuscript documented good long-term outcomes with 50% of those undergoing repair and 68% of those undergoing reconstruction returning to their previous level of play. Furthermore, the authors found that prior surgery significantly reduced the likelihood of a successful outcome.
- **Citation:** Rohrbough JT, Altchek DW, Hyman J, Williams RJ III, Botts JD. Medial collateral ligament reconstruction of the elbow using the docking technique. *Am J Sports Med.* 2002;30(4):541-548. doi:10.1177/03635465020300041401.
    - **Recommended for:** change in management
    - **Summary:** Following the success of Jobe in reconstructing the UCL, perfecting the surgical technique became the primary purpose. Rohrbough et al attempted to address some

concerns of the modified Jobe technique by developing the *docking technique*. In this paper, they describe the docking technique and present results of 36 cases at a minimum of 2 years. The technique described in this paper used a single humeral tunnel and routine elbow arthroscopy. In addition, the authors did not perform routine ulnar nerve transposition or detachment of the flexor origin. Using the docking technique, they reported 92% return to previous level of sports.

- **Citation:** Dugas JR, Walters BL, Beason DP, Fleisig GS, Chronister JE. Biomechanical comparison of ulnar collateral ligament repair with internal bracing versus modified Jobe reconstruction. *Am J Sports Med.* 2016;44(3):735-741. doi:10.1177/0363546515620390.
    - **Recommended for:** change in management
    - **Summary:** Jobe's work on valgus instability in the overhead athlete provided a means for return to play previously impossible for many athletes with incompetent UCLs. Since the first successful reconstruction in 1974, UCL reconstruction has become the gold standard for treating such patients. Dugas et al used a cadaveric model to determine whether an augmented repair was biomechanically similar to reconstruction. They found that repair of a transected UCL augmented with a tape anchored to the humerus and ulna had decreased gapping compared with reconstruction with the modified Jobe technique. There was no difference in failure metrics. This study formed the basis for a potential change in management of those patients with a repairable UCL.

Financial Disclosures

Dr. Joseph A. Abboud receives research support from DePuy, OREF, Orthospace, Tornier, and Zimmer; receives royalties from Integra; holds stock in Aevumed and Mininvasive; and is a consultant for Cayenne, DJO Surgical, and Globus.

Dr. Alexander W. Aleem has no financial or proprietary interest in the materials presented herein.

Dr. Luke Austin, MD has no financial or proprietary interest in the materials presented herein.

Dr. Wayne W. Chan has no financial or proprietary interest in the materials presented herein.

Dr. Talia Chapman has not disclosed any relevant financial relationships.

Dr. Michael C. Ciccotti has no financial or proprietary interest in the materials presented herein.

Dr. Michael G. Ciccotti has no financial or proprietary interest in the materials presented herein.

Dr. Jason L. Codding has no financial or proprietary interest in the materials presented herein.

Dr. Daniel E. Davis has no financial or proprietary interest in the materials presented herein.

Dr. Vahid Entezari has no financial or proprietary interest in the materials presented herein.

Dr. Seth Gamradt has no financial or proprietary interest in the materials presented herein.

Dr. Charles L. Getz receives royalties from Zimmer Biomet and is a speaker for Mitek and Zimmer Biomet.

Dr. Benjamin Hendy has no financial or proprietary interest in the materials presented herein.

Dr. J. Gabriel Horneff III has not disclosed any relevant financial relationships.

Dr. Jason E. Hsu has no financial or proprietary interest in the materials presented herein.

Dr. Asif Ilyas has not disclosed any relevant financial relationships.

Dr. Jason S. Klein has no financial or proprietary interest in the materials presented herein.

Dr. Mark D. Lazarus has not disclosed any relevant financial relationships.

Dr. Christopher McDowell has not disclosed any relevant financial relationships.

Dr. Surena Namdari receives royalties from Aevumed, DJO Surgical, and Miami Device Solutions; receives stock or stock options from Aevumed, Force Therapeutics, MD Live, MD Valuate, Orthophor, Parvizi Surgical Innovations, RubiconMD, and Tangen; receives research support from Arthrex, DePuy, DJO Surgical, Integra, and Wright Medical Technology; is a consultant for DePuy, DJO Surgical, Flexion Therapeutics, and Miami Device Solutions; is a paid speaker for DJO Surgical and Miami Device Solutions; and is a board member for Bone & Joint 360 and the Philadelphia Orthopaedic Society.

Dr. Reza Omid receives royalties from Integra and Medacta and is a consultant for both.

Dr. Eric M. Padegimas is a paid speaker for DJO Global.

Dr. Nilay A. Patel has no financial or proprietary interest in the materials presented herein.

Dr. E. Scott Paxton is a consultant for Miami Device Solutions, Wright Medical Technology, and Tornier and receives research support from Arthrex, Smith and Nephew and Wright/Tornier.

Dr. Matthew L. Ramsey has no financial or proprietary interest in the materials presented herein.

Dr. John Scolaro is an educational consultant for Smith and Nephew, Stryker, and Zimmer Biomet, has done product design for Globus Medical, and receives research support from AO Trauma North America and the Foundation for Orthopaedic Trauma.

Dr. Kalpit N. Shah has not disclosed any relevant financial relationships.

Dr. Michael A. Stone has received honoraria from DJO Surgical.

Dr. Jared R. Thomas has no financial or proprietary interest in the materials presented herein.

Dr. Nicholas A. Trasolini has no financial or proprietary interest in the materials presented herein.

Dr. Alexis Williams has no financial or proprietary interest in the materials presented herein.

Dr. Gerald R. Williams Jr has not disclosed any relevant financial relationships.

Dr. Benjamin Zmistowski has no financial or proprietary interest in the materials presented herein.

Index